NEUROLOGIC PROBLEMS

Executive Editor: Richard A. Weimer
Production Editor: Michael J. Rogers
Art Director: Don Sellers, AMI
Illustrators: Joe Vitek, Mary Angle, Nancy Obloy

NEUROLOGIC PROBLEMS

A Critical Care Nursing Focus

Mariah Snyder, R.N., Ph.D.
Associate Professor
University of Minnesota
Minneapolis, Minnesota

Mary Jackle, R.N., M.S.
Director of Community Education
Metropolitan Medical Center
Minneapolis, Minnesota

9 2 5 1

ROBERT J. BRADY CO.
A Prentice-Hall Publishing and Communications Company
Bowie, Md. 20715

Neurologic Problems: A Critical Care Nursing Focus

Library of Congress Cataloging in Publication Data

Snyder, Mariah.
    Neurologic problems, a critical care nursing focus.
    1. Neurological nursing.   2. Intensive care nursing. I. Jackle, Mary, joint author. II. Title.
[DNLM: 1. Nervous system diseases—Nursing. 2. Neurology—Nursing texts. WY160 S992n]
RC350.5.S69   610.73'68   80-11229
ISBN 0-87619-713-6

Prentice-Hall International, Inc., London
Prentice-Hall of Australia, Pty., Ltd., Sydney
Prentice-Hall of India Private Limited, New Delhi
Prentice-Hall of Japan, Inc., Tokyo
Prentice-Hall of Southeast Asia Pte. Ltd., Singapore
Whitehall Books, Limited, Petone, New Zealand

Printed in the United States of America

81 82 83 84 85 86 87 88 89 90 10 9 8 7 6 5 4 3 2 1

To Mary, Catherine, Angela, and Ruth
M.S.

To The Benedictines of St. Bede Priory, Eau Claire, WI
M.J.

CONTENTS

Dedication   v

Preface   ix

Introduction   x

Section 1   Cranial Problems   1

    Chapter 1   The Brain and Cranial Nerves   3

        Part I   Macroscopic Anatomy   5

        Part II   Microscopic Anatomy   27

        Part III   Review of Basic Neurophysiology   32

    Chapter 2   Increased Intracranial Pressure   37

        Part I   Anatomic Basis for Increased Intracranial Pressure   38

        Part II   Metabolic Needs of the Brain   42

        Part III   Autoregulation of Cerebral Blood Flow   46

        Part IV   Cerebral Water Balance   49

        Part V   Effects of Increased Intracranial Pressure   51

    Chapter 3   Causes of Cranial Dysfunction   61

        Part I   Trauma   63

        Part II   Tumors   76

        Part III   Vascular Problems   89

        Part IV   Infectious Processes   102

    Chapter 4   Diagnostic Tests   107

        Part I   Non-Invasive Procedures   108

        Part II   Invasive Procedures   117

    Chapter 5   Nursing Assessment of Neurologic Function   129

        Part I   Describing the Baseline   130

        Part II   Determining Significance of Changes   169

        Part III   Monitoring Intracranial Pressure   177

    Chapter 6   Disuse Phenomena   185

        Part I   Effects of Immobility and Preventive Measures   186

        Part II   Psychologic Effects of Immobility   210

Chapter 7   Alterations in Temperature Regulation   215

    Part I   Causes of Fever   216

    Part II   Hypothermia Units   220

    Part III   Nursing Care   224

Chapter 8   Nursing Management of Patients With Altered Behavior and Communication   227

    Part I   Perceptual Problems   228

    Part II   Communication Problems   235

Chapter 9   Seizures   243

    Part I   Causes   244

    Part II   Partial Seizures   246

    Part III   Generalized Seizures   248

    Part IV   Nursing Care   251

Chapter 10   Case Study: Brain Tumor, Craniotomy   257

    Part I   Pre-operative Period   258

    Part II   Craniotomy   272

    Part III   Post-operative Period   274

Chapter 11   Case Study: Closed Head Injury   279

    Part I   Critical Phase   280

    Part II   Recovery Phase   285

Section 2   Spinal Cord Problems   297

Chapter 12   The Spinal Cord   299

    Part I   Protective Structures   300

    Part II   Blood Supply   312

    Part III   Nerve Tracts   315

    Part IV   Autonomic Nervous System   329

Chapter 13   Causes of Spinal Cord Dysfunction   335

    Part I   Direct Trauma to the Cord   336

    Part II   Fractures of the Cervical Spine   338

    Part III   Tumors   345

    Part IV   Herniated Intervertebral Discs   350

    Part V   Interruption of Blood Supply   351

Chapter 14   Spinal Cord Injury: Nursing Assessment and Intervention   353

    Part I   Disruption of Motor and Sensory Tracts   354

Part II   Respiratory Status   366

Part III   Control of Internal Environment   370

Part IV   Psychologic Reactions   380

Chapter 15   Stabilization of the Spine   385

Part I   Skeletal Traction   386

Part II   Turning Frames   393

Part III   Hyperextension   400

Part IV   Surgical Fusion   401

Chapter 16   Case Study: Spinal Cord Injury   403

Part I   Initial Care   404

Part II   Intermediate Care   411

Appendix A Sample Nursing Care Plan   419

Appendix B Neurologic Clinical Flow Sheet   421

Index   422

Preface

In our years of nursing practice we frequently encounter nurses who are frightened and overwhelmed when assigned to care for critically ill neurologic patients. This may be due to the complexity of the nervous system and the many unknown aspects of its function. Many basic nursing programs devote minimal attention to this category of patients.

Since nursing care has a tremendous impact on the outcome of neurologic illness, nurses must be competent in managing a range of patient problems. We have selected content which provides the nurse with a sound basis for providing holistic care during the critical phase of neurologic illness. After completing the text, the reader will understand what is happening in selected neurologic problems, why it is occurring and what can be done to alter the process. Not all neurologic conditions are included, but transfer of knowledge to many situations will be possible.

The book is divided into two sections: the first centers on cranial problems, the second on the autonomic nervous system and spinal cord injury. Anatomy, physiology, pathology, assessment, and interventions for common nursing problems are presented. Each section concludes with a case study which allows for application of the knowledge to specific situations. Each chapter begins with an overview, a list of objectives and an outline of content. After each major section of the chapter, a summary is provided for review.

We would like to thank:

> Those who have taught us about the care of neurologic patients
> The many patients and families who have shared their lives with us and provided learning experiences which could never have been obtained from books
> Our colleagues at the University of Minnesota School of Nursing
> The administration and staff members at Metropolitan Medical Center, particularly Mary E. Jones, Director of Nursing; and John Cushing, Vice President for Corporate Development.
> Sheila Hall and Darlene Curtis for typing the manuscript through all the revisions, and
> Mr. and Mrs. Kent Heintzeman for their assistance.

Mariah Snyder
Mary Jackle

Introduction

You are about to begin studying a programmed text. This kind of instruction may be new to you, so please read the following directions.

The book is designed so that each chapter builds on the previous one, so start at the beginning of the book, at Frame One. Skipping around in the book would be confusing.

Each frame must be studied carefully because it represents one step in a series of concepts. Material is divided into small portions of information and explanations have been pared down so that the frames may be quickly understood. As you work on the book, cover the answer column with a strip of paper. Each frame will first give you information and then ask you questions about that information. You should check your answer with the one given. If you gave a wrong answer, you may have scanned the frame too quickly and missed details or subtle points. Return to the frame and study it again to see where your error occurred. You will also find information presented in the panels. The panels provide illustrations and a more detailed explanation of certain points. At the end of each major section of the chapter a summary frame will help to review your learning.

Once you have gotten used to the method you will be able to progress at a pace that is appropriate for you. Tests have indicated that our students learned the content well with an average of fifteen to twenty hours of study. Now it is your turn!

SECTION I
Cranial Problems

CHAPTER I

THE BRAIN AND CRANIAL NERVES

Knowledge of specific functions of areas of the brain and cranial nerves provides the nurse with a basis for planning nursing interventions for persons experiencing cerebral dysfunction.

There are several ways to describe the nervous system. The brain, cranial nerves, and spinal cord are called the central nervous system, while the spinal nerves and their branches to various parts of the body are called peripheral. Another division of the nervous system is the autonomic system which governs automatic adjustments of the internal body environment. This section will focus primarily on the cranial part of the central nervous system. This is information you will use while providing nursing care to patients with acute insults to the cerebral structures.

At the conclusion of this chapter you will be able to:

1. Recognize the three major divisions of the brain
2. Label the four cerebral lobes and the demarcations between the lobes
3. Recognize key functions associated with each cerebral lobe
4. Correctly use the terms ipsilateral and contralateral to describe dysfunction
5. Match each major area of the brain with its major functions
6. Match the cranial nerves with their chief functions
7. Label the coverings of the brain
8. Recognize the supratentorial and infratentorial areas of the brain
9. Describe the location, function, and normal components of cerebrospinal fluid
10. Label the internal carotid artery, basilar arteries, and the Circle of Willis
11. Recognize the chief functions of nerve cells
12. Differentiate the structure and function of axons and dendrites
13. Explain the function of the myelin sheath and neurilemma
14. Describe the structural features of synapses between neurons
15. Explain how nerve impulses are propagated along neurons and across synapses
16. Differentiate absolute and relative refractory periods.

Chapter outline

Macroscopic anatomy and associated functions
    Brain structure and function
        Cerebrum
        Cerebellum
        Brain stem
    Cranial nerve functions
    Meningeal structures
        Meningeal layers
        Tentorium cerebelli
    Cerebrospinal fluid and ventricular system
        Location
        Function
        Normal components
    Circulatory supply

Microscopic anatomy
    The neuron
    Supporting tissues
    Synapses

Review of basic neurophysiology
    Propagation of impulses
    Refractory periods
    Synaptic transmission

PART I
MACROSCOPIC ANATOMY

Brain Structure and Function

Frame 1

The brain is divided into three main areas—the cerebrum, the cerebellum, and the brain stem. Locate these areas on the side view of the brain in Figure 1.1.

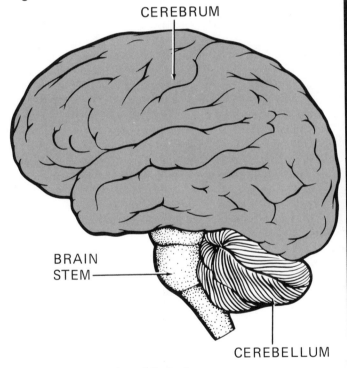

CEREBRUM

BRAIN STEM

CEREBELLUM

Figure 1.1. *Lateral view of the brain*

Frame 2

Each cerebral hemisphere is divided into four lobes that are named for the bones which lie over them. The surface of the brain is convoluted, and the shallow folds are called gyri. Deeper grooves called sulci and fissures divide the lobes. Find the lobes and prominent dividing lines in Figure 1.2.

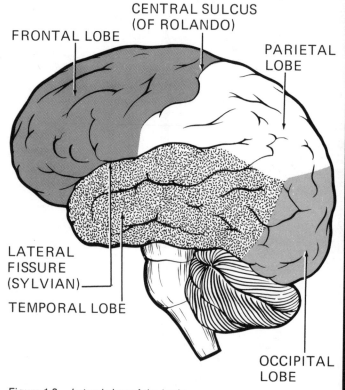

Figure 1.2. *Lateral view of the brain*

The next figure is a basal view of the cerebrum (looking up from the base of the skull). Locate the visible lobes and the longitudinal fissure which divides the right and left hemispheres.

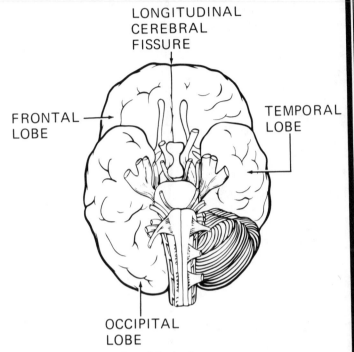

LONGITUDINAL
CEREBRAL
FISSURE

FRONTAL
LOBE

TEMPORAL
LOBE

OCCIPITAL
LOBE

Figure 1.3. *Rostral view of the brain*

Frame 3

Association areas combine input from several sensory modalities such as sight, touch, and sound during a conversation. They also compare immediate input with stored information. For example, association of a change in another person's expression and tone of voice and stored information about the meaning of these changes, result in the perception of anger. The major association areas and their functions are:

Pre-frontal area: abstract thinking, foresight, mature judgment, tactfulness, forbearance.

Post central gyrus, parietal lobe: somesthetic area for touch, position sense, and body image.

Temporal lobe: hearing, memory storage.

Occipital lobe: vision.

Figure 1.4 in Frame 5 shows the location of these areas.

Frame 4

Voluntary movement of the body is controlled by the part of the brain anterior to the central sulcus. This area is called the precentral gyrus or motor strip, and is arranged sequentially from toe to head. See Figure 1.4 in Frame 5.

Frame 5

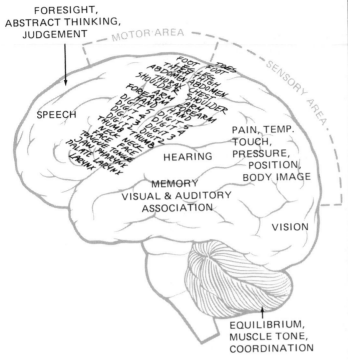

Figure 1.4. *Functional areas of the brain*

Match each lobe with its chief functions. (If you need to review locations of lobes, see Figure 1.2.)

1. Frontal lobe
2. Parietal lobe
3. Temporal lobe
4. Occipital lobe

a. vision
b. voluntary movement of body
c. thinking
d. hearing
e. touch, position sense
f. memory

1. b, c
2. e
3. d, f
4. a

5. The (central/lateral) sulcus separates the frontal and parietal lobes.

5. central

6. The motor area is (anterior/posterior) to the central sulcus.

6. anterior

7. Sensation is on the (same/opposite) side of the central sulcus as the motor area.

7. opposite

8. Damage to cells in the pre-frontal area would result in difficulty with (judgment/memory).

8. judgment

9. Damage to the (frontal/parietal) lobe may result in altered body image.

9. parietal

10. The shallow folds covering the surface of the brain are (gyri/fissures).

10. gyri

Frame 6

Figure 1.5 is an enlarged view of the motor–sensory areas. The body parts that have more intricate functions constitute a proportionately larger area of the motor strip than do other areas. The sensory area of the parietal lobe corresponds to the motor area in the frontal lobe, but there are less discrete delineations (i.e., a larger lesion is needed to disrupt sensory functions).

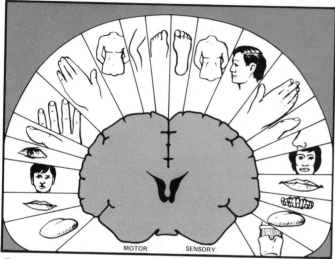

Figure 1.5. *Sequence of functions, motor and sensory strips*

1. The (face/leg) takes up a proportionately larger area of the motor strip.

2. The sensory area in the parietal lobe has (more/less) specific demarcations of functions than is found in the motor area of the frontal lobe.

1. face

2. less

Frame 7

Figure 1.6 shows the two areas of the brain thought to control speech. Traditionally it has been held that damage to Wernicke's center in the temporal lobe results in receptive aphasia, the inability to comprehend speech. Expressive aphasia, the inability to express oneself in speech, occurs when Broca's area of the motor strip in the frontal lobe is damaged. The speech center of a right-handed person is located in the left hemisphere 87% of the time.

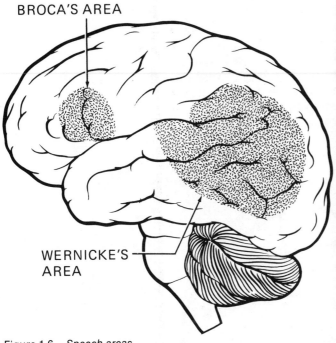

BROCA'S AREA

WERNICKE'S AREA

Figure 1.6. *Speech areas*

1. Mr. Richards is unable to understand verbal commands. He has _____ aphasia.

2. Mr. Richards has probably suffered damage to _____ area.

3. Expressive aphasia results from damage to _____ area.

4. Mr. James, who understands speech but cannot speak, has _____ aphasia.

1. receptive

2. Wernicke's

3. Broca's

4. expressive

Frame 8

In Figure 1.7 the brain has been sectioned through the center, and you are looking at it from the front rather than the side views in previous figures. Find the longitudinal fissure and lateral sulci. Notice that fibers from the cells in the motor area of the cerebrum cross to the opposite side of the body on their way through the brain stem.

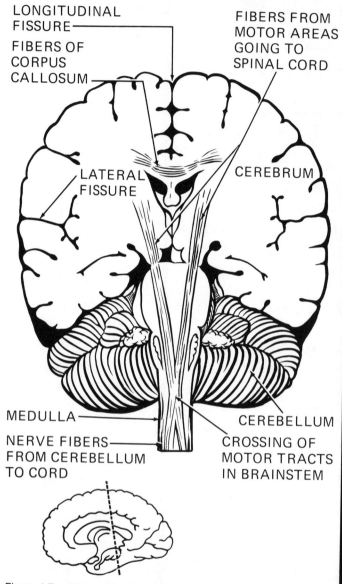

LONGITUDINAL FISSURE

FIBERS OF CORPUS CALLOSUM

FIBERS FROM MOTOR AREAS GOING TO SPINAL CORD

LATERAL FISSURE

CEREBRUM

MEDULLA

NERVE FIBERS FROM CEREBELLUM TO CORD

CEREBELLUM

CROSSING OF MOTOR TRACTS IN BRAINSTEM

Figure 1.7. *Motor and cerebellar tracts*

1. Because of the crossing of motor fibers, the right cerebral hemisphere would control the _____ side of the body.

   1. left

2. The left hemisphere controls movements on the _____ side.

   2. right

The word used to describe dysfunction on the opposite side of the body from the lesion is *contralateral*.

Frame 9

Now look at the nerve fibers coming from the cerebellum in Figure 1.7.

1. Do they cross to the opposite side?

   1. no

2. Therefore, damage to the right cerebellum would most likely result in dysfunction on the (right/left) side of the body.

   2. right

The term used to describe dysfunction on the *same* side as the lesion is *ipsilateral*.

3. *Cerebral* dysfunction results in symptoms being located (ipsilateral/contralateral) to the affected side of the brain.

   3. contralateral

4. Cerebellar damage results in (ipsilateral/contralateral) dysfunction.

   4. ipsilateral

Frame 10

Look at Figure 1.7 to see that nerve fibers also connect the right and left cerebral hemispheres. These connecting fibers form the corpus callosum. The corpus callosum provides for integration of sensory and motor activities of the two hemispheres.

1. The corpus callosum contains fibers linking which functions?

   1. a, b, c

   a. thinking
   b. sensation
   c. voluntary movement
   d. control of blood pressure

2. Mrs. Allen is not able to use both hands together to pick up large objects. Choose the possible reason.

   2. b

   a. damage to the thalamus
   b. damage to the corpus callosum
   c. increased intracranial pressure

Frame 11

Nerve fibers carrying information to the brain from the rest of the body are called *afferent*.

Fibers leading from the brain to the periphery are *efferent* nerves.

1. Sensations from the skin are carried to the brain by _____ fibers.

2. Impulses for voluntary movement travel along _____ nerves.

3. _____ means to the brain.

4. _____ means away from the brain.

1. efferent

2. afferent

3. Efferent

4. Afferent

Frame 12

The cerebellum is divided into a right and a left hemisphere with a structure called the vermis connecting the two hemispheres. Each cerebellar hemisphere is connected to adjacent brain structures by cerebellar peduncles which contain efferent and afferent nerve fibers. The cerebellum has often been compared to an automatic control device due to the many feedback and controlling functions of the cerebellum.

Three main functions of the cerebellum are:

> muscle synergy (coordination) throughout the body
> maintenance of equilibrium
> maintenance of muscle tone.

1. Jane Harris was in an accident and injured one cerebellar hemisphere. You would expect the resulting problems to be:

   a. contralateral
   b. ipsilateral

2. Choose the problems Jane might have:

   a. lack of sensation
   b. loss of muscular coordination
   c. disturbance of equilibrium
   d. memory lapses
   e. poor muscle tone

1. b

2. b, c, e

Frame 13

The brain stem contains structures that are essential to life and to maintenance of consciousness. There are three divisions in the brain stem, but the structures are actually continuous. Figure 1.8 shows the midbrain, pons, and medulla which compose this part of the brain. Note the location in relation to other cerebral areas.

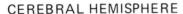

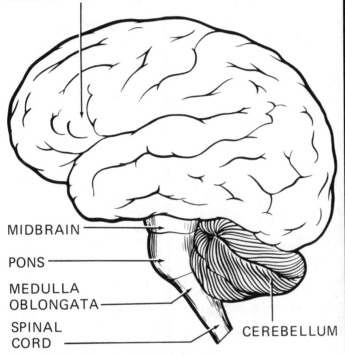

Figure 1.8. *Lateral view of the brain*

All areas of the central nervous system connect with the brain stem. The ascending and descending pathways to the spinal cord are located here. See Chapter 12 for a discussion of these pathways.

Frame 14

The reticular activating system (RAS) comprises a large portion of the brain stem.

An important function of the RAS is to maintain alertness. Pressure on the brain stem results in decreased alertness and possible loss of consciousness.

Locate the reticular activating system on Figure 1.9. It is the shaded area. The arrows depict connections with other cranial areas.

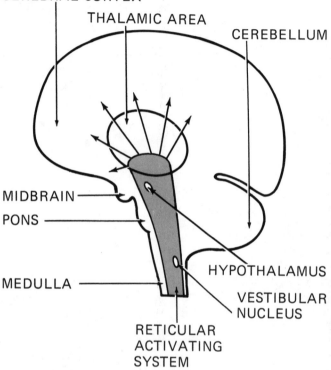

CEREBRAL CORTEX
THALAMIC AREA
CEREBELLUM
MIDBRAIN
PONS
MEDULLA
HYPOTHALAMUS
VESTIBULAR NUCLEUS
RETICULAR ACTIVATING SYSTEM

Figure 1.9. *Reticular activating system*

1. The three divisions of the brain stem are _____, _____, and _____.

   1. medulla, pons, midbrain

2. The _____ is the middle division.

   2. pons

3. The reticular activating system is primarily concerned with _____.

   3. level of alertness

Frame 15

Centers for many vital body activities are also located in the brain stem. Included are:

inhibitory cardiovascular center (medulla)
inspiratory respiratory center (medulla)
excitatory cardiovascular center (medulla and pons)
pneumotaxic center for normal respiratory patterns (pons).

1. Located in the brain stem are five centers relating to essential body functions. The centers are related to the function of which systems?

   a. circulatory
   b. respiratory
   c. integumentary
   d. skeletal

1. a, b

2. Choose the functions that are controlled by structures in the brain stem.

   a. emotions
   b. thinking
   c. voluntary movements
   d. alertness
   e. respirations

2. d, e

Cranial Nerve Functions

Frame 16

All of the cranial nerves except the olfactory and optic nerves originate in the brain stem. Locate the origin of the cranial nerves in Figure 1.10.

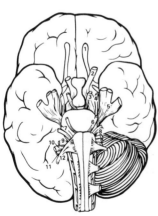

1 OLFACTORY NERVE
2 OPTIC NERVE
3 OCULOMOTOR NERVE
4 TROCHLEAR NERVE
5 TRIGEMINAL:
    OPHTHALMIC DIV.
    MAXILLARY DIV.
    MANDIBULAR DIV.
6 ABDUCENS NERVE
7 FACIAL NERVE
8 VESTIBULOCOCHLEAR
    (ACOUSTIC)
9 GLOSSOPHARYNGEAL NERVE
10 VAGUS NERVE
11 SPINAL ACCESSORY NERVE
12 HYPOGLOSSAL NERVE

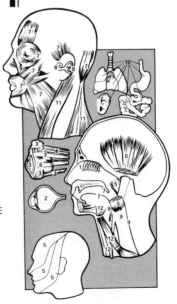

Figure 1.10. *Cranial nerve functions*

Cranial nerves carry sensations from the periphery to the brain, and transmit messages from the brain to the viscera. Study Figure 1.10 to review functions of the cranial nerves.

Reflexes—Six important parasympathetic reflexes are dependent upon a functional vagus system which includes cranial nerve X and portions of VII, IX, and XI. Each of these nerves have some fibers that affect the following reflexes:

> gag reflex
> vomiting reflex
> cough reflex
> salivary—taste reflex
> carotid sinus reflex (slow heart rate and vasodilation)
> carotid body reflex (responds to changes of pO_2 and pCO_2 in blood.)

Refer to Figure 1.10 to answer these questions.

1. The three cranial nerves that control the external eye muscles are the _____, _____, and _____.

2. The _____ nerve carries visual sensations to the brain.

3. The oculomotor nerve, CN number _____, contains parasympathetic fibers for pupil constriction.

4. The sensory fibers to the tongue are supplied by the _____ and _____ cranial nerves.

5. If the trigeminal nerve was damaged, the muscles needed for _____ would not be innervated. Sensation would not be felt in what areas?

6. The gag reflex is dependent upon a functional _____ system.

7. The vagal system is also known as the _____ system.

8. The muscles for facial expression are innervated by fibers from the _____ cranial nerve.

1. oculomotor, abducens, trochlear

2. optic

3. III

4. VII and IX

5. chewing
mouth, nose, orbit, anterior half scalp

6. vagal

7. parasympathetic

8. VII

Frame 17

The hypothalamus, located anterior to the brain stem, controls appetite, sexual function, temperature, and water balance. It also exerts influence on emotions.

The thalamus, located adjacent to the hypothalamus, is the crucial structure for the perception of sensation. It receives sensory input from throughout the body and relays it to higher areas of the brain.

In addition, the optic chiasm is located just above the midbrain. This is the area in which the fibers of the two optic nerves come together.

1. Perception of sensory stimulation is mediated by the _____.

   1. thalamus

2. The hypothalamus _____ appetite, sexual function, body temperature, and water balance.

   2. controls

Meningeal Structures

Frame 18

In addition to the protection supplied to the brain by the bony skull, three coverings encase the brain to soften blows to the head.

Find the three meningeal layers: dura mater, arachnoid membrane, and pia mater, in Figure 1.11. Note that the dura mater is the thickest of the membranes.

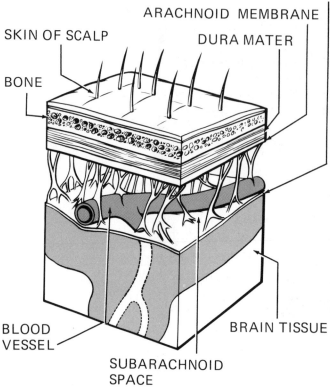

PIA MATER

ARACHNOID MEMBRANE

SKIN OF SCALP   DURA MATER

BONE

BLOOD VESSEL   BRAIN TISSUE

SUBARACHNOID SPACE

Figure 1.11.   *Meningeal layers*

Cerebrospinal fluid flows into the space between the arachnoid and pia mater. This is called the subarachnoid space. A potential space exists between the dura and arachnoid.

The meningeal layers contain nerve endings which are sensitive to displacement and to foreign substances.

1. Cerebrospinal fluid circulates in the (epidural/subarachnoid) space.

2. The dura mater is the (outermost/innermost) meningeal layer.

3. The meninges are (sensitive/insensitive) to stimulation and pain.

4. The (dura/pia mater) is the thickest protective layer.

1. subarachnoid

2. outermost

3. sensitive

4. dura

Frame 19

The enfoldings of the meninges divide the structures of the brain into anatomic compartments. The tentorium is a fold that divides the cerebral hemispheres from the cerebellum. The cerebral hemispheres are above the tentorium (supratentorial) and the cerebellum is below (infratentorial).

The falx separates the right and left cerebral hemispheres. These two meningeal folds (falx and tentorium) help to stabilize the cranial structures.

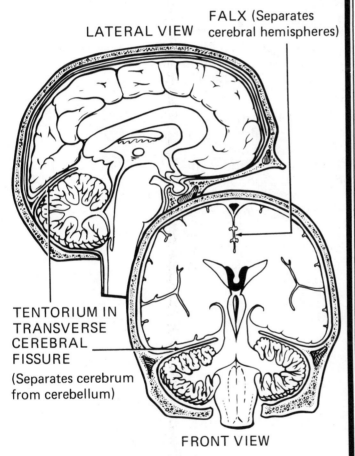

FALX (Separates cerebral hemispheres)
LATERAL VIEW

TENTORIUM IN TRANSVERSE CEREBRAL FISSURE

(Separates cerebrum from cerebellum)

FRONT VIEW

Figure 1.12. *Falx cerebri and tentorium*

1. The cerebrum is located in the

    a. supratentorial space
    b. infratentorial space

1. a

2. The cerebellum is located

   a. supratentorially
   b. infratentorially

3. The falx

   a. separates the cerebrum and cerebellum
   b. connects the two cerebral hemispheres
   c. separates the right and left cerebral hemispheres

2. b

3. c

Cerebrospinal Fluid and Ventricular System

Frame 20

The cerebrospinal fluid (CSF) that flows in the subarachnoid space, serves to cushion the brain and the spinal cord. Cerebrospinal fluid is manufactured in the choroid plexes. These are found primarily in the lateral ventricle and, to some extent, in the third ventricle.

The CSF flows from the ventricles through the Foramen of Magendie and Luschka into the subarachnoid space. A portion of the CSF circulates slowly upward, until it reaches the arachnoid villi and is incorporated in the venous blood stream. Another portion circulates down into the subarachnoid space surrounding the spinal cord.

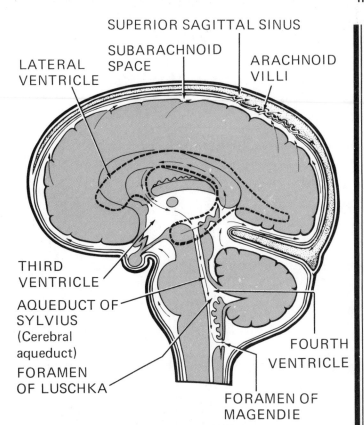

SUPERIOR SAGITTAL SINUS

SUBARACHNOID
SPACE

LATERAL
VENTRICLE

ARACHNOID
VILLI

THIRD
VENTRICLE

AQUEDUCT OF
SYLVIUS
(Cerebral
aqueduct)

FORAMEN
OF LUSCHKA

FOURTH
VENTRICLE

FORAMEN OF
MAGENDIE

Figure 1.13. *Ventricular system and CSF flow*

1. The _____ ___ _____ connects the third and fourth ventricles.

2. Most of the production of CSF takes place in the choroid plexus of the _____ ventricle.

1. Aqueduct of Sylvius

2. lateral

Frame 21

About 400–500 ml of CSF are manufactured each day, but reabsorption keeps the circulating amount at approximately 135 ml. Normal CSF contains small amounts of protein, sugar, chlorides, and a few lymphocytes.

1. About how much CSF is produced daily?

    a. 50 ml
    b. 135 ml
    c. 200 ml
    d. 400 ml

1. d

2. What is the circulating amount of CSF?

    a. 50 ml
    b. 135 ml
    c. 400 ml

3. CSF is absorbed

    a. into the brain
    b. into the 3rd ventricle
    c. into the venous circulation

4. The purpose of CSF is

    a. to cushion the brain
    b. to bring oxygen and nutrients to brain cells
    c. to increase intracranial pressure

5. Which of the following substances would you find in normal CSF?

    a. small amounts of sugar
    b. large amounts of chloride
    c. many lymphocytes
    d. small amounts of protein
    e. small amounts of blood

2. b

3. c

4. a (b is a function of the blood)

5. a, d

Circulatory Supply

Frame 22

Now review the blood supply of the brain. Trace the cranial circulation on Figure 1.14.

Blood reaches the brain via two main pathways:

    Right and left internal carotid arteries
    Basilar artery formed by the joining of the two vertebral arteries.

At the base of the brain, these structures are connected via communicating arteries to form the Circle of Willis.

The Circle of Willis, to some extent, promotes circulation to all cerebral structures even if one channel is blocked.

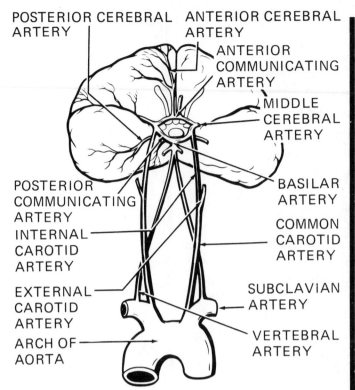

POSTERIOR CEREBRAL ARTERY

ANTERIOR CEREBRAL ARTERY

ANTERIOR COMMUNICATING ARTERY

MIDDLE CEREBRAL ARTERY

POSTERIOR COMMUNICATING ARTERY

INTERNAL CAROTID ARTERY

EXTERNAL CAROTID ARTERY

ARCH OF AORTA

BASILAR ARTERY

COMMON CAROTID ARTERY

SUBCLAVIAN ARTERY

VERTEBRAL ARTERY

Figure 1.14. *Circle of Willis*

True or false:

1. _____ The main channels for blood from the aorta to the brain are the common carotid arteries and the vertebral arteries.

2. _____ The anterior communicating artery is part of the Circle of Willis.

3. _____ The Circle of Willis is located within the cerebral hemispheres.

4. _____ The posterior communicating arteries connect the internal carotid and the basilar arteries.

5. _____ The Circle of Willis promotes collateral circulation.

1. True

2. True

3. False, at the base of the brain

4. True

5. True

Frame 23

On the lateral view of the brain in Figure 1.15 note the pattern of blood supply to the lateral surface of the brain.

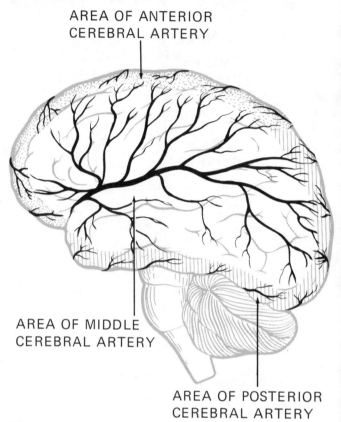

AREA OF ANTERIOR
CEREBRAL ARTERY

AREA OF MIDDLE
CEREBRAL ARTERY

AREA OF POSTERIOR
CEREBRAL ARTERY

Figure 1.15. *Cerebral arteries*

True or False:

1. _____ Disruption of blood supply in the middle cerebral artery could damage the speech areas in the brain.

2. _____ The area nourished by the posterior cerebral artery is associated with vision.

3. _____ Lack of circulation to the cerebral cortex could cause problems with logic and judgment.

1. True (See Frame 7.)

2. True

3. True

PART II
MICROSCOPIC ANATOMY

The unique properties of nerve cells make their three fundamental functions possible:

Receive and react to stimuli
Transmit impulses rapidly
Coordinate the reactions of other body systems.

The Neuron

Frame 24

The neuron is the basic unit of the nervous system.

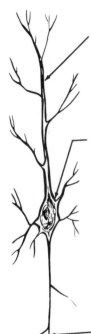

DENDRITES: THESE SHORT, BRANCHED PROCESSES RECEIVE STIMULATION FROM OTHER CELLS AND CONDUCT IMPULSES TOWARD THE CELL BODY. CELLS CAN HAVE ONE OR MORE DENDRITES.

CELL BODY: THIS STRUCTURE IS RICH IN POTASSIUM IONS ESSENTIAL TO NERVE IMPULSE TRANSMISSION AND IS ABLE TO SYNTHESIZE LARGE AMOUNTS OF PROTEIN TO MAINTAIN ITS INTEGRITY AND PERFORM ITS FUNCTIONS. THE MITOCHONDRIA ARE THE POWERHOUSES WHERE ENERGY IS PRODUCED FROM CARBOHYDRATE AND OXYGEN.

AXON: THIS PROCESS CONDUCTS IMPULSES AWAY FROM THE CELL BODY. MOST NERVE CELLS HAVE ONLY ONE AXON.

Figure 1.16.   *Nerve cell*

1. The differences between axons and dendrites are

   a. Axons carry impulses to the cells and dendrites carry them away from the cells.
   b. Dendrites are usually shorter than axons and have tree-like branches.

   c. Cells usually have only one axon but many dendrites.

   d. Dendrites are the powerhouses of the cell and axons are nerve fibers.

1. b, c

2. Energy for cell function is produced in the

   a. Axon
   b. Mitochondria
   c. Golgi bodies
   d. Cell membrane

2. b

3. Choose the chief functions of nerve cells

   a. Transmit stimuli quickly through the system
   b. Secrete hormones into the bloodstream
   c. Sense and respond to external stimuli
   d. Coordinate the reactions of body systems to maintain homeostasis

3. a, c, d

Supporting Tissues

Frame 25

There are several other kinds of cells in the nervous system.

Neuroglia (glial cells) provide repair, support, and protection for delicate nerve cells.

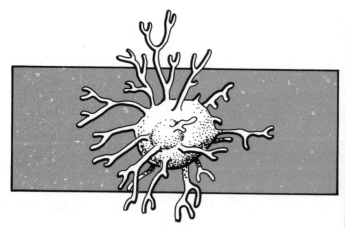

Figure 1.17. *Neuroglia*

Microglia cells act as phagocytes and clear away the debris occurring in normal cellular disintegration.

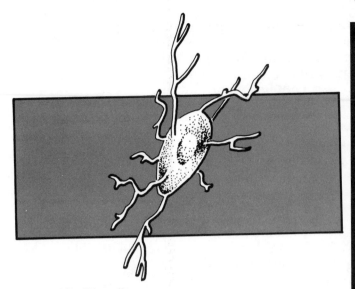

Figure 1.18. *Microglia*

Match the cells found in the nervous system with their function

1. microglia	a.	conduction of nerve impulses	1. c
2. neuron	b.	support and repair of tissue	2. a
3. neuroglia	c.	phagocytic action	3. b

Frame 26

The axons of many nerve cells are surrounded by a layer of fatty tissue called the myelin sheath.

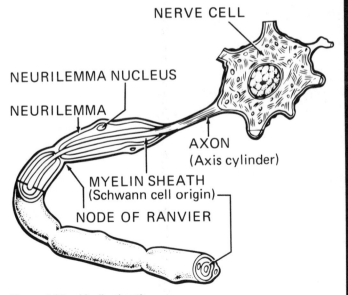

Figure 1.19. *Myelin sheath*

The myelin sheath acts as an effective electric insulator. The Nodes of Ranvier are areas where the stimulus can be "boosted" for faster conduction along the fiber. Some fibers, such as those in the autonomic nervous system, do not have a myelin sheath.

The myelin sheath is covered by a delicate membrane, called the neurilemma. After injury to a nerve, the neurilemma functions as a scaffold along which new nerve fibers can regenerate. Some nerve fibers do not have a neurilemma. Thus, injury to these nerves is permanent.

1. The main function of the myelin sheath is:

2. The neurilemma is important in:

3. The Nodes of Ranvier affect the speed of:

1. insulating the fiber electrically

2. nerve fiber regeneration

3. stimulus conduction along the nerve

Synapses

Frame 27

The synapse is the contact site of one neuron with another. A space called the synaptic cleft exists between the neurons at the synapse. This space can be seen only with an electron microscope.

Note in Figure 1.20 that synapses occur between:

    A. An axon and another neuron's cell body
    B. Two axons
    C. An axon and the dendrite of another neuron
    D. An axon and a gland cell (or sensory endings and muscles)

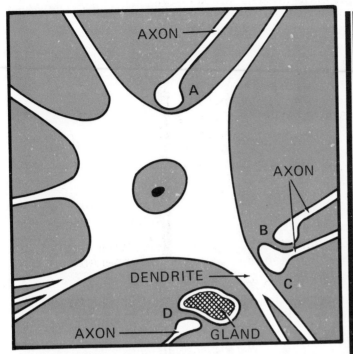

Figure 1.20. *Four kinds of synapses*

A specific synapse might not be a permanent structure. It can be replaced by a new synapse.

The axon of one neuron may have only a few synapses, or many thousands. Dendrites can receive synaptic contacts from as many as 15,000 different neurons.

True or False:

1. _____ Nerve fibers of various cells are connected physically so impulses can be transmitted.

2. _____ A large number of dendrite synapses would bring many impulses into the cell.

3. _____ The synaptic structure of the nervous system is fixed and unchanging.

1. False (there is a synaptic cleft)

2. True

3. False (new synapses can be formed)

PART III
REVIEW OF BASIC
NEUROPHYSIOLOGY

Propagation Of Impulses

Frame 28

The cell membrane acts as a thin boundary between the cytoplasm inside the cell and the extracellular fluid outside the cell. The cytoplasm contains electrolytes that have more negative charges, while extracellular fluid tends to have a positive charge.

The resting neuron is a charged cell that is not conducting an impulse.

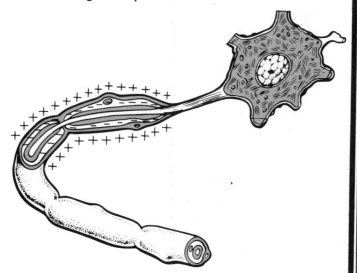

Figure 1.21.   *Polarized nerve cell*

1. The resting neuron is polarized. This means that the outer surface of the cell membrane is electrically _____ while the inner surface is _____.

2. The cell membrane is a boundary between the _____ fluid outside the cell and the _____ inside the cell.

1. positive
   negative

2. extracellular
   cytoplasm (or
   intracellular fluid)

Frame 29

The nerve impulse is not an electric current like one passing through a wire; rather, it is a series of ionic changes along the membrane. (Recall that particles such as sodium and potassium have positive electrical charges. These charged particles are called ions.)

Figure 1.22 shows that when a nerve is stimulated, the cell membrane allows positive sodium (Na+) ions to rush into the cell, producing a positive charge at the site. This is called *depolarization*. Potassium (K+) then moves out of the membrane to restore the resting potential at the site. This process is *repolarization*. Later, the small amount of sodium which entered the cell is pumped out. The other ion changes are slight and do not need to be corrected.

APPLICATION OF STIMULUS

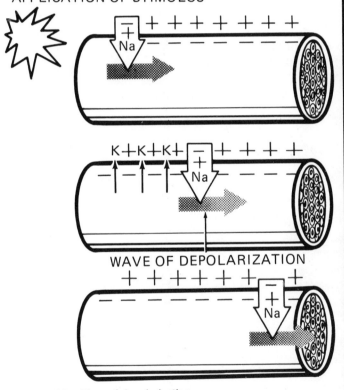

Figure 1.22. *Wave of depolarization*

The wave of polarization and depolarization moves along the membrane and the ionic changes can be measured as an electrical event.

True or False:

1. _____ Nerve impulses are conducted by ionic changes along the cell membrane of the nerve.

2. _____ During depolarization, potassium rushes into the cell making the inside of the membrane electrically positive.

3. _____ Repolarization means returning the membrane to its resting state.

4. _____ The resting potential of a fiber is an equal number of positive and negative ions on both sides of the membrane.

5. _____ The nerve impulse is a wave of metabolic activity that can be measured as an electrical event traveling along a neuronal membrane.

1. True

2. False (sodium does this)

3. True

4. False, (outside is positive, inside is negative)

5. True

Refractory Periods

Frame 30

A nerve cell is not excitable for a millisecond after the initiation of an impulse, no matter how strong the stimulus is. This interval is called the *absolute* refractory period. Immediately following this period is an interval during which the nerve fiber can be stimulated only by an exceptionally strong stimulus. This is called the *relative* refractory period.

The total polarization-depolarization cycle takes less than one second, so the nerve is capable of almost continuous transmission.

1. How does the absolute refractory period differ from the relative refractory period?

1. absolute—no new impulse can be transmitted relative—a very strong impulse can initiate an impulse

Synaptic Transmission

Frame 31

Now review how impulses move across synapses.

Figure 1.23 shows the synaptic knob at the end of the axon. The pre-synaptic vesicles contain precursors of chemical substances which are neurotransmitters. When the neurotransmitters are secreted, they diffuse across the synaptic cleft and cause the synaptic membrane of the next neuron to depolarize. The impulse wave then starts down the next neuron.

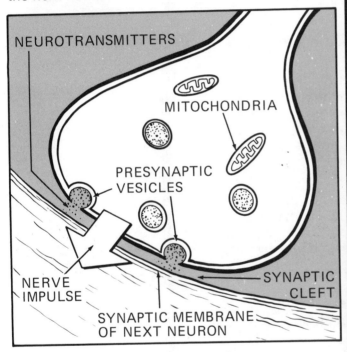

Figure 1.23. *Impulse transmission across the synapse*

The synapse will repolarize in a few milliseconds as the neurotransmitter is inactivated by enzymatic action. It is then ready for another impulse. The best known neurotransmitters are acetylcholine, norepinephrine, serotonin, and dopamine, but there are many others.

The synapse differs from nerve fibers in that it is fatigable. If the store of neurotransmitter chemicals is depleted, the synapse will not transmit the impulse.

1. Impulses cross the synaptic cleft by which mechanism:

   a. electrical "jumping"
   b. chemical substances causing depolarization of the next neuron
   c. direct contact of two fibers

2. Neurotransmitters are secreted by the:

   a. mitochondria
   b. plasma membrane
   c. presynaptic vesicle

3. Study figure 1.23 to determine: how do impulses move across a synapse?

   a. in one direction only
   b. in both directions

4. Why is this an advantage in the organization of the nervous system?

   a. Prevents impulses from traveling backwards through the axon to the cell body and dendrites
   b. Permits impulse flow only through a functional sequence of neurons
   c. Requires more energy for impulse transmission

5. Medications, anesthetics, and insufficient blood supply can interfere with the production and/or action of neurotransmitters. What would be the effect of such interference?

   a. depletion of neurotransmitters in the synapses
   b. fatigue of the axons
   c. increased excitation of the post synaptic membrane

1. b

2. c

3. a (pre-synaptic vesicles that secrete neurotransmitter on one side only)

4. a, b

5. a

CHAPTER 2

INCREASED INTRACRANIAL PRESSURE

Increased intracranial pressure (ICP) is found in many neurologic patients. Although the causes of increased pressure may vary, the mechanisms involved in the increasing pressure are similar.

At the conclusion of this chapter you will be able to:

1. Explain the anatomic basis for the occurrence of increased intracranial pressure
2. Relate the effects of increased intracranial pressure on cranial contents and body functions
3. Correlate metabolic findings and patient status
4. Select compensatory mechanisms utilized when intracranial pressure increases
5. Trace the evolution of cerebral edema
6. Locate sites of herniation in increased supratentorial and infratentorial pressure
7. Explain the effects of ↑ICP and herniation on brain cells.

Chapter outline

Anatomic basis for increased intracranial pressure (↑ICP)
    Cranial components
    Adjustments to volume changes
Metabolic needs of the brain
    Extent of metabolic demand
    Interference with nutrient supply
    Conditions affecting metabolism
        Lack of oxygen
        Lack of glucose
        Fever
Autoregulation of cerebral blood flow
    Systemic arterial pressure changes
    Cerebral vasodilation
Cerebral water balance
Effects of increased intracranial pressure
    Tissue damage
    Herniation
        Supratentorial
        Infratentorial

PART I
ANATOMIC BASIS FOR INCREASED INTRACRANIAL PRESSURE

Cranial Components

Frame 1

The brain is tightly enclosed within the cranial cavity. Both the bony skull and the meningeal covering form boundaries which prevent expansion. There are three major intracranial components—brain tissue, cerebrospinal fluid, and intravascular blood. The amounts of the three components fluctuate, but they essentially remain within certain limits.

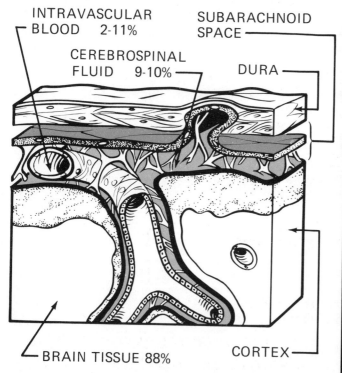

Figure 2.1. *Intracranial contents*

The cerebrospinal fluid is nearly constant in volume, and the cranial contents are nearly non-compressible. If one component increases, it does so at the expense of the other components. This shift is possible only within narrow limits without damaging cranial tissue.

1. The reason that an increase in cranial contents causes symptomatology, while this does not occur as readily in other body compartments, is that the brain is enclosed in a _____.

   1. non-expansible bony structure

2. The three cranial components are _____, _____, _____.

   2. blood, CSF, brain tissue

3. The cranial component which has the widest range of variability is the _____.

   3. intravascular blood

Frame 2

The relationship of the capacity of the container (skull) to the contents (intravascular blood, CSF, tissue), is the primary determinant of ICP.

If the three cranial contents exceed the established boundaries, increased intracranial pressure results.

	(water) mm H_2O	(mercury) mm Hg
Normal intracranial pressure	110–140	0–15
Increased intracranial pressure	200	15

1. If the intracranial pressure measures 30 mm Hg., this indicates (normal / increased) pressure.

   1. increased

2. If the cranial contents increase in volume the intracranial pressure (decreases/increases).

   2. increases

Adjustments To Volume Changes

Frame 3

The cranial compartments adjust to changes in volume in the following ways:

Expansion of *brain tissue* due to tumor causes

→more absorption of CSF into venous sinuses

→escape of blood into the systemic vascular system

Similarly:

Increase in *CSF* → blood moves into the systemic system

Increase in *blood volume* → ↑CSF absorption

If these changes do not reduce the pressure, the brain tissue may be displaced through available openings in the cranium. Figure 2.2 shows three common sites for displacement: across the midline, through the tentorial notch, and through the foramen magnum.

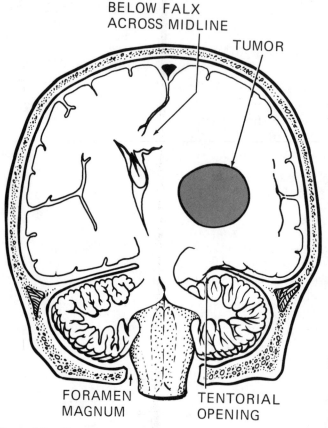

BELOW FALX
ACROSS MIDLINE

TUMOR

FORAMEN
MAGNUM

TENTORIAL
OPENING

Figure 2.2. *Sites of brain herniation*

True or False:

1. _____ A patient's intracranial pressure is measured at 207 mm H_2O. This is high normal.

2. _____ If brain tissue expands, blood is displaced from the brain to make room.

3. _____ The main determinant of intracranial pressure is the relationship between the volume of the skull and the cranial contents.

4. _____ CSF volume remains the same regardless of shifts in intracranial pressure.

1. False (See Frame 2.)

2. True

3. True

4. False (CSF can be reabsorbed into venous sinuses)

5. _____ Displacement of brain tissue through skull openings is a response to low intracranial pressures.

5. False

You will learn about monitoring intracranial pressure in Chapter 5.

Frame 4

Summary:

The primary determinant of intracranial pressure is the relationship between skull capacity and the volume of intracranial contents: brain tissue, intravascular blood, and CSF.

	mm H_2O	mm Hg
Normal intracranial pressure	110–140	0–15
Increased intracranial pressure	> 200	> 15

Cranial components adjust to increased pressure by redirection of blood into systemic circulation, absorption of CSF into venous sinuses, and displacement of brain tissue through skull openings.

PART II
METABOLIC NEEDS OF THE BRAIN

Extent Of Metabolic Demand

Frame 5

The brain comprises only 2% of the body weight, but astoundingly, the brain consumes 20% of the body's oxygen consumption and 25% of the body's glucose.

Maintenance of an adequate supply of *oxygen* and *glucose* is essential for the functioning of the brain. Here are some facts you should know:

—The brain's demand for nutrients remains constant even if the body is at rest.
—The vital centers of the brain stem are particularly sensitive to decreased nourishment.
—The brain has a minimum capacity for storage of oxygen and glucose, and needs a steady supply.

Interference With Nutrient Supply

Anything that interferes with the circulatory transport of oxygen and glucose to the brain can hinder brain cell metabolism and cause damage to cells. While increased intracranial pressure is not the sole cause of interference with transport of oxygen to the brain, it is one of the most important.

1. Which conditions would interfere with continuous delivery of adequate oxygen and glucose to brain cells?

   1. all

   a. shock
   b. increased intracranial pressure
   c. cerebral arteriosclerosis
   d. intracranial hemorrhage

2. Why does the brain need a constant supply of oxygen and glucose?

   a. because it can't store these nutrients
   b. because metabolic demand is not affected by activity and rest

c. CSF quickly removes these from the blood

3. Which brain structure is particularly sensitive to decreased levels of oxygen and glucose?

a. meninges
b. brain stem
c. frontal lobe
d. temporal lobe

2. a, b

3. b

Conditions Affecting Metabolism

Frame 6

Oxygen is essential for normal brain metabolism.

Lack of oxygen for 10 seconds, and/or a cerebral oxygen tension below 30 mm Hg, results in loss of consciousness (coma).

Lack of oxygen for 4–5 minutes usually results in brain death at normal body temperature.

1. Essential nutrients for the brain cells are _____ and _____.

1. oxygen
   glucose

2. Coma occurs if the brain has been without oxygen for _____ seconds or if the cerebral oxygen tension is below _____ mm Hg.

2. 10
   30

3. If the brain is deprived of oxygen for 4–5 minutes _____ occurs.

3. brain death

Frame 7

In addition to oxygen, the brain also requires glucose. The normal range of blood glucose is 80-120 mg/100 ml, by the most common method of measurement. With this range as a standard, arterial glucose levels below 70 mg/100 ml result in confusion. Coma occurs when arterial glucose levels fall below 20 mg/100 ml.

1. Mr. Dee has a blood glucose level of 50 mg/100 ml. You could expect (coma/confusion).

    1. confusion

2. A later finding on Mr. Dee shows an arterial oxygen tension of 20 mm Hg and a blood glucose level of 10 mg/100 ml. He (would/would not) be easily aroused.

    2. would not

Frame 8

Fever greatly increases the usage of oxygen and glucose, and thus the flow of blood to the brain. Each 1°C rise in temperature increases the metabolic demands by 10%. For example, when the temperature increases from 37°C to 41°C, there is a 40% increase in oxygen consumption.

A temperature above 42°C causes a collapse in cerebral blood flow and a decrease in the systemic arterial pressure.

1. Ann has a temperature of 39.5°C. By how much are her oxygen consumption needs increased?

    1. 25% (39.5 − 37 = 2.5 × 10%)

2. There is a collapse of the cerebral vascular system when a temperature rises above _____ °C.

    2. 42°C

Frame 9

Glucose and oxygen are transformed into energy needed for cerebral metabolism. The greater share of this energy is used to reestablish the electrochemical gradients needed for excitation of the neurons and the transmission of impulses. Energy is also needed for the biosynthesis of transmitter substances and for maintenance of cellular integrity. If not enough energy is available for impulse transmission, coma results.

1. List three of the processes requiring energy expenditure in the brain.

    a. _____
    b. _____

    1. a. electrochemical gradients for impulse transmission
    b. biosynthesis of transmitter substances

c. _____

c. maintenance of cellular integrity

Frame 10

Summary:

The brain's need for oxygen and glucose is constant and vital, and there is no storage capacity.

Coma—lack of O_2 for 10 seconds, cerebral O_2 tension <30 mm Hg
—arterial glucose level <20 mg/100 ml

Confusion—arterial glucose level <70 mg/ 100 ml

Brain death—lack of O_2 for 4–5 minutes

Fever increases metabolic demands 10% for each degree Centigrade.

PART III
AUTOREGULATION OF
CEREBRAL BLOOD FLOW

Systemic Arterial Pressure Changes

Frame 11

You can now appreciate the important role of the cerebral circulation in supplying adequate oxygen and glucose to the brain. This formula demonstrates the relationship of the factors affecting cerebral blood flow:

$$\text{Cerebral perfusion pressure} = \frac{\left[\text{Mean systemic arterial pressure}\right] - \left[\text{Mean intracranial pressure}\right]}{\text{Cerebral vascular resistance}}$$

1. If intracranial pressure rises and the systemic arterial pressure stays the same, cerebral blood flow will (rise/fall).

2. If both the intracranial pressure and the systemic arterial pressure rise proportionately, cerebral blood flow would (rise/fall/stay about the same).

1. fall

2. stay about the same

Frame 12

This, in fact, is one way the body protects the brain's supply of oxygen and glucose. If the intracranial pressure rises, the systemic arterial pressure also rises to maintain cerebral blood flow.

This autoregulatory process can only be increased to a certain point. If the intracranial pressure continues to rise, a point is reached where the systemic blood pressure can no longer provide sufficient blood to the brain.

Mr. Williams is hospitalized for treatment of a head injury suffered while playing basketball. Here are his mean arterial pressures at:

1:00   100
1:20   104
1:35   106
1:45   110

True or False:

1. _____ Mr. Williams' arterial pressure could be rising to protect the cerebral blood flow as his intracranial pressure rises.

2. _____ The patient's blood pressure will continue to rise as long as the intracranial pressure increases.

1. True

2. False

Cerebral Vasodilation

Frame 13

Cerebral vascular resistance is the hindrance to blood flow caused by the walls of the blood vessels. Vessels of large diameter offer less resistance to flow than small ones. Look again at the formula in Frame 11 to answer these questions.

1. If the cranial arteries dilate, there will be (more/less) cerebral vascular resistance.

2. If cerebral vascular resistance drops, cerebral blood flow will (increase/decrease).

1. less

2. increase

Frame 14

Now you can see why cerebral vasodilation is another compensatory mechanism in increased intracranial pressure.

When the cerebral oxygen tension falls below 50 mm Hg, the cerebral arteries dilate to increase blood flow and oxygen delivery.

If this mechanism fails to raise the oxygen tension, the brain cells will not have enough oxygen to produce energy. They will then produce energy by means of a chemical process that does not require oxygen (anaerobic metabolism). A byproduct of this process is lactic acid that accumulates and makes the blood more acidic. More acid in the blood causes vasodilation and greater cerebral blood flow.

1. If Mr. Williams' intracranial pressure rises enough to compromise cerebral blood flow, what effects will be seen?

    1. b, c

    a. increased cerebral oxygen tension
    b. impaired delivery of glucose to brain cells
    c. decreased oxygen supply to brain cells

2. If his brain has an inadequate oxygen supply, anaerobic pathways are used to produce energy resulting in a build up of what substance?

    2. c

    a. oxygen
    b. carbon dioxide
    c. lactic acid
    d. none of the above

3. What are the two chemical changes causing vasodilation and increased cerebral blood flow?

    3. b, d

    a. increased ATP production
    b. lowered blood pH (more acid)
    c. low CO_2 tension
    d. O_2 tension below 50 mm Hg

Summary:

When increased intracranial pressure interferes with cerebral blood flow, the following autoregulatory mechanisms operate to protect blood flow to the brain:

Increase in mean systemic arterial pressure
Cerebral vasodilation caused by
↓O_2 tension
↓ blood pH due to anaerobic metabolism with accumulation of lactic acid.

PART IV
CEREBRAL WATER BALANCE

Frame 15

A phenomenon often seen in increased intracranial pressure is cerebral edema. Cerebral edema is an increase in tissue fluid content and, hence, an increase in tissue volume. It may be the primary cause of increased intracranial pressure or it may accompany other causes of increased pressure.

Why does edema occur? When you bang your leg against a door, there is tissue damage and subsequent edema. The skin allows for expansion without undue pressure on the underlying structures. However, when edema occurs intracranially there is little extra room and increased pressure occurs.

Almost all forms of insult to the brain affect cerebral water balance and lead to edema. Included are trauma, ischemia and anoxia, tumors, and arterial hypertension.

1. Which intracranial components are indicated in this schematic diagram?

   1. A. brain tissue
      B. CSF
      C. intravascular blood

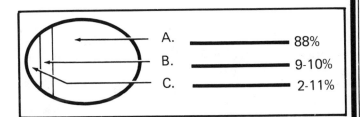

Figure 2.3. *Percentage of cranial components*

2. Cerebral edema refers to increased volume of which component?

   2. brain tissue

3. What effect does cerebral edema have upon intracranial pressure?

   3. increases

4. What are some causes of cerebral edema?

   4. trauma, ischemia, anoxia, tumors, hypertension.

49

Frame 16

The endothelial lining of capillaries in the brain is different from capillaries in the rest of the body. The cells are tightly joined and form a barrier to diffusion.

Fat-soluble substances dissolve in the lipid layer of the membrane and then diffuse into the brain. An example of this is a fat-soluble vitamin.

Electrolytes, glucose, and amino acids are thought to pass through special pores in the membrane, or are taken up by chemical "pumps."

This feature of the capillary membrane is called the blood-brain barrier, and protects the brain cells from many substances in the blood that could damage the sensitive nerve cells. This mechanism also has a disadvantage. Since medications vary in solubility, not all will cross the blood-brain barrier in concentrations adequate for therapeutic use.

Factors associated with cerebral edema and increased intracranial pressure alter the permeability of this barrier, leaving the brain more vulnerable to toxic damage.

True or False:

1. _____ Cerebral edema indicates an increase in CSF.

2. _____ Glucose is able to pass the blood-brain barrier.

3. _____ The blood-brain barrier is the special ability of the cerebral capillary membrane to regulate diffusion of molecules into the brain.

4. _____ You would expect to see some cerebral edema with an intracerebral inflammatory process.

5. _____ Tissue fluid decreases following trauma.

6. _____ The blood-brain barrier may become less protective in ↑ICP.

1. False

2. True

3. True

4. True

5. False

6. True

PART V
EFFECTS OF INCREASED INTRACRANIAL PRESSURE

Tissue Damage

Frame 17

Increased intracranial pressure may take a spiral pattern unless interventions are initiated to interrupt the process. Initial trauma causes tissue damage resulting in cerebral edema.

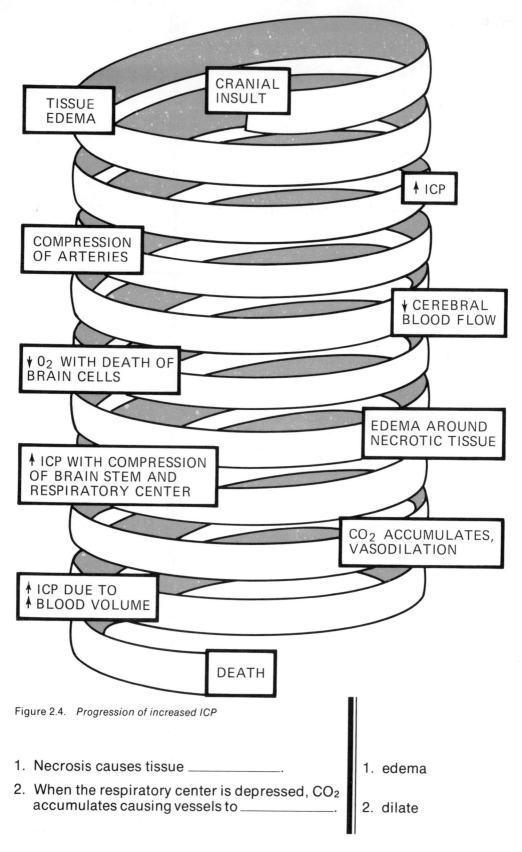

Figure 2.4. *Progression of increased ICP*

1. Necrosis causes tissue _____.

2. When the respiratory center is depressed, CO_2 accumulates causing vessels to _____.

1. edema

2. dilate

Frame 18

A brief review:

1. There is little room for expansion of the three cranial components because

   a. the skull is rigid
   b. the meningeal folds create compartments within the cranium
   c. there are no methods of compensation for ↑ volume

2. The meningeal fold which divides the cranial vault into upper and lower compartments is the

   a. falx
   b. central sulcus
   c. tentorium

3. The supratentorial space contains the

   a. cerebellum
   b. cerebral hemispheres
   c. brain stem
   d. all of the above

1. a, b

2. c (See Frame 19, Chapter 1.)

3. b

Frame 19

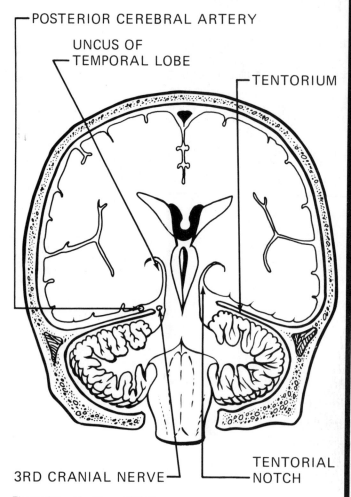

POSTERIOR CEREBRAL ARTERY

UNCUS OF
TEMPORAL LOBE

TENTORIUM

3RD CRANIAL NERVE

TENTORIAL
NOTCH

Figure 2.5. *Position of CN III*

Note in Figure 2.5 that the tentorium extends only part of the way across the base of the cerebrum. The opening is called the tentorial notch.

Now observe that the 3rd cranial nerve is present in the tentorial notch. A fold of the temporal lobe, called the uncus, lies above the tentorial notch.

1. What are the functions of the 3rd cranial nerve? (Hint: See Frame 16, Chapter 1.)

1. pupillary constriction and eye movement.

Herniation

Frame 20

Lesions and/or edema in the supratentorial compartment tend to push the uncus of the temporal
lobe through the tentorial notch. This is called
uncal or tentorial herniation. The downward pressure of the uncus compresses the oculomotor
nerve and the posterior cerebral artery. With increasing pressure, the midbrain is compressed
against the opposite side of the tentorium.

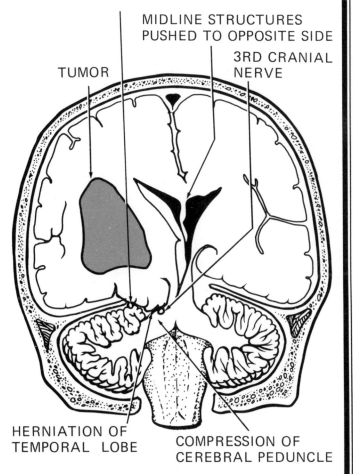

POSTERIOR CEREBRAL ARTERY

MIDLINE STRUCTURES
PUSHED TO OPPOSITE SIDE

3RD CRANIAL
NERVE

TUMOR

HERNIATION OF
TEMPORAL LOBE

COMPRESSION OF
CEREBRAL PEDUNCLE

Figure 2.6.   *Uncal herniation*

Increasing supratentorial pressure and continuing herniation may cause obstruction to cerebrospinal fluid flow in the ventricular system, adding to the volume of cranial contents.

Ischemia and hemorrhage in the brain stem likewise follow tentorial herniation. Both the initial direct downward pressure, and finally the actual displacement of the brain stem downward, causes the ischemia and tissue damage.

Compression of the brain stem results in decreased levels of consciousness and eventual coma.

1. Continuing supratentorial increased ICP results in _____ herniation.

2. Mary Miller has a lesion in the right cerebral hemisphere. The lesion would cause initial compression of the third cranial nerve on her _____ side.

3. The midbrain is pushed against the tentorium on her _____ side.

4. Increased pressure is made worse by obstruction of flow of _____ _____ _____.

5. If the Aqueduct of Sylvius is obstructed, CSF will pool in the _____ and _____ ventricles. (Hint: See Frame 20, Chapter 1.)

1. uncal or tentorial

2. right

3. left

4. cerebrospinal fluid

5. lateral third

Frame 21

Infratentorial masses and pressure may push the cerebellar tonsils and the medulla through the foramen magnum, which is the opening at the base of the skull.

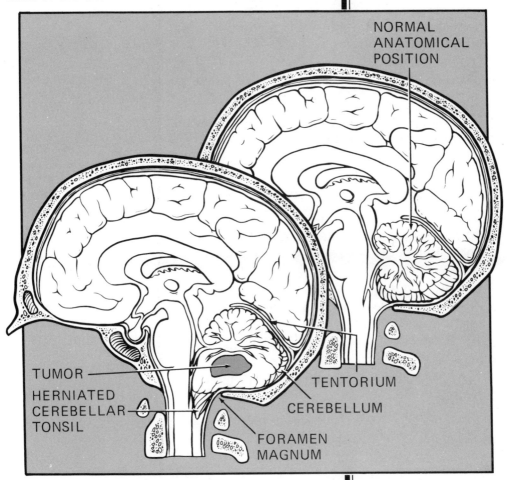

Figure 2.7. *Foramen magnum herniation*

Because the bony encasement of the cervical vertebrae does not allow for expansion, compression of the medulla often results in respiratory arrest. The anoxia resulting from respiratory and circulatory changes causes coma and eventual death.

A less common finding is infratentorial herniation. Lesions in the infratentorial compartment may press cerebellar tissue upwards through the tentorial notch.

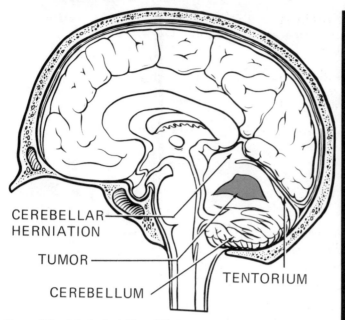

Figure 2.8. *Infratentorial herniation*

1. Increased intracranial pressure resulting from infratentorial lesions most frequently results in herniation of the cerebellar tonsils through the _____ _____.

1. foramen magnum

2. When herniation occurs from a lesion in the infratentorial compartment, compression of the medulla results in _____ _____.

2. respiratory arrest

You will learn to assess signs and symptoms of increased intracranial pressure and herniation in Chapter 5.

Frame 22

Summary:

Cerebral edema is an increase of tissue fluid in the brain caused by trauma, anoxia, tumors, and hypertension. It increases intracranial pressure, and alters the permeability of the blood-brain barrier.

The vicious circle of events in ↑ICP are:
—decreased cerebral blood flow with compensatory mechanisms to increase blood volume and ICP
—cell anoxia, edema, and necrosis with increased ICP

—compression of the brain stem and respiratory center which contributes to more anoxia, edema, and ↑ICP

Increased supratentorial pressure can cause herniation of the uncus of the temporal lobe through the tentorial notch. This results in:

—compression of the 3rd cranial nerve
—compression of the posterior cerebral artery
—compression of the midbrain
—obstructed flow of CSF out of the lateral and third ventricle

Increased infratentorial pressure can cause
—herniation of the cerebellar tonsils and medulla through the foramen magnum
—herniation through the tentorium

Herniated and compressed brain tissue becomes anoxic, edematous, and necrotic.

CHAPTER 3

CAUSES OF CRANIAL DYSFUNCTION

You have learned the mechanisms of increased intracranial pressure. In this chapter you will study the most important causes of ↑ICP. While the specific causative factor is important in the treatment and prognosis, the symptoms and much of the accompanying nursing care are related to the area of the brain in which the lesion is located. Five main types of dysfunction are included: trauma, tumors, vascular problems, infectious processes, and ventricular system problems. These five do not always cause pronounced ↑ICP, but almost all of them produce some ↑ICP. Nearly all of the causes of insult to the brain upset the cerebral water balance, which causes cerebral edema.

At the conclusion of this chapter you will be able to:

1. Associate commonly found symptom complexes with the cause
2. Compare symptoms found in rapidly and slowly increasing lesions
3. Differentiate various types of brain tumors
4. Differentiate symptoms found in subdural, epidural, and intracranial hematomas
5. Recognize the focal symptoms caused by lesions in particular anatomic areas
6. Differentiate between cerebral infarcts and intracerebral hematomas
7. Describe the symptomatology found in meningeal irritations
8. List common causes of infectious processes
9. Identify causes for interference in the ventricular system resulting in ↑ICP.

Chapter outline

Trauma
    Epidural hematoma
    Subdural hematoma
    Cerebral edema
    Concussion and contusion

Tumors
    Types
    Symptoms
        Pathologic mechanisms
        Generalized symptoms
        Location-related symptoms
            Pituitary gland tumor
            Parietal lobe
            Cerebellar tumors

Vascular problems
  Aneurysm
  Arteriosclerotic vascular disease
    Infarction
    Hematoma
  Arteriovenous malformation

Infectious processes
  Course
  Symptoms

PART I
TRAUMA

Three patients in the neuro ICU have suffered head trauma, but all have different problems. Matt Bly has an epidural hematoma resulting from being hit on the head by a club; Jack Witt's subdural hematoma followed a fall in which he hit his head; Mary Sue Davis is recovering from a closed head injury with brain stem trauma following an auto accident. These are three typical types of head trauma.

Epidural Hematoma

Frame 1

Hematomas may occur in any area of the cranial vault. A frequently used nomenclature refers to the anatomical location (parietal, temporal etc.) and the relationship of the hematoma to the dura.

Mr. Bly had an epidural hematoma in the temporal area. The blow to his head was to the left temporal bone. X-rays showed a fracture of the left temporal bone. The middle meningeal artery enters the cranium through the foramen spinosum found in the temporal bone. A fracture through the temporal bone may sever or damage this artery resulting in bleeding into the temporal fossa. The blood clot is *outside* the meningeal layer of dura (epi- or extra-dural).

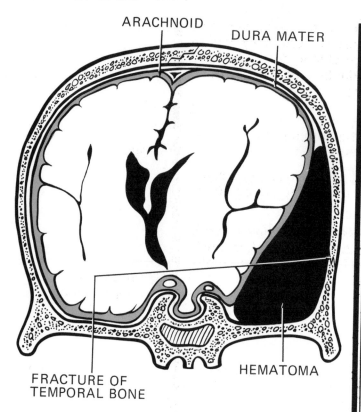

Figure 3.1   *Epidural hematoma*

Because the bleeding is arterial, the hematoma accumulates quite rapidly and pushes the brain away from the skull. Epidurals may form in other cranial areas, but the lateral temporal fossa is the most common site.

1. Epidural hematomas form (between the dura and the brain/between the dura and the skull).

2. The artery lacerated in the temporal area causing the epidural hematoma is the _____.

3. The hematoma pushes the brain (toward/away from) the skull.

1. between dura and skull

2. middle meningeal artery

3. away from

Frame 2

Initially Mr. Bly felt dazed after being struck on the head. This resulted from interference with the normal transmission of neural impulses. He had a severe headache. As the hematoma increased in size, it pushed the brain from the skull causing stretching and tearing of the pain-sensitive meninges and blood vessels. Clinically it was noted that Mr. Bly was irritable and then became less responsive. Some dilation of the left pupil was also seen at this time.

1. Mr. Bly's epidural hematoma was in the (supra/infra) tentorial space.

2. The dilation of his left pupil is due to pressure on the (second/third) cranial nerve located in the tentorial notch.

3. Pressure on this nerve and on the brain stem is caused by herniation of the (cerebellar tonsil/ uncus of the temporal lobe) through the tentorial notch.

1. supra

2. third

3. uncus of the temporal lobe

Frame 3

Hematomas add a fourth component, extravascular blood, to the cranial contents. As the clot increases in size, the underlying or adjacent brain is compressed. Edema accompanies the tissue compression further increasing the extravascular fluid and increasing intracranial pressure.

Because Mr. Bly's fracture was in the temporal area and caused serious clinical findings, he was taken to surgery and the clot was evacuated. Had the clot not been removed, he may have suffered irreparable damage to the brain stem.

Choose the pathology in Column II which is the most likely cause of the symptoms in Column I.

	Column I	Column II
1. ___	Decreased consciousness	a. uncal herniation
2. ___	Ipsilateral pupil dilation	b. traction on meninges
3. ___	Headache	c. interference with neural transmission
4. ___	Dazed—momentary lapse of consciousness	

1. a or c
2. a
3. b
4. c

True or False:

5. _____ Epidural hematomas in the temporal fossa do not require surgical intervention.

6. _____ Arterial bleeding results in rapid formation of hematomas.

7. _____ Epidural hematoma refers to hematoma in the temporal fossa.

5. False

6. True

7. False

Subdural Hematoma

Frame 4

Jack Witt, age 66, fell three weeks ago hitting his head on the sidewalk. A skull x-ray at the time revealed no fractures. Jack was observed overnight in the hospital and then sent home. During the three weeks at home his family noted increasing confusion and drowsiness. Just prior to admission, Jack noted weakness on his right side.

A diagnostic test was done revealing a subdural hematoma in the left frontal region. In subdural hematomas the blood accumulates between the dura and the arachnoid layers.

1. Which diagram depicts where Mr. Witt's hematoma was located? (A/B/C)

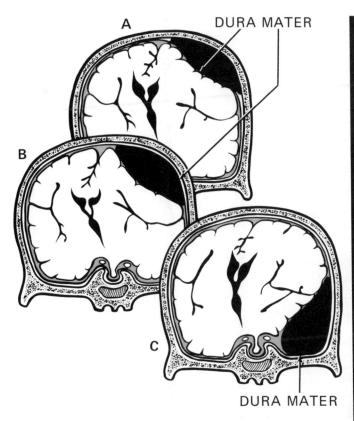

A DURA MATER

B

C

DURA MATER

Figure 3.2. *Hematoma sites*

1. B is correct, A is a frontal epidural hematoma, and C is a temporal subdural hematoma

2. Mr. Witt's hematoma was in the left frontal area. Motor weakness would be on the (left/right) side.

2. right

3. Mr. Witt's hematoma was distant from the central gyrus. You would therefore expect him to have (more/less) difficulty with motor function than with a frontal lesion closer to the central gyrus.

3. less

Frame 5

Subdural hematomas usually result from venous bleeding and accumulate less rapidly than hematomas occurring from arterial sources. Veins in the space between the dura and arachnoid are damaged, and blood slowly seeps from them. Normally only small amounts of a lymph-like material are present in the subdural space. The uninjured subdural vessels have little capacity to reabsorb the blood, despite the slow pace at which it accumulates.

In the older population, many persons have cerebral atrophy, creating a larger subdural space with lack of support for the venous network. Therefore, trauma to the head is more likely to result in a hematoma.

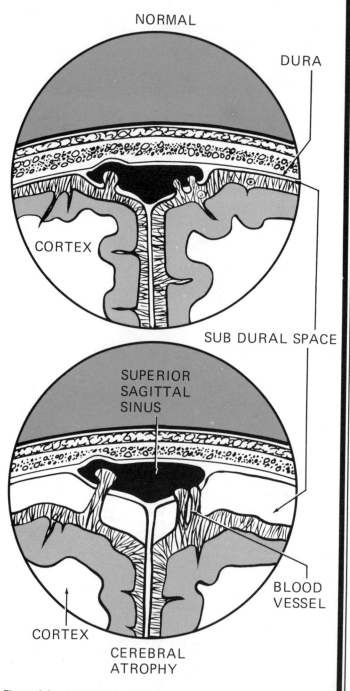

Figure 3.3. *Cerebral atrophy*

Chronic alcoholics are also prone to cerebral atrophy and subsequent subdural hematoma formation.

In addition to being in the older age group with a higher risk for subdural hematoma, Jack Witt was on anticoagulant therapy. Following minor trauma, a damaged vessel will normally seal the defect by clot formation. Anticoagulant therapy delays this process.

1. From the following list, select the individuals who would be likely to develop a subdural hematoma following trauma.

   a. 83-year-old who has unsteady gait
   b. 36-year-old on antihypertensives
   c. 48-year-old who is an alcoholic
   d. 53-year-old on anticoagulants
   e. 25-year-old on insulin

1. a, c, d

2. Subdural hematomas are located

   a. between the dura and skull
   b. between the dura and the arachnoid layer
   c. in the subarachnoid space

2. b

Frame 6

Like epidural hematomas, subdural hematomas may occur any place in the cranium. Arterial bleeding in the subdural space may also cause hematoma formation; symptoms occur more rapidly from arterial bleeding than from venous sources. In addition to location, subdurals are classified as chronic and acute. In acute subdurals symptoms develop rapidly and prompt surgical intervention is required. Chronic subdurals may be present for weeks or months while the person's condition fluctuates. Medical treatment may not be sought promptly.

Indicate whether the following statements are true or false.

1. _____ Subdurals are usually the result of arterial bleeding.

1. False

2. _____ Subdurals occur only in the supratentorial area.

2. False

3. _____ Chronic subdurals may be present for months.

3. True

Trauma may also cause intracerebral hematomas. Intracerebral hematomas are often associated with penetrating injuries: gun shot wounds, depressed bone fractures. We will consider this type of hematoma with the vascular causes of cerebral dysfunction.

Frame 7

Summary:

Epidural hematoma
—rapidly forming arterial blood clot between the dura and the skull
—progressive change in consciousness: dazed → irritable → lethargic, with interference in normal neural transmission
—headache due to stretching of meninges and blood vessels
—ipsilateral pupil dilation due to uncal herniation and pressure on third cranial nerve
—is a real emergency
—treatment—evacuation of the clot

Subdural hematoma
—usually venous blood clot, between dura and arachnoid; acute—rapidly developing symptoms, prompt surgery required; chronic—fluctuating symptoms for weeks or months
—symptoms depend on function of brain area affected
—populations at higher risk: elderly, alcoholics, patients on anticoagulants

Cerebral Edema

Frame 8

Mary Sue Davis was recovering from a closed head injury. She was a passenger in a car which collided with another car. Mrs. Davis was unconscious when the ambulance arrived and remained comatose for three days following the accident.

The rapid acceleration/deceleration of the head causes brain tissue damage with resultant cerebral edema. In edema there is an increase in interstitial and intracellular fluid which may result in interference with microcirculation. Problems then occur with the transport of oxygen and nutrients to the cell and the removal of metabolic wastes.

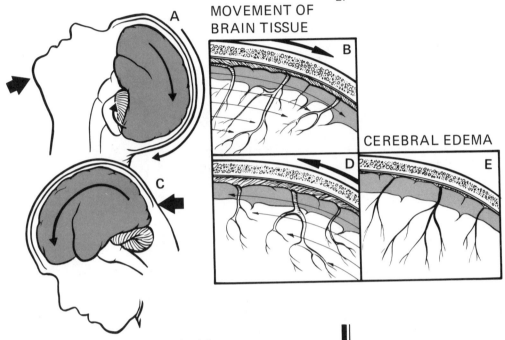

Figure 3.4. *Acceleration/deceleration injury*

A, C Forceful extension and flexion of the neck

B, D Movement of the brain within the skull

E Cerebral edema

Frame 9

The brain stem is quite firmly fixed in the internal area of the cranium. Rapid acceleration/deceleration forces other cranial contents against it. The brain stem itself may be torn by the force of these movements.

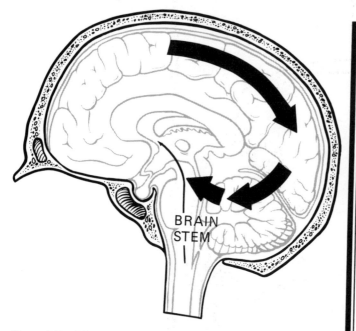

Figure 3.5.   *Effect of acceleration/deceleration on the brainstem*

True or False:

1. _____ Rapid acceleration and deceleration pushes the cranial contents against each other causing injury.

2. _____ Forces from opposite directions can tear tissue in the brain stem.

1. True

2. True

Concussion And Contusion

Frame 10

Two terms used in describing closed head injuries are concussion and contusion.

A *concussion* is a transient neuronal dysfunction causing loss of consciousness. The brain shows no visible damage. However, a sharp rise in intra-cranial pressure occurs. The pressure seeks to be dissipated through the foramen magnum in the skull. Thus, the brain stem receives the greatest pressure.

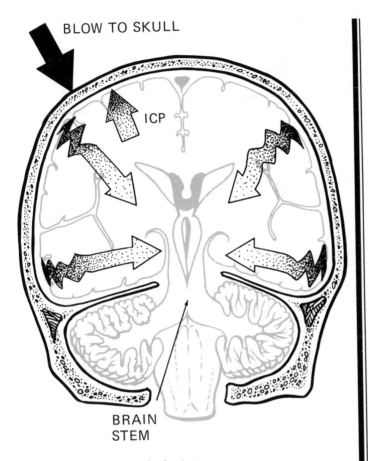

BLOW TO SKULL

ICP

BRAIN
STEM

Figure 3.6. *Pressure on brain stem*

1. Which of these functions is controlled by the brain stem?

    a. thinking
    b. consciousness
    c. visual association
    d. motor coordination

1. b

It is thought that excess acetylcholine is produced following brain injury, and that this interferes with the transmission of nerve impulses.

2. Loss of consciousness during a period of ↑ICP could be related to which factor(s)?

    a. pressure on brain stem areas controlling consciousness
    b. ↑ acetylcholine production which blocks neural transmission
    c. cerebral edema causing an increase in cranial contents.

2. a, b, c

3. A concussion of the brain is associated with which factor(s)?

   a. visible damage to brain cells
   b. increased intracranial pressure
   c. no loss of consciousness
   d. trauma to the head

3. b, d

Frame 11

Mary Sue Davis had a contusion of the brain stem with cerebral edema. A *contusion* is injury to the brain with small, diffuse venous hemorrhages. Both white and grey matter may have a bruised, discolored appearance.

Cell function is hindered by
   ↓pH with lactic acid accumulation
   ↓oxygen consumption.

Contusions can occur any place in the cranium but are most frequently found near bony prominences of the skull.

Figure 3.7 shows common sites for contusions. In addition, the brain stem may be injured when forced against nearby structures.

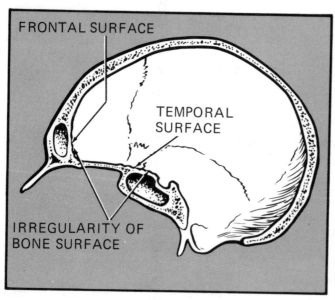

FRONTAL SURFACE

TEMPORAL SURFACE

IRREGULARITY OF BONE SURFACE

Figure 3.7. *Common sites for contusions*

Contusions may result in permanent tissue damage and scarring. Signs and symptoms depend on the severity and location of the injury.

1. Indicate whether the following findings would be more likely found in a contusion or a concussion.

   a. purplish discoloration of the brain _____
   b. increase in acetylcholine _____
   c. decrease in pH _____
   d. increase of lactic acid in tissue _____
   e. no visible tissue involvement _____

2. List three common sites for contusions.

1. a. contusion
   b. concussion
   c. contusion
   d. contusion
   e. concussion

2. brain stem
   frontal lobe
   temporal lobe

Frame 12

Summary:

Accidents causing rapid acceleration/deceleration of the head result in brain tissue damage due to cerebral edema. These movements can also cause a shearing injury to the brain stem.

Concussion is a brain injury associated with
—loss of consciousness
—no visible damage to tissue
—↑ICP with pressure on the brain stem
—↑acetylcholine interfering with impulse transmission.

Contusion is injury to the brain with
—small, diffuse venous hemorrhages
—↓pH and accumulation of lactic acid
—↓oxygen consumption
—signs and symptoms dependent on severity and location.

PART II
TUMORS

Types

Frame 13

Tumors are a major cause of increased intracranial pressure. Here are the terms used to describe the chief kinds of brain tumors.

Primary	originate in structures inside the cranial vault. The name depends on the type of tissue from which the tumor originated. Table I lists the various types.
Metastatic	originate in tissues outside the cranial vault, most commonly lung and breast tissue.
Benign	cells are well differentiated and the tumor is surgically accessible
Malignant	either surgically inaccessible or cells are not differentiated

TABLE 1. Histological Classification of Primary Brain Tumors.

Tissue	Tumor	Percentage of type
Glial (connective tissue)	Gliomas	43
Astrocyte	Astrocytoma (Grades I, II, III, IV)	
Oligodendrocyte (myelin sheath of cranial axons)	Oligodendrocytoma	
Ependymal cells	Ependymoma	
Meninges (leptomeningeal tissue)	Meningioma	16
Pituitary (adenohypophyseal)	Adenoma	8
	Chromophobe	
	Chromophil	
Schwann cells (cranial nerve sheath covering)	Neurofibroma	6
Ganglion	Medulloblastoma	1
Metastatic		13
Other		3

Common locations of these tumors are shown in the next figure.

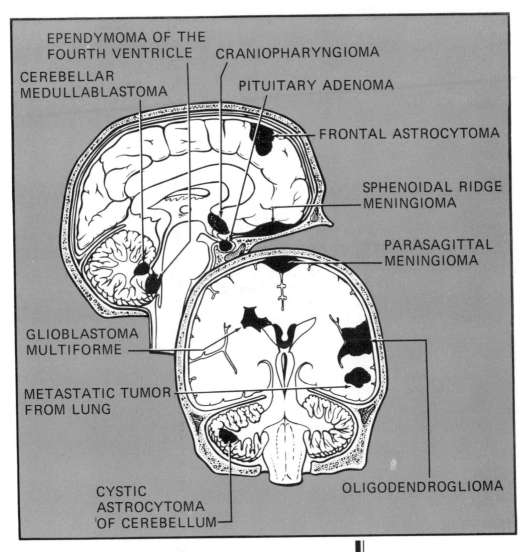

Figure 3.8. *Location of selected brain tumors*

1. A primary brain tumor originates from tissues located in the _____.

2. The three types of brain tumors originating from glial or connective tissue are _____, _____, and _____.

3. A tumor originating from the dura mater is called a _____.

4. Malignant brain tumors are characterized by being surgically _____ and having _____ cells.

1. cranium

2. astrocytomas
   oligodendrocytomas
   ependymoma

3. meningioma

4. inaccessible
   non-differentiated

Symptoms

Frame 14

Tumors cause symptoms by:

—taking up space within the skull, causing increased intracranial pressure and cerebral edema

—compressing cerebral spinal fluid channels; continued CSF formation causes ↑ ICP

—pressing on a portion of the brain causing irritation or damage to structures

—destroying brain tissue by its own unregulated growth which competes for space and nourishment.

Generalized symptoms related to increased ICP are: headache, nausea and vomiting unrelated to eating and mental cloudiness.

Frame 15

Specific symptoms are caused by the *location* of the tumor rather than by its histological classification.

> Some kinds of tumors are found only in one area, and therefore produce the same symptoms, e.g. pituitary tumors.

> Tumors vary in rapidity of growth. Malignant tumors, such as gliomas, grow rapidly. Signs of ↑ICP as well as specific, functional or *focal* signs appear sooner. When tumors grow slowly the brain is able to compensate more readily, and the tumor may be large before symptoms appear. Meningiomas are typical of slow growing tumors.

> Tumors in the motor strip are noted earlier than those occurring in the parietal lobe.

True or False:

1. _____ Symptoms produced by a tumor depend upon its histological type rather than its location.

2. _____ A slow growing tumor may become very large before causing symptoms.

3. _____ Tumors affecting the motor strip of the brain are often the last to be recognized.

Consider now some examples of tumors in specific locations, and their focal signs.

1. False

2. True

3. False

Frame 16

Michael O'Hara, age 32, was admitted for neurologic evaluation of visual difficulties and enlargement of his hands and feet. A pituitary tumor was suspected.

Review these facts about the pituitary gland (or hypophysis):

The pituitary gland has two lobes: the adenohypophysis and neurohypophysis.

Functions:

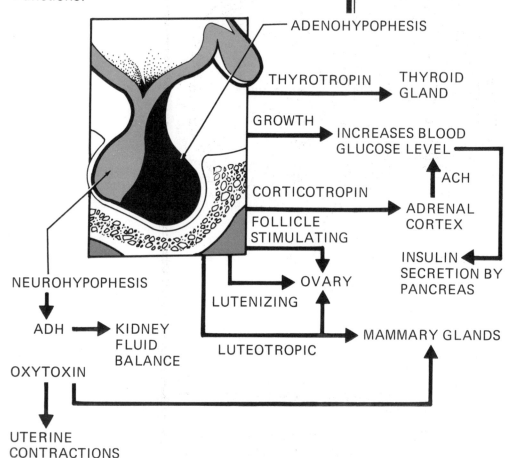

Figure 3.9. *Pituitary functions*

Location:

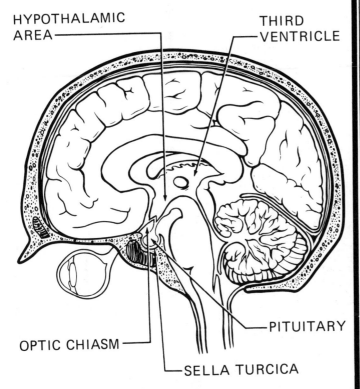

HYPOTHALAMIC AREA

THIRD VENTRICLE

PITUITARY

OPTIC CHIASM

SELLA TURCICA

Figure 3.10. *Location of the pituitary*

True or False:

1. _____ The pituitary gland is located at the base of the brain, near the floor of the third ventricle.

2. _____ Tumors of the pituitary could also affect the hypothalamus because of its proximity.

3. _____ Endocrine disturbances would be an unlikely result of a pituitary tumor.

4. _____ Visual problems may occur as a result of pressure on the optic nerves by a pituitary tumor.

1. True

2. True

3. False

4. True

Michael's enlarged feet and hands (acromegaly) were a result of the tumor stimulating production of growth hormone.

Frame 17

Because of the proximity of the hypothalamus to the pituitary gland, tumors or surgery in this area may cause dysfunction of the hypothalamus. Surgery in the area of the pituitary can also cause a deficiency in secretion of antidiuretic hormone (ADH). Lack of ADH results in excessive excretion of urine which can approach 20 liters/day. Fluid and electrolyte imbalances result.

1. Diabetes insipidus is caused by (increase/decrease) in ADH.

2. In a person with diabetes insipidus, the urine output would more likely be

    a. 500 ml/day
    b. 1000 ml/day
    c. 2000 ml/day
    d. 6000 ml/day

If this condition persists, it is treated by the administration of vasopressin (Pitressin), a pituitary hormone which causes the renal tubules to retain water.

1. decrease

2. d

Frame 18

Another problem caused by a pituitary tumor is a visual field defect. Note that the crossing of the optic nerve fibers (optic chiasm) is just above the pituitary gland.

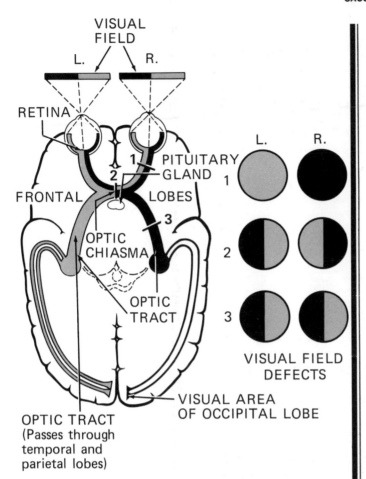

Figure 3.11. *Visual field defects*

Study figure 3.11 and follow input from the left visual field in both eyes (colored black in both eyes). Note that stimulation is sensed by the right side of the retina in both eyes. Nerve tracts from this part of the retina in the left eye cross over to the right optic tract at the chiasm. (The nerve tracts from the nasal side of the right eye also cross to the left here.)

The circles on the right show the areas of blindness corresponding to damage at various levels of the visual pathway.

1. At point 1, there is loss of the whole visual field in the _____ eye.

2. At point 2, there is damage to the _____ half of the visual field in both eyes. This would be expected in a tumor of the _____ gland.

1. right

2. outer (temporal)
   pituitary

3. At point 3, the _____ half of both visual fields cannot be seen.

3. left

4. The most likely visual field defect caused by a pituitary tumor would be at points _____ and _____.

4. 2, 3

5. A patient with a defect at point 3 would not see someone approaching from his _____ side.

5. left

6. If the optic chiasm were damaged, the patient would have no _____ vision.

6. peripheral or lateral

Note: Visual field defects can also be caused by hemorrhage or trauma which affect the optic tracts.

Frame 19

Olaf Davidson was admitted to the hospital for diagnostic tests because he had problems with sensation on his right side, especially in his lower body and leg. A tumor in the left parietal lobe was located.

Recall the functions of the parietal lobe.

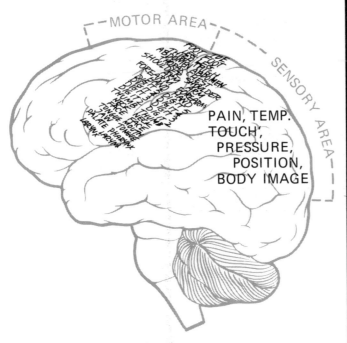

MOTOR AREA

SENSORY AREA

PAIN, TEMP.
TOUCH,
PRESSURE,
POSITION,
BODY IMAGE

Figure 3.12. *Parietal lobe functions*

Some common symptoms associated with parietal lobe lesions include:

apraxia—difficulty in performing voluntary acts

agnosia—inability to recognize objects, due to loss of *comprehension* of auditory, visual, or other stimuli

astereognosis—inability to recognize familiar objects by touch

homonymous hemianopsia—loss of one half of the visual field

(Frame 18, Figure 3.11, point 3)

The tumor found in surgery was a grade IV astrocytoma, a rapidly growing tumor, which had become large enough to cause focal symptoms.

1. Mr. Davidson's sensory problems were worse in the lower part of his body and his leg. Why?

1. Because the tumor probably involves part of the sensory strip related to these areas

2. Why were these symptoms noted on the right side?

2. Because of the crossing of nerve fibers (Tumor is on the left.)

3. Mr. Davidson did not notice the foods on the right side of his meal trays. What is this problem called?

3. homonymous hemianopsia (field cut)

4. This patient could not differentiate a half dollar from a dime without looking at the coins. What is the term for this?

4. astereognosis

5. Mr. Davidson also had problems with body image. He did not realize that his own right hand was caught in the wheel chair spokes. Integration of body image is the function of which part of the brain?

5. parietal lobe

6. When asked to put his right hand on the tray table, Mr. Davidson was unable to do it correctly. What is this called?

6. apraxia (motor)

Frame 20

Anita Billings had a metastatic tumor removed from her left cerebellar hemisphere. The rapid growth of the tumor had forced tissue against the Aqueduct of Sylvius, preventing the normal flow of CSF. Two mechanisms for increased intracranial pressure were present: increased tissue from the rapidly growing tumor, and an increase in CSF in the ventricles due to blockage of the outflow channel. Because of the increased intracranial pressure, Anita experienced a bursting headache before surgery.

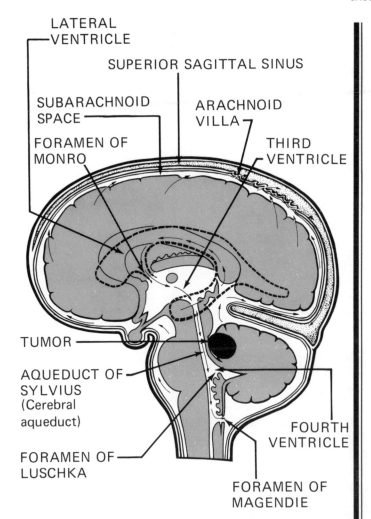

LATERAL VENTRICLE

SUPERIOR SAGITTAL SINUS

SUBARACHNOID SPACE

ARACHNOID VILLA

FORAMEN OF MONRO

THIRD VENTRICLE

TUMOR

AQUEDUCT OF SYLVIUS (Cerebral aqueduct)

FOURTH VENTRICLE

FORAMEN OF LUSCHKA

FORAMEN OF MAGENDIE

Figure 3.13.   *Cerebellar tumor*

Locate the site of CSF blockage in tbe diagram.

1. Where would CSF tend to back up?

2. What was the cause of the patient's headache?

1. In the third ventricle and lateral ventricle

2. ↑ICP

Frame 21

Ms. Billings had a left cerebellar hemisphere tumor. Her symptoms also included muscular incoordination (ataxia), inability to maintain a stable posture with her eyes closed, and difficulty with accuracy in bringing her hand to her mouth to feed herself.

The symptoms were more pronounced on her left side. Removal of the tumor temporarily relieved the blockage of flow of CSF and decreased Ms. Billing's headache and other symptoms. However metastatic tumors carry a poor prognosis.

1. Tumors in a cerebellar lobe cause (ipsilateral/ contralateral) symptoms.

2. To test for cerebellar involvement, stability in maintaining posture is checked by asking the person to keep her eyes (open/closed) while standing.

3. Muscular incoordination is called (agnosia/ ataxia).

1. ipsilateral

2. closed

3. ataxia

Frame 22

Summary:

Types of cranial tumors:

Primary—originates in cranial tissues
Metastatic—originates elsewhere in the body and migrates to the brain.
Benign—have well differentiated cells and are surgically accessible.
Malignant—cells not differentiated or are surgically inaccessible.

Tumors cause symptoms by adding volume to the skull contents, compressing CSF channels, pressure, and irritation to brain cells, as well as outright destruction of tissue.

Generalized symptoms are due to ↑ICP; specific symptoms are due to location rather than type of tumor.

Focal symptoms related to location:
Pituitary tumor: endocrine problems, visual field cuts.

Parietal lobe tumor: Problems with performing voluntary acts (apraxia), recognition of objects (agnosia and astereognosis), visual field problems, loss of sensation contralaterally.

Cerebellar tumor: CSF blockage, muscular incoordination ipsilaterally.

PART III
VASCULAR PROBLEMS

You have learned that head trauma can cause disruptions in the vascular system. Several additional vascular lesions may also cause brain dysfunction and possibly raise intracranial pressure. In most instances not only is the immediate area involved because of localized pressure and edema, but vast areas of the brain may be affected because of interruption of the vascular system.

Frame 23

Martha Thompson was admitted to the hospital with a severe headache in the occipital area. She described the headache as "just suddenly happening" after she had shoveled snow. Physical examination showed:

nuchal rigidity (pain when the neck is moved)

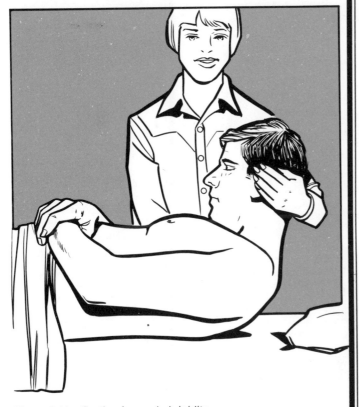

Figure 3.14. *Testing for nuchal rigidity*

photophobia (sensitivity to light)

a positive Kernig's sign (patient cannot fully extend leg when hip is flexed)

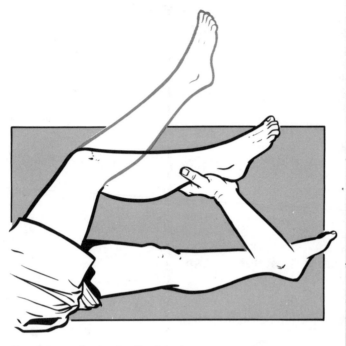

Figure 3.15.   *Testing for Kernig's sign*

These signs indicate meningeal irritation. (Remember the meninges have many pain sensitive structures.) The CSF fluid specimen from the lumbar puncture contained fresh blood with a RBC count of 190,000/ml present. A diagnosis of ruptured intracerebral aneurysm was made.

1. Which of the following signs are indicative of meningeal irritation?

    a. photophobia
    b. headache
    c. nuchal rigidity
    d. positive Babinski's sign
    e. positive Kernig's sign

2. The amount of blood in Ms. Thompson's CSF indicates

    a. bleeding into the subarachnoid space
    b. bleeding caused by the lumbar puncture
    c. problems with normal blood clotting

1. a, b, c, e

2. a

Aneurysm

Frame 24

An aneurysm results from a weakness in the arterial wall. Arterial vessels are composed of three layers—the endothelial lining, smooth muscle, and connective tissue.

A defect in the smooth muscle layer allows the endothelial lining to bulge through, forming an aneurysm.

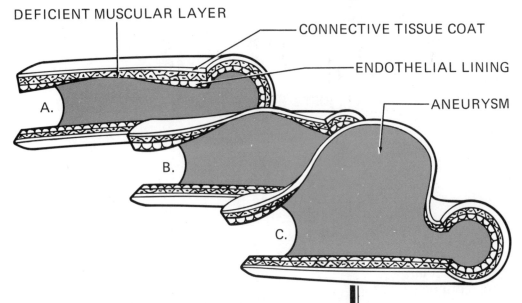

DEFICIENT MUSCULAR LAYER

CONNECTIVE TISSUE COAT

ENDOTHELIAL LINING

ANEURYSM

A.

B.

C.

Figure 3.16.   *Stages in development of an aneurysm*

Intracranial aneurysms may be found on any vessel, but the most common sites are shown in Figure 3.17. Aneurysms frequently occur where arteries branch.

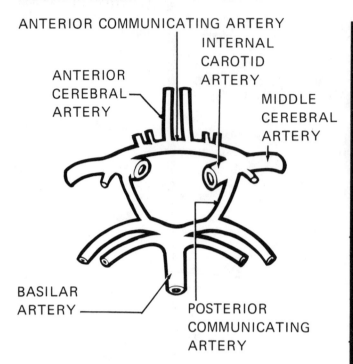

ANTERIOR COMMUNICATING ARTERY

INTERNAL CAROTID ARTERY

ANTERIOR CEREBRAL ARTERY

MIDDLE CEREBRAL ARTERY

BASILAR ARTERY

POSTERIOR COMMUNICATING ARTERY

Figure 3.17.   *Common aneurysm sites*

1. Aneurysms result from a defect in which layer of the artery wall?

   a. endothelial
   b. muscular
   c. connective tissue

2. Which of the following is an aneurysm on the anterior communicating artery?

1. b

2. A

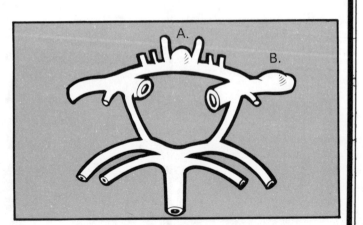

Figure 3.18.   *Aneurysms in Circle of Willis*

Frame 25

Hypertension or an increase in cerebral blood pressure due to such activities as the Valsalva maneuver, coitus, or sudden exertion may put undue stress on the aneurysm causing it to rupture. The exertion from Ms. Thompson's snow shoveling caused the aneurysm on her anterior communicating artery to rupture. The blood seeped into the subarachnoid space. (If the ruptured aneurysm were on a vessel located within brain tissue, an intracerebral hematoma would occur.) Aneurysms on vessels in certain areas may cause focal symptoms due to pressure on adjacent structures.

Surgical repair of Ms. Thompson's aneurysm was carried out and she recovered fully from the surgery.

1. An (increase/decrease) in blood pressure causes aneurysms to rupture.

   1. increase

2. If an aneurysm ruptures on an artery that is surrounded by brain tissue, you would expect to find an (intracerebral/epidural) hematoma.

   2. intracerebral

Arteriosclerotic Vascular Disease

Frame 26

Arteriosclerotic vascular disease (ASVD) is a frequent cause of cranial pathology. Due to aging, the arterial walls become hardened and inelastic.

Atherosclerosis is a process in which patchy deposits of cholesterol begin to destroy the internal lining of blood vessels. These two processes can occur simultaneously.

Figure 3.19 demonstrates some of the problems caused by these changes. In B, the vessel becomes narrowed by plaque formation, and in C, an embolus obstructs the artery. The effect of such obstruction is a cerebral infarct. The brain cells supplied by the artery receive little or no blood and the surrounding tissue becomes necrotic.

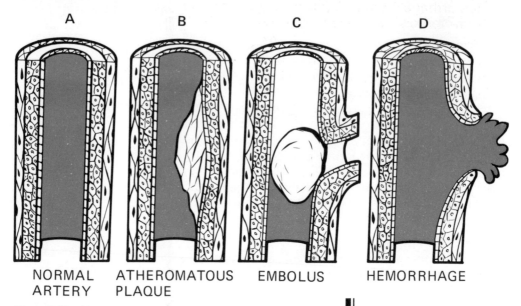

NORMAL ARTERY   ATHEROMATOUS PLAQUE   EMBOLUS   HEMORRHAGE

Figure 3.19. *Vascular changes preventing blood flow*

An increase in blood pressure can cause weakened arteries to rupture (D). Bleeding occurs in cerebral tissue, and a clot of hematoma forms. The manifestations depend on the location of the hematoma. ICP is increased if the clot is large.

1. Interruption of circulation to brain cells can be caused by which arterial changes?

   a. rupture of an artery
   b. obstruction by a blood clot
   c. narrowing due to plaque information
   d. all of the above

   1. d

2. Obstruction of cerebral arteries by plaques and emboli results in

   a. decreased cellular demand for O_2 and glucose
   b. cell death due to inadequate supply of nutrients
   c. damage to cells by bleeding into the tissue

   2. b

3. Hemorrhage from a ruptured aneurysm and from vessels weakened by ASVD are both caused by

    a. hypertension
    b. sudden exertion
    c. Valsalva maneuver
    d. all of the above

3. d

Frame 27

Sam Hansen had arisen at night to go to the bathroom and collapsed at the bedside. On admission, the nurse noted the following signs:

    right hemiplegia
    unresponsiveness to stimuli
    blood pressure: 70/40
    feeble, rapid pulse
    apneustic breathing (inhales, holds breath, exhales)

Diagnostic tests revealed an intracerebral clot in the left frontal lobe just anterior to the Rolando fissure. The vessel which ruptured was the left anterior cerebral artery. Cerebral edema was noted surrounding the clot.

Figure 3.20 shows the part of the brain supplied by the anterior cerebral artery.

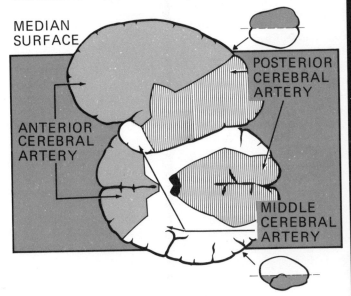

MEDIAN SURFACE

POSTERIOR CEREBRAL ARTERY

ANTERIOR CEREBRAL ARTERY

MIDDLE CEREBRAL ARTERY

Figure 3.20. *Arterial supply areas in the brain*

1. Arteries rupture in ASVD because the walls of the vessel are (thick/weakened).

2. The brain area affected by Mr. Hansen's hematoma controls (motor/sensory) function on the (ipsilateral/contralateral) side of the body.

3. Cerebral edema causes increased intracranial pressure which is directed downward toward the (parietal lobe/brain stem).

4. Mr. Hansen's apneustic breathing indicates pressure on the respiratory regulating center. This structure is located in the (cerebellum/brain stem).

5. Apneustic breating is a change in the (pattern/adequacy) of respiration.

1. weakened

2. motor, contralateral

3. brain stem (Review Figure 3.6.)

4. brain stem

5. pattern

Frame 28

In contrast to Mr. Hansen, who had a sudden onset of symptoms, Sara Sage's symptoms appeared gradually. She suffered an infarct of the right middle cerebral artery. As the vessel became more occluded, the symptoms became more pronounced. In infarcts, the patient often states that the symptoms have been transient in the past.

The middle cerebral artery supplies parts of the parietal and temporal lobes, the sensory and motor strips, and Broca's area.

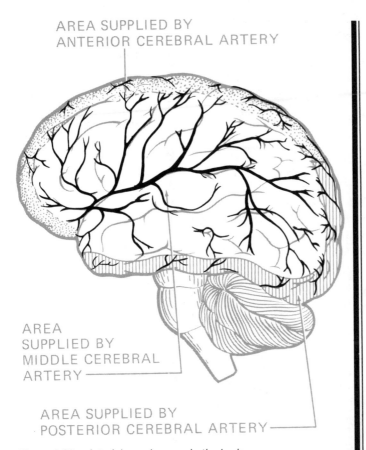

AREA SUPPLIED BY
ANTERIOR CEREBRAL ARTERY

AREA
SUPPLIED BY
MIDDLE CEREBRAL
ARTERY

AREA SUPPLIED BY
POSTERIOR CEREBRAL ARTERY

Figure 3.21. *Arterial supply areas in the brain*

Mrs. Sage had paralysis of her left arm and leg. The left side of her face drooped. She also had sensory deficits on her left side. Homonymous hemianopsia was present. Mrs. Sage could not move her eyes (conjugate gaze) to the left. Mrs. Sage's lack of awareness of the left side of her body was typical of lesions in this area.

True or False:

1. _____ Symptoms in an infarct occur more suddenly than in an intracerebral hematoma.

2. _____ In an infarct of the right middle cerebral artery, there are symptoms on the right side of the body.

3. _____ The middle cerebral artery extends to both the motor and sensory strips.

1. False

2. False, left

3. True

4. _____ Homonymous hemianopsia is loss of vision in one eye.

    4. False (Review Frame 18.)

5. _____ Aphasia (the inability to produce and understand speech) is not a common finding in lesions of the middle cerebral artery.

    5. False

Frame 29

One main area supplied by the middle cerebral artery is the internal capsule. Afferent and efferent fibers from all segments of the cerebral cortex converge in the internal capsule.

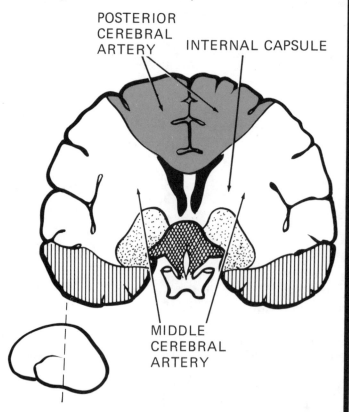

POSTERIOR CEREBRAL ARTERY   INTERNAL CAPSULE

MIDDLE CEREBRAL ARTERY

Figure 3.22. *Arterial supply areas of the brain*

An infarct of even a small branch of the middle cerebral artery affects the motor and sensory abilities of one side of the body.

1. The artery supplying the internal capsule is a branch of the _____ _____ artery.

    1. middle cerebral

2. The internal capsule contains fibers for all
_____ and _____ functions.

2. motor, sensory

Frame 30

Severe cerebral edema frequently follows infarcts. Initially Mrs. Sage had no movement or
sensation of her left side. Gradually she regained
some use of her arm and leg as the cerebral
edema subsided.

Another factor that contributes to the recovery of
function is the establishment of collateral circu-
laticn. An adequate Circle of Willis, well-devel-
oped cerebral arteries free of atherosclerosis, and
meningial, choroidal, and capillary anastomoses
are needed for providing blood to the deprived
tissue. Retrograde blood flow may also supply
blood to the ischemic tissue.

1. List two conditions that result in improvement
of a patient's condition following an infarct.

1. decreased edema,
establishment of
collateral
circulation

Arteriovenous Malformation

Frame 31

An arteriovenous (AV) malformation is another
vascular condition which may cause cerebral
dysfunction. Arteriovenous malformations are
congenital defects with an abnormally large
number of vessels in one surface area of the brain.
The most common site for AV malformations is
the parietal lobe. Seizures are a common finding
in AV malformations due to irritation of underlying brain tissue. Rupture of the involved vessels
often results in subarachnoid hemorrhage.

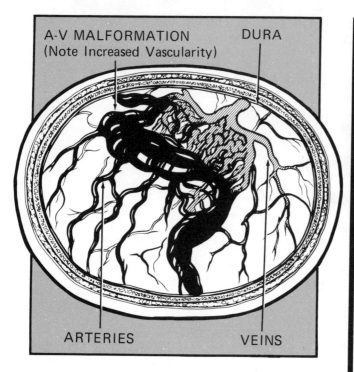

Figure 3.23. *AV malformation*

True or False:

1. _____ In AV malformations the blood supply to the area is decreased.

2. _____ Arteriovenous malformations occur due to a congenital defect.

1. False

2. True

Frame 32

Summary:

Vascular lesions causing cerebral dysfunction are:

Aneurysm—ballooning of an artery at a point of weakness in the muscular wall
—causes pressure on cranial structures
—can rupture into brain tissue or subarachnoid space

ASVD —hardening of arterial walls with plaque formation
—causes occlusion of the lumen by plaque
—can rupture from ↑ BP

Emboli —blood clots formed on roughened intimal lining of arteries or brought to brain from another part of the system
—cause occlusion of artery

Arterio-venous mal-forma-tions —congenital defect with a large collection of vessels on surface of the brain
—can cause pressure or can rupture

These lesions can damage brain tissue by:

Bleeding into the tissue → damage to cells, hematoma formation with ↑ ICP
Interrupting the constant supply of O_2 and glucose needed for metabolism → cell death
Cerebral edema with ↑ ICP

Symptoms caused by hemorrhage and infarct depend on the area of the brain affected

sudden onset—hemorrhage
gradual onset—occlusion of arteries

Improvement in symptoms can occur when cerebral edema subsides and/or collateral circulation is established to the area.

PART IV
INFECTIOUS PROCESSES

Infectious processes also account for cranial dysfunction and/or increased intracranial pressure. While brain abscesses still occur, meningitis is the most frequent infectious process affecting the brain. There are many causes of meningitis.

Course

Frame 33

Tom Allison was admitted following trauma in which he sustained a skull fracture which involved the frontal bone and sinuses. Figure 3.24 shows a fracture of the frontal bone. If fractures tear the dura, an opening between the brain and the nasal passages is created.

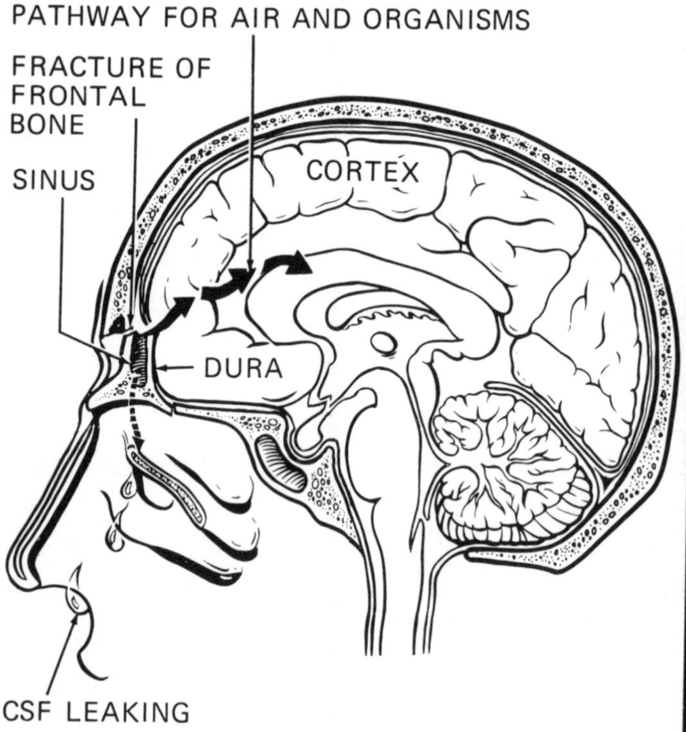

PATHWAY FOR AIR AND ORGANISMS

FRACTURE OF FRONTAL BONE

SINUS

CORTEX

DURA

CSF LEAKING

Figure 3.24. *Frontal bone fracture*

Use Figure 3.24 to decide if these statements are true or false:

1. _____ A fracture at the base of the brain may tear the tough covering of the brain, the dura.

2. _____ Cerebrospinal fluid can escape through the torn dura and drain into the nose.

3. _____ Tom Allison is at no greater risk of intracranial infection than the patients discussed previously who had vascular problems.

4. _____ Air could enter the brain through the nose and sinuses.

1. True

2. True

3. False, organisms can move from the nose to the brain

4. True

Frame 34

The nurse who admitted Mr. Allison noticed clear fluid drainage from his nose. She used testape to determine whether the drainage was CSF, as CSF contains glucose while nasal discharge does not. The testape was positive for glucose, so she documented this finding as cerebrospinal rhinorrhea. (CSF drainage from the ear is called otorrhea.) The physician ordered antibiotics and bedrest with the head elevated. He cautioned Mr. Allison against activities involving straining and the Valsalva maneuver, and told him not to blow his nose. Increased pressure forces fluid from the nasal passages into the brain.

1. Rhinorrhea is CSF leakage through the _____.

2. A test which determines if drainage is CSF is _____.

3. Meningitis is possible following a basilar skull fracture if the _____ is torn.

4. Actions which would decrease the chances for meningitis when rhinorrhea is present include:

1. nose

2. testape for glucose

3. dura

4. head elevated, bedrest, antibiotics, instruct patient not to pick or blow nose

Despite all of these precautions, Mr. Allison developed meningitis.

Symptoms

Frame 35

Meningitis is an inflammation of the protective coverings of the brain. Organisms causing meningitis include *meningococcus, pneumococcus,* fungi *(cryptococcus), streptococcus,* and influenza virus. Symptoms are related to meningeal irritation and inflammation.

Do you recall the findings typical of meningeal irritation?

1. Flexion of the head causes _____. This is called _____ _____.

2. Inability to extend the leg fully when the hip is flexed is a positive_____ _____.

3. Photophobia is increased sensitivity to _____.

4. Because of the inflammation you would expect _____ temperature.

5. Inflammation of sensitive meningeal nerve endings would cause _____ and _____.

1. pain
   nuchal rigidity

2. Kernig's sign

3. light

4. elevated

5. pain, stiffness

Frame 36

Intracranial infections present a major treatment problem. The intact blood-brain barrier serves to keep organisms out of the brain, but also prevents the transfer of many antibiotics from the blood stream to the brain tissue. The physician chooses antibiotics which are most likely to pass the blood-brain barrier.

Frame 37

Summary:

Types of infectious processes—brain abscess, meningitis

Basilar skull fractures carry an increased risk of infection as organisms can enter the brain from the nose or ear.

CSF can drain from the nose (rhinorrhea) or ear (otorrhea)
Straining and blowing the nose are contraindicated.
Testape can be used to identify CSF drainage

Signs and symptoms: nuchal rigidity, + Kernig's sign, photophobia, fever, pain, stiffness

The blood-brain barrier may prevent transfer of antibiotics to brain tissue.

CHAPTER 4

DIAGNOSTIC TESTS

The brain is a complex organism; therefore, detection of a specific dysfunction is difficult. The enclosure of the brain within the protective bony skull prevents the use of diagnostic methods used in examining other parts of the body. The development of diagnostic tests has greatly aided the advancement of neurology and neurosurgery. The diagnostic process for neurologic dysfunctions can be like a detective story.

At the conclusion of this chapter you will be able to:

1. Describe the procedure for electroencephalogram (EEG), computerized axial tomography (CAT), angiogram, and lumbar puncture
2. When given a situation, select the appropriate nursing interventions for a patient having the diagnostic tests
3. Identify complications associated with cerebral angiograms.

Chapter Outline

Non-invasive procedures
    CAT scan
    Electroencephalogram

Invasive procedures
    Cerebral angiogram
        Procedure
        Complications
        Patient care
    Lumbar puncture
        Procedure
        Patient care

PART I
NON-INVASIVE
PROCEDURES

Computerized Axial Tomography

Frame 1

Jake Thompson, age 67, was admitted to the ICU after a car accident in which he sustained a head injury. Routine skull x-rays revealed a hairline fracture of the temporal bone, and a suspicious area which could be a brain tumor. Mr. Thompson's neurologic signs soon returned to normal and he was scheduled for further evaluation by computerized axial tomography (CAT).

CAT scans give a detailed picture of the entire brain (or whatever area of the body is being studied). This is accomplished by a machine that combines an x-ray beam and a computer.

Ordinary skull x-rays usually present two views: anterior—posterior and lateral. In computerized tomography, x-rays are taken at 180 different positions. The computer calculates the densities of cranial components according to their varying absorption of the x-ray beam. The computer then prints out a picture of the components: air, CSF, blood, brain tissue, bone, calcifications, tumors, edema.

The CAT scan is highly accurate in picking up abnormalities, particularly in areas such as the brain which are not readily accessible to other diagnostic methods.

Mark these statements about CAT scans true or false.

1. _____ A contrast media is needed to detect densities of tissue.

2. _____ X-rays are taken at many angles.

3. _____ Brain tumors are the only abnormalities that can be detected.

1. False

2. True

3. False

Frame 2

The test has many advantages. Foremost is the absence of complications from the procedure. CAT scans are painless, requiring only that the patient remain quiet in the supine position. The test takes 20 to 40 minutes to complete. No specific preparation of patients is required, and they may eat and drink prior to the procedure. It is recommended that the hair be washed if hair spray has been used.

Hair pins and ornaments should be removed. The procedure itself requires no special observations or care.

1. In preparing Mr. Thompson for the CAT scan, which measures would you use?

    a. Determine if he has back pain when lying flat
    b. Inform him that the procedure takes approximately one-half hour
    c. Do not give food or fluids after midnight
    d. Arrange to have his head shaved

1. a, b

Frame 3

For the CAT scan, the patient's head is placed in a rubber cap which extends into a water-filled lucite cube. The patient lies flat on a table.

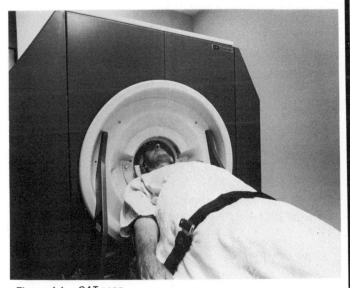

Figure 4.1. *CAT scan*

It is necessary that the patient remain quiet during the test, but conversation with the attending staff is permitted. The staff are shielded from radiation in a lead-lined booth so the patient is alone in the room.

True or False:

1. _____ The patient is in a sitting position for the test.

2. _____ The technician is at the patient's side during the procedure.

3. _____ It is difficult to do a CAT scan on a restless patient.

1. False

2. False

3. True

The CAT scan showed a lesion in Mr. Thompson's left parietal area, and the possible presence of a second lesion.

Electroencephalogram

Frame 4

Subsequently, Mr. Thompson was scheduled for an electroencephalogram. The principle underlying the EEG is that fluctuations in the electrical activity of the brain can be noted and recorded by electrodes attached to the scalp. The varying differences in electrical potential are measured by electrodes attached to two points on the scalp.

Panel 1
Characteristics of the EEG tracing.

Waves
The recorded electrical potential changes in a rhythmic, repeating fashion. These changes are recorded as waves.

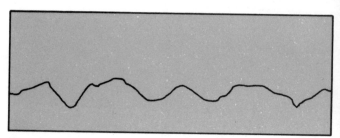

Figure 4.2. *EEG wave*

Frequency

The pattern of waves, or rhythm, is called the frequency, and is expressed in cycles per second. Here are the four most common normal frequencies.

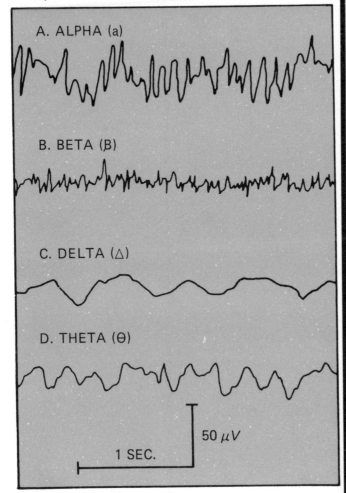

A. ALPHA (α)

B. BETA (β)

C. DELTA (Δ)

D. THETA (θ)

50 μV

1 SEC.

Figure 4.3. *EEG frequencies*

Form

Waves vary in shape, therefore different shapes, or forms, can be described.

Amplitude

This is the peak to peak measurement of repeated waves.

Velocity

The rate of ascent and descent of waves is called velocity. A slow wave ascends and descends gradually. (Look at the Delta frequency.) A rapid wave has a more vertical ascent and descent. (Look at the Alpha waves.)

A spike is a fast wave with steep slopes on each side that may appear randomly or in bursts. It is an abnormal sign which can indicate the location of pathology.

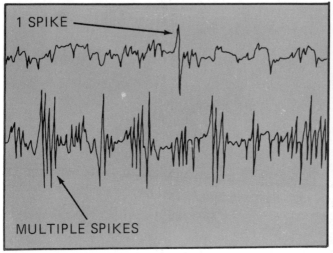

Figure 4.4. *EEG spikes*

Incidence
Changes in EEG waves can be:
transient—a single wave differs from the pattern
paroxysmal—there is a sudden burst of change in the recording, which then returns to normal

What do you remember about EEG waves?

1. Which of the frequencies is the most rapid (greatest number of waves/second)?

2. Which is the slowest frequency?

3. Label the following frequencies.

1. Beta

2. Delta

3. A. alpha
   B. delta

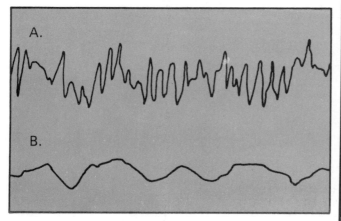

Figure 4.5. *Practice tracing*

4. Label the characteristics indicated A and B

4. A. wave
   B. spike

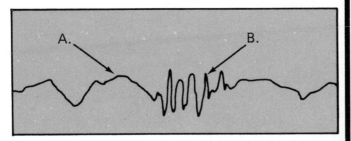

Figure 4.6. *Practice tracing*

Frame 5

In a normal, awake adult, the following EEG characteristics are present:

  alpha rhythm posterior (occipital-parietal)
  alpha activity is found in other parts of the brain, particularly on both the left and right of the midline
  beta activity is intermittent, but tends to be in the central regions
  theta activity may also be present in the central area
  delta is not normal in an awake adult

1. What type of activity would you expect to find in:

    a. left occipital area
    b. central area
    c. right upper parietal

1. a. alpha rhythm
   b. beta and theta
   c. alpha activity

2. Which type of wave is not normally seen when the patient is awake:

    a. Alpha
    b. Beta
    c. Delta
    d. Theta

2. c

Frame 6

The EEG is done with the patient lying down or seated in a chair. Eighteen electrodes are pasted to the scalp (occasionally small needles are used instead) in various locations.

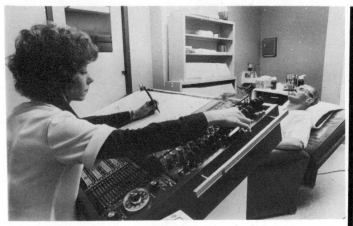

Figure 4.7. *Patient having EEG*

The test takes approximately 45–60 minutes. It is necessary that the patient remain quiet during the test as muscular activity will cause distortions in the recording.

During the procedure two stimuli may be used. The patient may be asked to hyperventilate for a period of three minutes because, in susceptible individuals, activity indicative of absence seizures or other types of seizures will occur. Photic stimulation with short, rhythmic flashes of a high-intensity strobe light is also used. Again the stimulus may elicit activity indicative of a seizure disorder.

True or False:

1. _____ Small holes are drilled in the scalp for attaching the electrodes.

2. _____ Hyperventilation may elicit activity indicative of seizures.

3. _____ Muscular activity does not affect EEG tracings.

1. False

2. True

3. False

Frame 7

Before the EEG the nurse informed Mr. Thompson about the test: length, position, electrode placement, stimuli, and that it is relatively pain-free. If his hair were oily or dirty, it would have been shampooed.

If the patient is on anticonvulsant medication, specific medical orders should be obtained regarding administration before the test.

Post-procedure care involves removal of paste left by the electrodes. The patient may also have questions concerning the procedure. No limitations on activity or special care are required because of the EEG.

True or False:

1. _____ The test takes approximately 1 hour.

2. _____ A strobe light is used to elicit the presence of meningitis.

3. _____ After the EEG the patient should remain on bedrest for eight hours.

4. _____ Oily hair should be shampooed prior to the test.

1. True

2. False

3. False

4. True

Frame 8

EEGs are most useful in diagnosing seizure disorders. Cortical lesions (those near the surface) are detected more readily by EEG than are deep lesions. Deep lesions usually cause bursts of synchronous slow wave activity in both cerebral hemispheres. Supratentorial lesions cause focal EEG changes as the cortical neurons or the thalamocortical projections are affected. Slow activity is more prominent with rapidly growing tumors. Infratentorial lesions are detected on EEG's only when the reticular system becomes involved.

1. An EEG would be of more diagnostic use in (supratentorial/infratentorial) lesions.

2. A rapidly growing tumor in Mr. Thompson's parietal lobe would cause (fast/slow) EEG activity.

3. The condition most clearly diagnosed by an EEG is (epilepsy/meningitis).

1. supratentorial (cortex is above the tentorium)

2. slow

3. epilepsy

Frame 9

Summary: Non-invasive diagnostic tests

The CAT scan uses x-rays and computer calculations to picture varying densities of cranial components in 180 positions. There are no complications, and no specific pre- or post-procedure care.

The EEG is a measurement of electrical activity of the brain by electrodes fastened to the scalp.

Brain waves vary in frequency, amplitude, velocity, and form. During the test, stimulation is obtained by strobe light and hyperventilation to detect seizure activity.

Preparation: patient's hair should be clean, explain the procedure. Check anticonvulsant order. No special care is required after the EEG.

PART II
INVASIVE PROCEDURES

Cerebral Angiogram

Frame 10

Another diagnostic test, an angiogram, was ordered for Mr. Thompson to confirm and clarify the findings from the CAT scan.

In an angiogram, a needle or catheter is placed in a selected artery such as the carotid, femoral, brachial, or vertebral. A contrast media is injected and a series of rapid x-rays are taken. The two most common contrast medias are 60% methyl-gucamine (Renografin) and 50% sodium dia-trizoate (Hypaque).

There is some risk of allergic reactions to these substances. Symptoms include:

flushing of the skin
hives
laryngeal stridor
seizures

If an allergic reaction is suspected, the patient will be given epinephrine (Adrenalin).

Write whether you agree or disagree with these actions.

1. During an angiogram a patient complains of itching on his back and dyspnea. The staff asks him to lie quietly for a few more moments until the test is finished.

   1. disagree, signs of allergy should be treated immediately

2. A nurse explains to Mr. Thompson that a needle will be placed in one of his arteries, and a dye will be injected. The dye shows up brightly on the x-ray and outlines the arteries that supply his brain.

   2. agree

117

Frame 11

From midnight before the angiogram, Mr. Thompson was not given fluids and food in case a general anesthetic would be required. Usually local anesthesia is used if the patient is quiet and cooperative. The physician explained that the test would take about an hour and described the purposes and risks, to enable Mr. Thompson to give informed consent. A sedative was administered before the test to help allay anxiety and help Mr. Thompson to cooperate by lying quietly. The radiology staff is with the patient at all times, except when x-rays are being taken. Figures 4.8 and 4.9 show Mr. Thompson positioned for the test, and the carotid artery site for injection of the contrast media.

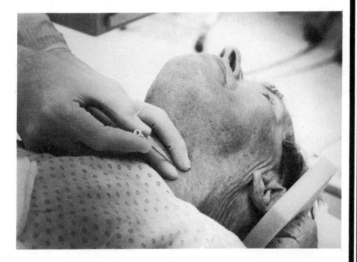

Figure 4.8. *Patient positioned for cerebral angiography*

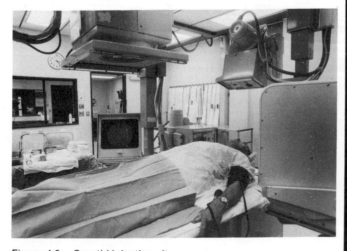

Figure 4.9. *Carotid injection site*

When the dye is injected the patient experiences a warm, flushed feeling in the head, and occasionally a headache and a salty taste in the mouth. He hears the x-ray frames sliding into place for repeated pictures.

1. The catheter for Mr. Thompson's angiogram is placed in the _____ artery.

   1. carotid

2. _____ anesthesia is usually used for angiograms.

   2. Local

3. The patient must lie quietly for about _____ minutes.

   3. 60

4. The noise the patient hears is due to the _____ machine.

   4. x-ray

5. Side effects of the dye injection are _____, _____ and _____.

   5. headache, flushing, salty taste

6. How would you gain the patient's cooperation during the test?

   6. Explain beforehand what he will experience, explain procedure as it is done, tell him what he can do to help, give feedback about how well the procedure is going

Frame 12

Repeated injections of dye are made to visualize anterior-posterior and lateral vessels on one or both sides. Angiograms give the following information

—the rate of filling of the vessels: delay can indicate a pathologic state
—patency of vessels: stenosis, infarct, and plaques can be seen
—displacement of vessels from their normal location due to a lesion
—increased vascularity in one area: may be due to AV malformation or tumors
—abnormality of structure, such as an aneurysm

1. Which of the following problems could be detected by an angiogram?

a. infarct of middle cerebral artery
b. tumor in the temporal lobe
c. AV malformation
d. subdural hematoma

1. a, b, c, d

Frame 13

Mr. Thompson's angiogram went smoothly, but complications occur in about one out of a hundred procedures. The most common complications are:

Dislodgment of plaque occurring in older patients who have ASVD. The pressure of the injection can free some plaque which embolizes and lodges in a smaller vessel causing an infarct. Manifestations depend on the brain area affected. Motor weakness and speech problems are the most common problems and may be transient or permanent.

Arterial spasm due to irritation from the dye. Spasm decreases blood flow to the adjacent area of the brain. Motor and speech symptoms are transient and are alleviated by the administration of papaverine HCl, an antispasmodic drug which acts on the smooth muscle of the blood vessel to increase blood flow.

1. Complications of angiograms occur in about _____ per cent of the patients.

1. 1%

2. The two most common complications in addition to allergic reaction are _____ and _____.

2. spasm, emboli

3. Papaverine is administered to relieve _____.

3. arterial spasm

4. You would expect to find more complications of angiograms in (younger/older) patients.

4. older

Frame 14

After the needle/catheter is removed from the artery, direct pressure is applied for 5 minutes to prevent hemorrhage. A pressure dressing is then applied.

When Mr. Thompson returned to his room, he was carefully observed by the nurse and kept quiet for 12–18 hours. An ice pack was placed on his neck to reduce pain and swelling.

1. Which observations are important in Mr. Thompson's care after carotid angiography?

    a. signs of new bleeding on the dressing
    b. ability to move all extremities
    c. speech which is clear and appropriate

1. a, b, c

2. There is hematoma formation and edema at the injection site. What nearby structure could be adversely affected by the increased pressure?

    a. mandible
    b. trachea
    c. trigeminal nerve

2. b

3. What observations need to be made about Mr. Thompson's respiratory status?

    a. rate of respirations
    b. presence of dyspnea
    c. skin color

3. a, b, c

Frame 15

Care differs if the injection site was the femoral or brachial artery.

> After femoral angiogram the patient's hip is kept extended.

> Pulses distal to the injection site are assessed for adequacy as spasm or hematoma could obstruct the vessel.

1. A patient asks to sit up in the chair soon after having a femoral angiogram. Should the nurse allow this?

1. No, hip should not be flexed

2. After a brachial site is used for an angiogram, which pulses should be checked?

2. radial and/or ulnar

Frame 16

Summary:

The *angiogram* uses contrast media to outline the cranial vessels on x-ray. Dye is injected into carotid, femoral, brachial, or vertebral arteries.

Complications: allergic reaction to dye, arterial spasm, emboli

Pre-procedure preparation: nothing by mouth after midnight, explanation of procedure, consent form, sedation

Post procedure care:

Observations: hemorrhage from injection site, neurologic integrity, respiratory adequacy when carotid site is used, pulses distal to femoral or brachial sites

Care: pressure dressing on site, ice pack to reduce edema and pain, bedrest for 12–18 hours, no hip flexion when femoral site is used.

Lumbar Puncture

Frame 17

Lumbar puncture (LP) is a common procedure for neurosurgical and neuromedical diagnosis. The purposes are:

Diagnostic:

A. To obtain CSF for examination
B. To measure CSF pressure
C. To perform tests for blockage of CSF flow in the spinal column
D. To inject air or dye for x-ray visualization of the ventricular system and subarachnoid space

Therapeutic:

E. To inject medications and anesthetics
F. To reduce intracranial pressure and allow for meningeal healing in cases of CSF leakage
G. To drain CSF during neurosurgery for better visualization of the cranial structures

Use purposes A through E to explain why lumbar puncture would be indicated in these situations.

1. _____ Suspected subarachnoid hemorrhage

2. _____ Cerebrospinal fluid rhinorrhea following basal skull fracture

3. _____ Organisms causing a brain abscess are sensitive to an antibiotic that will not cross the blood-brain barrier

1. A (maybe B)

2. F

3. E

4. _____ Myelogram

5. _____ X-ray shows compressed vertebrae in thoracic area

4. D

5. C (maybe D)

Frame 18

The space between the 3rd and 4th, or 4th and 5th lumbar vertebrae is chosen for the LP since the spinal cord ends at L2. Using the vertebral space below the cord lessens the chances of damage to the cord. Figure 4.10 shows the relationship of the cord, the vertebrae, and anatomical landmarks.

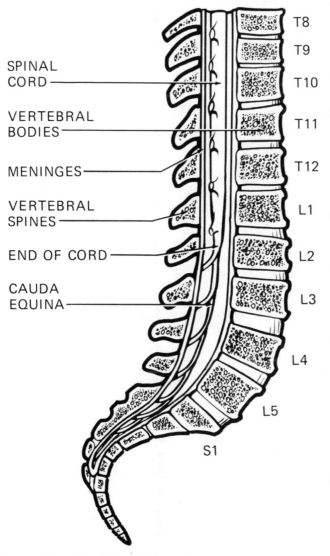

Figure 4.10. *Lateral view of lower spine*

1. Locate the end of the spinal cord.

2. Draw brackets to show the area where the needle can be positioned in a lumbar puncture.

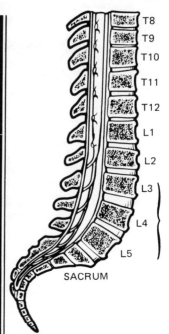

Figure 4.11   *LP needle sites*

Panel 2
Procedure for Lumbar Puncture

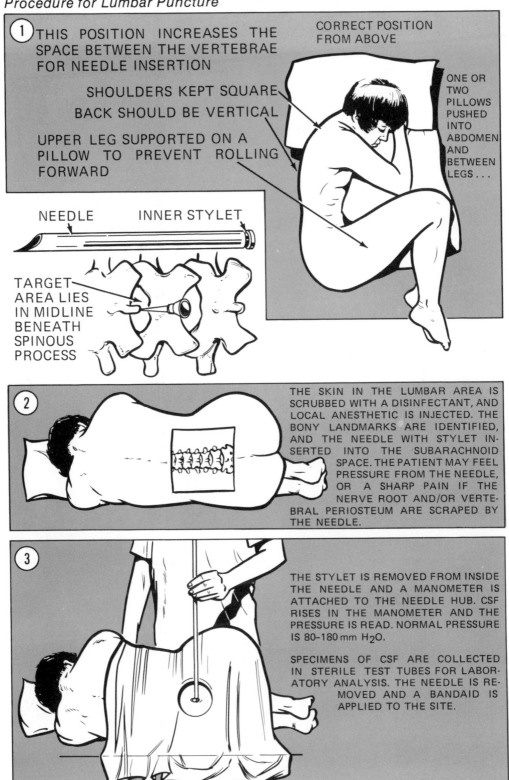

1. THIS POSITION INCREASES THE SPACE BETWEEN THE VERTEBRAE FOR NEEDLE INSERTION

SHOULDERS KEPT SQUARE

BACK SHOULD BE VERTICAL

UPPER LEG SUPPORTED ON A PILLOW TO PREVENT ROLLING FORWARD

CORRECT POSITION FROM ABOVE

ONE OR TWO PILLOWS PUSHED INTO ABDOMEN AND BETWEEN LEGS . . .

NEEDLE   INNER STYLET

TARGET AREA LIES IN MIDLINE BENEATH SPINOUS PROCESS

2. THE SKIN IN THE LUMBAR AREA IS SCRUBBED WITH A DISINFECTANT, AND LOCAL ANESTHETIC IS INJECTED. THE BONY LANDMARKS ARE IDENTIFIED, AND THE NEEDLE WITH STYLET INSERTED INTO THE SUBARACHNOID SPACE. THE PATIENT MAY FEEL PRESSURE FROM THE NEEDLE, OR A SHARP PAIN IF THE NERVE ROOT AND/OR VERTEBRAL PERIOSTEUM ARE SCRAPED BY THE NEEDLE.

3. THE STYLET IS REMOVED FROM INSIDE THE NEEDLE AND A MANOMETER IS ATTACHED TO THE NEEDLE HUB. CSF RISES IN THE MANOMETER AND THE PRESSURE IS READ. NORMAL PRESSURE IS 80–180 mm H_2O.

SPECIMENS OF CSF ARE COLLECTED IN STERILE TEST TUBES FOR LABORATORY ANALYSIS. THE NEEDLE IS REMOVED AND A BANDAID IS APPLIED TO THE SITE.

Figure 4.12.   *Lumbar puncture procedure*

Frame 19

Use Panel 2 to answer these questions:

1. The patient is placed _____ of the bed or table for an LP.

2. The fetal position _____ the space between the vertebral bones.

3. Pain will be felt if the needle touches a _____ or the vertebral _____.

4. Normal CSF pressure is _____ – _____ mm H_2O.

5. The LP site is covered with a _____.

1. on the edge

2. opens, enlarges

3. nerve periosteum

4. 80, 180

5. bandaid

Frame 20

Queckenstedt test for blockage of CSF flow:

> With the manometer attached to the needle, the jugular veins are compressed for 10 seconds.

> CSF pressure rises.

> Pressure on the jugular veins is released.

> Time required for CSF pressure to return to pre-test level is measured.

> Blockage of CSF channels by tumor or other pathology results in slow decrease of CSF pressure.

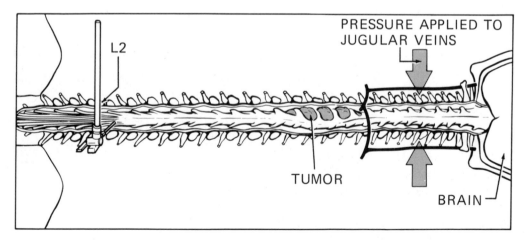

Figure 4.13. *Queckenstedt test*

1. A patient has lumbar CSF pressure of 165. This (is/is not) within normal limits.

   1. is

2. The compression of jugular veins tests for CSF (volume/blockage).

   2. blockage

3. The needle for an LP is placed between the (first and second/third and fourth) lumber vertebrae.

   3. third and fourth

4. If the spinal subarachnoid space is blocked, CSF pressure will (rapidly/slowly) return to normal after compression of jugular veins.

   4. slowly

Frame 21

Contraindications to LP are:

Increased intracranial pressure—removal of fluid from below the skull greatly accelerates the process of downward pressure and herniation of brain contents through the foramen magnum.

Septicemia or infection at the LP site—risk of introducing infection.

Use of anticoagulants—risk of bleeding.

1. Mr. Wilson has cerebral edema following a closed head injury. He (should/should not) be scheduled for an LP.

   1. should not

2. Infection in the lumbar area (is/is not) a significant risk in LPs.

   2. is

Frame 22

CSF is removed and sent to the laboratory. Refer to Chapter 1, Frame 21 for normal characteristics of CSF. Findings from CSF help to diagnose subarachnoid hemorrhage, meningitis, and demyelinating conditions.

Frame 23

Post-procedure care includes keeping the patient flat in bed for 8–12 hours. Because of the needle hole in the dura, some CSF leaks from this opening. In the recumbent position there is less CSF pressure in the lower spine area, thus the escape of fluid is decreased.

Headache is a frequent after-effect of the LP found in 10–20% of the patients. The headache may be due to the shift in pressure of the CSF and the traction on the pain-sensitive meningeal veins. Codeine is used to relieve the pain.

Voiding should be checked after the procedure. The nerve root or the filum terminale may have been traumatized by the insertion of the needle resulting in temporary problems in voiding. This is almost always a transient problem.

Frame 24

Summary:

In lumbar puncture a needle is inserted below the end of the spinal cord to obtain CSF for diagnosis, to check CSF pressure, or to inject medication and contrast media

Contraindications are: increased intracranial pressure, infection at the site and systemic anticoagulation.

After LP:

Flat bedrest for 8–12 hours
Analgesia for headache
Check urinary output

CHAPTER 5

NURSING ASSESSMENT OF NEUROLOGIC FUNCTION

Assessing is an important element of nursing, but it is especially vital in caring for neurologic patients. The nurse is with the patient frequently and is often the first to note subtle changes in the patient's condition. Early detection of these changes in neuro patients allows for prompt interventions which may mean the difference between recovery or permanent damage.

At the conclusion of this chapter you will be able to:

1. Identify the physiologic/pathologic basis for the components of the neuro assessment
2. Describe the proper technique for doing each component of the assessment
3. Describe indicators of compensation, decompensation, and cerebral death
4. Identify the major parts of the intracranial screw
5. Describe the procedure for insertion of the screw
6. Recognize significant changes in pressure readings
7. When given a situation, select appropriate nursing actions for a patient on intracranial monitoring
8. When given a situation, select actions to take when alterations from normal are found
9. When given a situation, record the findings from the assessment.

Chapter outline

Describing the baseline
   Vital signs
   Pupils, visual field
   Level of consciousness
   Motor and sensory function
   Homeostatic balance

Determining significance of changes
   Stage of compensation
   Decompensation
   Cerebral death

Monitoring intracranial pressure
   Purposes
   Equipment
   Nursing care

PART I
DESCRIBING THE
BASELINE

Jenny Olson, age 19, is admitted to the ICU for observation following a car accident. She had received a severe blow on her head.

On admission the nurse, Karl Evans, uses a clinical flow sheet to chart a baseline assessment and further observations. This provides a graphic picture of the patient's progress which clearly demonstrates significant variations.

A sample of a neuro flow sheet is provided in Appendix B. This may be xeroxed and used in any way you wish. Now review the observations and charting done for Ms. Olson.

Vital Signs

Frame 1

Vital signs are a major component of a neurologic assessment. Blood pressure, pulse, and respirations are included with each check. Temperature is taken frequently if elevated. On this clinical flow sheet, the temperature will be recorded in the Fahrenheit scale.
Ms. Olson's vital signs on admission are charted in Figure 5.1.

NEUROLOGIC   CLINICAL FLOW SHEET

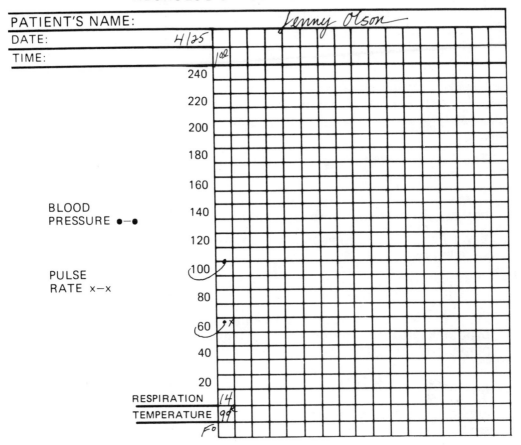

Figure 5.1.   *Vital signs*

If Ms. Olson's intracranial pressure increases, the systolic blood pressure will rise. The pulse will slow as the heart contracts more forcefully to overcome increased pressure within the skull. These mechanisms keep the brain supplied with blood.

1. If Ms. Olson had increasing intracranial pressure, you would find which of the following changes in BP:

   1. b

   a. change from 110/66 to 90/60
   b. change from 110/66 to 140/70
   c. change from 110/66 to 150/110

2. What would you expect to happen to her pulse rate:

   2. b

   a. remain at 68
   b. decrease below 68
   c. rise above 68

Frame 2

Ms. Olson's body temperature is now normal. The temperature control center is located in the hypothalamus. Damage to this area can cause marked hyperthermia (fever).

However, a more common cause of fever in neurologic patients is infection. Pneumonia and bladder infections often complicate neurologic illness.

1. The hypothalamus is located (above/within) the brain stem.

   1. above

2. Damage to the base of the brain (would/would not) affect the temperature regulating center.

   2. would

3. Fever (is/is not) an immediate result of brain stem injury.

   3. is not

4. The most common cause of fever in neurologic patients is ($\uparrow$ ICP/infection).

   4. infection

5. Mr. R. had a gunshot wound that damaged the hypothalamic area. You would expect his temperature to be (high/normal/low).

   5. high

Frame 3

A number of factors must be considered in assessing respirations. First consider rate, depth, and rhythm.

1. Which part of the brain controls respiratory rate and pattern?

   1. c

   a. cortex
   b. cerebellum
   c. brain stem

2. As increased intracranial pressure is transmitted downward toward the opening in the base of the skull, which part of the brain would be most affected?

   2. a

   a. brain stem
   b. frontal lobe
   c. lateral ventricles

3. Increased intracranial pressure causing uncal herniation would have what effect on respirations?

   3. b

   a. no change
   b. altered rate and pattern

In order to assess the respirations adequately, the nurse should have a clear view of the patient's chest and adequate light. Respirations should be counted for a full minute, and any changes in depth and rhythm are described on the chart.

Frame 4

The rate and depth of respirations normally vary widely in response to the body's needs.

If carbon dioxide levels in the blood increase, the respiratory control center in the brain stem increases both the rate and depth of respirations. This is the most powerful stimulus.

Accumulation of acids in the blood causes increased respiratory rate and depth to blow off carbon dioxide. This rids the body of extra acid.

Low oxygen levels also stimulate the respiratory center, but are weaker stimuli to breathing than an increased CO_2 load.

1. (Oxygen/CO_2) is the more powerful respiratory stimulus.

2. An increase in acid in the blood (increases/decreases) respiratory rate and length.

1. CO_2

2. increases

Frame 5

CHEYNE STOKES RESPIRATIONS (CSR)

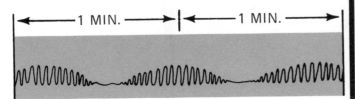

Figure 5.2. *CSR pattern*

Bilateral dysfunction of deep hemispheric structures or the upper brain stem can depress the respiratory center. At the beginning of the CSR pattern, the respirations are shallow and slow. CO_2 accumulates to a high level before the respiratory center is triggered to remove it. The respirations become faster and deeper to rapidly remove CO_2. When CO_2 falls below the stimulus level, respirations again become slow and shallow. There is sometimes a period of apnea between patterns.

1. The increased respiratory rate in CSR is due to an increase in (CO_2/O_2).

    1. CO_2

2. CSR is caused by dysfunction of the (frontal lobe/pons).

    2. pons

3. The slowing and stoppage of respirations in CSR is due to an inadequate (stimulus/musculature) for respiration.

    3. stimulus

Frame 6

CENTRAL NEUROGENIC HYPERVENTILATION (CNH)

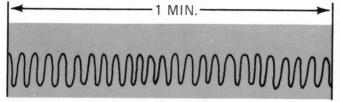

Figure 5.3. *CNH pattern*

CNH occurs when the midbrain and upper pons are involved. It is typified by sustained, regular, rapid, and fairly deep respirations.

A regular rhythm of hyperventilation can also occur in respiratory diseases such as pulmonary edema. Pulmonary edema is not uncommon in patients who have suffered cerebral trauma. If the breath sounds are moist, and arterial O_2 levels are below 70-80 mmHg, the cause is probably pulmonary rather than neurogenic.

True or False:

1. _____ CNH is characterized by shallow respirations.

    1. False

2. _____ Pulmonary edema can be differentiated from CNH by moist breath sounds.

    2. True

3. _____ CNH occurs when there is dysfunction in the pons.

    3. True

Frame 7

BIOT'S OR ATAXIC BREATHING

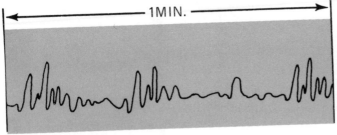

Figure 5.4. *Ataxic pattern*

Damage to the dorsomedial part of the medulla or lesions of the posterior fossa may cause ataxic breathing. Respirations are both deep and shallow with irregular pauses. This pattern may be mistaken for Cheyne Stokes. Recall that CSR has a more regular pattern.

1. Which of the following describes an ataxic breathing pattern?

   a. regularly occurring period of apnea
   b. shallow respirations
   c. irregular shallow and deep respirations

2. The nurse can distinguish ataxic breathing from CSR by its:

   a. irregularity
   b. deep and shallow respirations

1. c

2. a

Frame 8

APNEUSTIC BREATHING

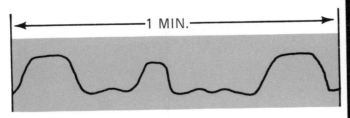

Figure 5.5. *Apneustic pattern*

Apneustic breathing occurs when there is damage to the respiratory control mechanism in the medulla. A prolonged inspiratory phase with a pause before expiration characterizes this pattern. A patient with apneustic breathing has a poor prognosis.

True or False:

1. _____ A patient inspires rapidly and expires slowly in a regular pattern. This is apneustic breathing.

2. _____ Apneustic breathing is caused by cortical damage.

1. False

2. False

Frame 9

Assessment of the respiratory function of neurologic patients should include:

A. Observing adequacy of ventilation
Is the airway patent? If O_2 is administered, is the flow rate and method effective? Are the chest muscles effective in ventilation?

B. Assessing adequacy of blood oxygenation
Is there any cyanosis of mucous membranes? Are the blood oxygen and carbon dioxide levels within the normal range? Can breath sounds be heard over all areas of the lung? If not, whole parts of the lung may not be contributing to oxygen and carbon dioxide exchange. This may be due to airway obstruction, alveolar collapse, infection, and consolidation.

C. Are there extra sounds which indicate pulmonary problems?
Rales or crackles—fizzing carbonated sounds usually heard on inspiration, caused by moisture in the small airways. Wheezes and rhonchi—more prominent on expiration, caused by narrowed airways due to secretions, spasm, stenosis, etc.

Frame 10

Here is a list of neurologic patients. Choose factor A or B to explain why each has inadequate respiratory function with changes in rate and depth of respirations.

A. Inadequate amount of air brought into the lungs.

B. Interference with O_2 and CO_2 exchange between the blood and alveoli.

1. _____ Mr. R. has a concussion and pulmonary edema.

    1. B

2. _____ Mrs. E. is unconscious following a craniotomy and her trachea is blocked by secretions.

    2. A

3. _____ Mrs. H. has paralysis of her chest muscles.

    3. A

4. _____ Mr. S. is undergoing neurologic tests, and he has congestive heart failure.

    4. B

Frame 11

Two hours after admission, Jenny Olson's neuro flow sheet showed these changes:

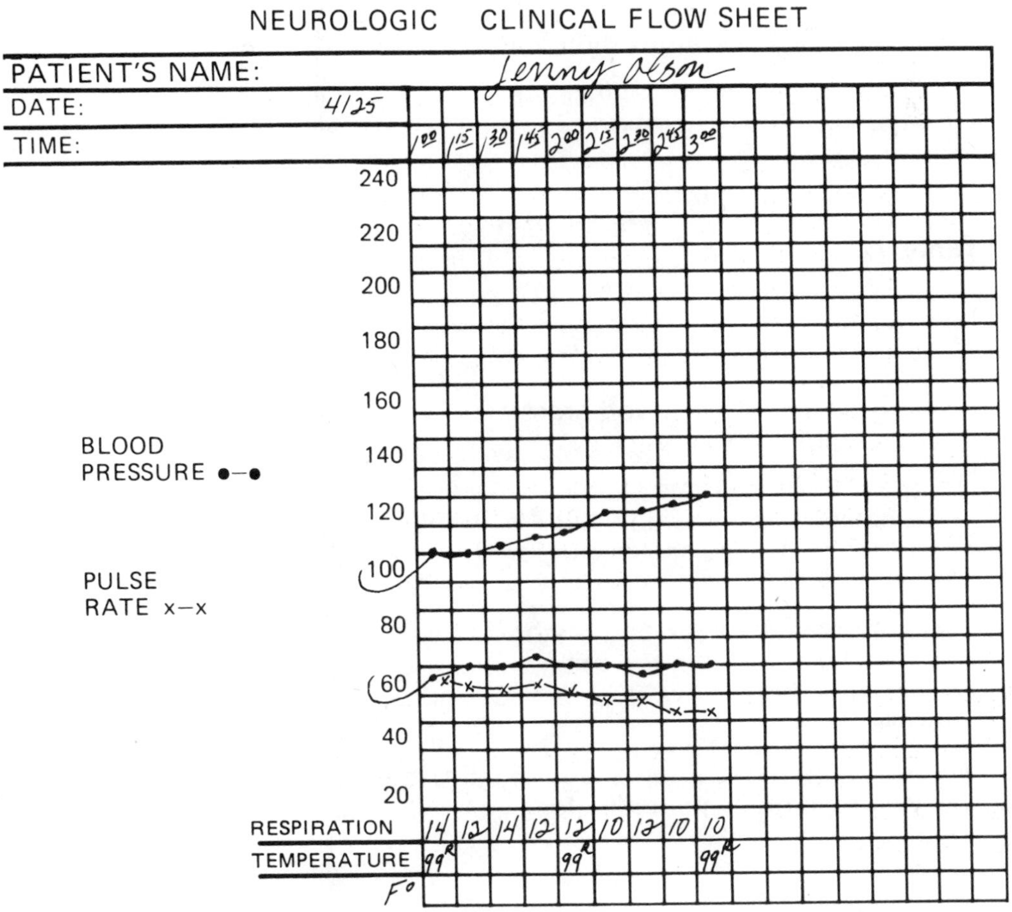

NEUROLOGIC CLINICAL FLOW SHEET

PATIENT'S NAME:	Jenny Olson
DATE:	4/25
TIME:	1⁰⁰ 1¹⁵ 1³⁰ 1⁴⁵ 2⁰⁰ 2¹³ 2³⁰ 2⁴⁵ 3⁰⁰

BLOOD PRESSURE ●—●

PULSE RATE x—x

240		
220		
200		
180		
160		
140		
120		
100		
80		
60		
40		
20		

RESPIRATION	14 12 14 12 12 10 12 10 10
TEMPERATURE F°	99⁸ 99⁸ 99⁸

Figure 5.6. *Vital signs*

Mr. Evans described the respirations in his notes as "slow ataxic respirations." Breath sounds were normal over the whole lung area, there was no cyanosis, and blood gases were within normal limits.

1. The changes in Ms. Olson's blood pressure indicate:

    a. normal recovery from the shock of her accident
    b. increased intracranial pressure
    c. inaccurate monitoring

2. The pulse rate is slower because:

    a. the heart is failing
    b. the heart is pumping more forcefully
    c. the control center in the brain is damaged

3. Ataxic respirations are:

    a. an irregular pattern of deep and shallow breaths
    b. characterized by an inspiratory pause
    c. also indicative of pulmonary edema

4. Jenny Olson's vital signs indicate:

    a. improvement since admission
    b. stability of her condition
    c. increased ICP

1. b

2. b

3. a

4. c

Frame 12

Summary:

↑ ICP causes:
   Increase in systolic blood pressure
   Slowing of pulse rate

Temperature elevations can be caused by:
   Damage to the hypothalamus
   Infection—particularly respiratory and urinary

Respiratory rate, depth, and rhythm are controlled by a center in the brain stem.
   The center is sensitive to blood CO_2 and O_2 levels.

Altered breathing patterns depend on the level of the brain stem affected.

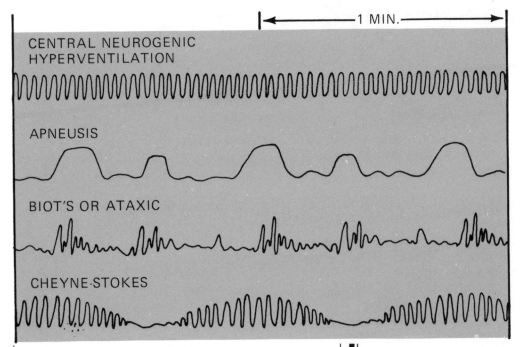

Figure 5.7. *Abnormal patterns of breathing*

General assessment of respiratory status includes:

—adequacy of ventilation: airway patency, O_2 administration, muscular effort
—adequacy of O_2/CO_2 exchange: cyanosis, blood O_2 and CO_2 levels, breath sounds.

Pupils and Visual Field

Frame 13

The size, equality, and reaction of the pupils are important indicators of neurologic status.

The pupil of the eye is supplied by sympathetic and parasympathetic fibers.

SYMPATHETIC FIBERS

Origin: ganglion of thoracic spinal cord T 1, 2, 3
Pathway: travels through the hypothalamus to eye muscles
Normal effect: stimulates muscles that dilate pupils (mydriasis)
Effect of damage: to the pons, hypothalamus → constriction of pupils

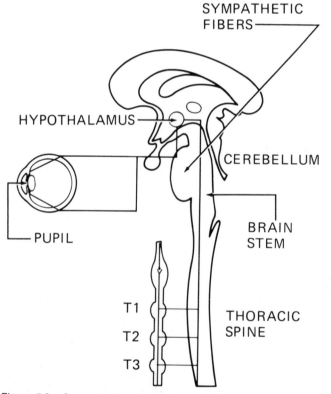

Figure 5.8.   *Sympathetic pathway for pupil dilation*

1. The effect of the sympathetic nerve fibers is to (constrict/dilate) the pupils.

1. dilate

2. Pupillary dilation is called (miosis/mydriasis).

2. mydriasis

3. Mr. F. has a tumor in the pons which has destroyed some of the nerve fibers. His pupils are constricted and will not dilate. The (sympathetic/parasympathetic) fibers to the pupil are not functioning.

3. sympathetic

Frame 14

PARASYMPATHETIC FIBERS

Origin: nuclei of the third cranial (oculomotor) nerve
Pathway: oculomotor nerve (CN III)
Normal effect: stimulates muscles that constrict the pupil (miosis)
Effect of damage: to CN III → dilation of pupils

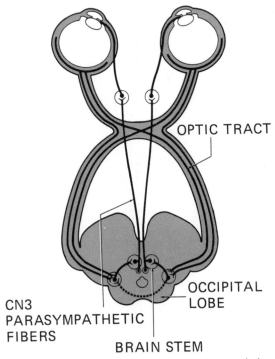

Figure 5.9. *Parasympathetic pathway for pupil constriction*

1. Pupil constriction in the presence of light is the function of _____ nerve fibers.

1. parasympathetic

2. The parasympathetic fibers are part of the _____ cranial nerve.

2. III, oculomotor

3. Mr. Z. has damage to the oculomotor nerve on the right side. You would expect his right pupil to be _____.

3. dilated

4. The term for pupil dilation is _____.

4. mydriasis

Frame 15

In the normally functioning eye, a balance exists between the sympathetic and parasympathetic fibers. However, if one or the other is impaired, the other set of fibers takes total control. In uncal herniation, the parasympathetic fibers are compressed, leaving the sympathetic fibers to control pupil reaction.

In Figure 5.10 you are looking down at the opening in the tentorium. Note the position of the third cranial nerve and the arterial blood supply in relation to the tentorium.

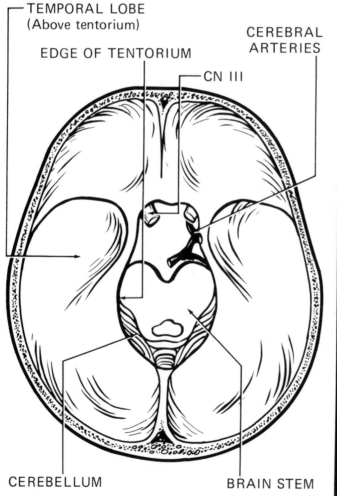

TEMPORAL LOBE
(Above tentorium)

EDGE OF TENTORIUM

CEREBRAL ARTERIES

CN III

CEREBELLUM

BRAIN STEM

Figure 5.10. *Tentorial opening*

1. Herniation of part of the brain through the tentorial opening (would/would not) cause pressure on the oculomotor nerve.

   1. would

2. Pressure on the oculomotor nerve causes (constriction/dilation) of pupils.

   2. dilation

Slight pressure causes minor dilation, whereas complete paralysis of the nerve causes full dilation. This reaction is ipsilateral to the damage.

3. Mr. Q. has left uncal herniation with paralysis of CN III. You would expect his (right/left) pupil to be (fully/partially) dilated.

   3. left, fully

Frame 16

If a lesion is unilateral, initially only the pupil on that side will be affected. If the lesion and/or ↑ICP continues without effective treatment, both pupils will dilate.

Bilateral, dilated fixed pupils are an ominous sign because they indicate that extensive supratentorial pressure is being exerted on the brain stem.

True or False:

1. _____ The pupil is initially dilated on the same side as the expanding lesion.

   1. True

2. _____ Bilateral dilated or fixed pupils indicate the patient's condition is improving.

   2. False

Frame 17

Wide use of drugs in today's society necessitates cautious interpretation of pupillary size. Drugs which cause dilation of the pupil include amphetamine and atropine.

Drugs which cause pupillary constriction are heroin and morphine.

Cycloplegic drops are used in eye exams, and many neuro patients have eye exams. These cause dilation of the pupil. A note should be placed on the chart to alert the staff if a patient has had eye drops.

Select from Column II the action of the drug named in Column I.

Column I	Column II	
1. heroin	a. dilation of	1. b
2. cycloplegic drops	pupil	2. a
3. atropine	b. constriction	3. a
4. amphetamines	of pupil	4. a

Frame 18

When Mr. Evans checked Ms. Olson's pupils, he began by observing *size* and *equality* in both eyes simultaneously. Size can be estimated by using a ruler, a guide on the clinical flow sheet, or a strip of EKG paper (each small box = 1 mm^2).

Then he dimmed the lights to darken the area. This allows maximum response to the test light. Mr. Evans flashed a small light into each eye to determine pupillary *reaction.* Ms. Olson's pupils constricted with light and dilated again when the light was removed. He noted whether this reaction was brisk (normal) or sluggish (indicating pressure on the nerve).

Pupillary reaction is described as:

    a. *direct*—constriction when light shines in the eye

    b. *consensual*—constriction when light shines in the *other* eye. The consensual response is caused by branching of CN III fibers in the optic chiasm. Ms. Olson had a normal consensual response in both eyes. Figure 5.11 shows the admission charting.

NEUROLOGIC   CLINICAL FLOW SHEET

PATIENT'S NAME: *Jenny Olson*																
DATE:			4/25													
TIME:				1⁰⁰												

REACTION		R	SIZE	2													
+ SLOW			REACTION	++													
++ BRISK			SIZE	2													
− NO REACTION c EYE CLOSED		L	REACTION	++													

PUPIL
SCALE

2mm
●

4mm
●

6mm
●

Figure 5.11. *Pupillary reaction*

True or False:

1. _____ Pupil size should be recorded as small, medium, or dilated.

2. _____ A fully dilated pupil indicates parasympathetic paralysis.

3. _____ Sluggish constriction to light is a normal pupillary response in a dark room.

4. _____ Ms. Olson's pupils are equal and normally reactive.

5. _____ The right pupil normally constricts when light is flashed into the left eye.

6. _____ A lesion of the oculomotor nerve would not affect the consensual response.

1. False
2. True
3. False
4. True
5. True
6. False

Frame 19

Match the drawings with the correct description or cause.

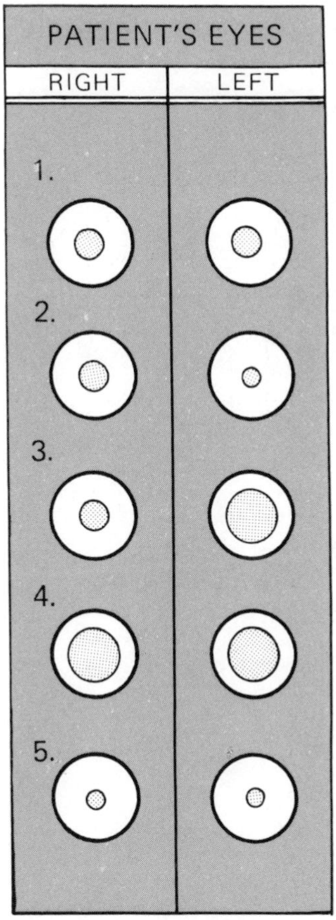

PATIENT'S EYES

RIGHT | LEFT

1.
2.
3.
4.
5.

Cause

a. paralysis of CN III and dangerous pressure on brain stem
b. compressed CN III on left side of brain
c. damage to pons, or heroin effect
d. pupils equal
e. loss of consensual response on the right

1. d
2. e
3. b
4. a
5. c

Figure 5.12. *Pupil sizes*

Frame 20

Figure 5.13 describes the changes in Ms. Olson's pupils during a two hour period after admission.

NEUROLOGIC   CLINICAL FLOW SHEET

PATIENT'S NAME:	*Jenny Olson*													
DATE:			4/25											
TIME:				1⁰⁰	1¹⁵	1³⁰	1⁴⁵	2⁰⁰	2¹⁵	2³⁰	2⁴⁵	3⁰⁰		

REACTION		R	SIZE	2	2	2	2	2	2	2	2	2		
+ SLOW ++ BRISK − NO REACTION c EYE CLOSED			REACTION	++	++	++	++	+	+	+	+	+		
		L	SIZE	2	2	2	2	3	3	3	4	4		
			REACTION	++	++	++	++	+	+	+	+	+		

PUPIL
SCALE

2mm
●

4mm
●

6mm
●

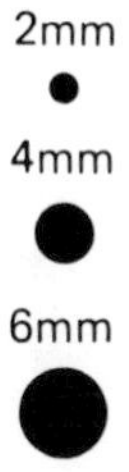

Figure 5.13. *Pupillary changes*

True or False:

1. _____ On admission Ms. Olson's pupils are equal and reactive.

   (The abbreviation for this is PERL, *P*upils *E*qual, *R*eact to *L*ight)

   1. True

2. _____ Ms. Olson's pupils remain within normal limits during the two hour period.

   2. False

3. _____ Ms. Olson's pupillary signs indicate pressure on the left oculomotor nerve.

   3. True

4. _____ Left pupil dilation and slow reaction to light indicates interference with parasympathetic nerve fibers.

   4. True

5. _____ Dangerously high ICP will not affect Ms. Olson's right pupil size and reactivity.

   5. False

Frame 21

Movements of the eye are also important. The third cranial nerve innervates most of the muscles for movement of the eye. The fourth and sixth CN are in close proximity in the brain stem to the third nerve. Together these nerves control external eye movements. Increasing intracranial pressure may cause pressure on these nerves resulting in the eye being "fixed" in place.

1. Name the three cranial nerves that control eye movement.

1. 3, 4, 6th oculomotor, trochlear, abducens

2. What causes a "fixed" eye?

2. paralysis of these nerves

Frame 22

In normal, awake, resting patients, the eyes are directed straight ahead and there are no involuntary movements.

Nystagmus is a term used to describe abnormal eye movements resulting from interference with the multiple factors involved in maintaining the eyes in position for normal vision. Involuntary to-and-fro oscillations of the eye occur. The movements may be:

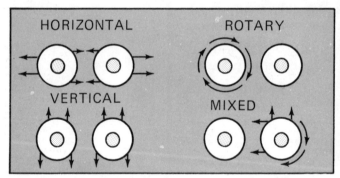

Figure 5.14. *Nystagmus*

1. vertical
2. rotary

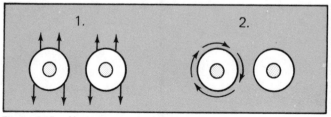

Figure 5.15. *Nystagmus*

148

3. Nystagmus refers to (voluntary/involuntary) movements of the eyes.

3. involuntary

Panel 1
Everything You Wanted to Know About Doll's Eyes Movements

Some reflex eye movements are elicited for diagnosis of neurologic problems.

Oculocephalic Reflex (Doll's eyes)

Patients with brain lesions may exhibit the oculocephalic reflex. If the head is turned one way, the eyes immediately look the other way.

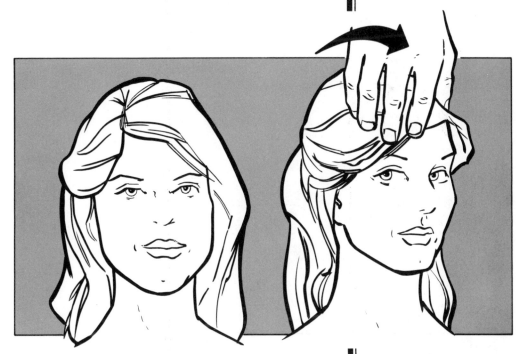

Figure 5.16. *Oculocephalic reflex*

Similarly, when the neck is flexed the eyes look up, and if the head is bent back the eyes look down.

Normally, this reflex is present to allow a person to voluntarily fix his vision on a point while his body is moving (watching the road while running, for example).

When the reflex appears involuntarily, it indicates damage to higher brain centers. Therefore it is tested only in comatose patients. As the patient's condition deteriorates further and the oculomotor nerve is paralyzed, the oculocephalic reflex disappears.

Oculovestibular Reflex (Cold Caloric)

To elicit this reflex, cold water is instilled into the external ear canal. In the normal, awake patient, there will be a slow movement of the eyes toward the irrigated ear and rapid movement back to the midposition.

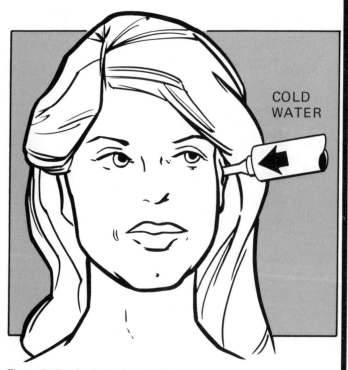

COLD WATER

Figure 5.17. *Oculovestibular reflex*

As consciousness is lost due to brain disease, the eyes tend to stay longer in position toward the irrigated ear.

The normal reflex depends upon intact nerve fiber connections between the brain and the vestibular *apparatus (semi-circular canals) in the ear that regulate equilibrium.*

Frame 23

Mr. Evans also examined Ms. Olson for any large visual field deficits. He asked her to close one eye, and look at his opposite eye. He brought his pen from beside her head on the opposite side into the center of her field of vision. He did this from several directions. Ms. Olson indicated when she saw the pen. This was repeated for the other eye. Ms. Olson did not have any obvious field cuts. More sophisticated testing is necessary if field cut problems are suspected. If you need to review the pathologic cause of field defects, see Chapter 3, Frame 18.

True or False:

1. _____ Lesions of the optic nerve (CNII) pathway can result in visual field defects.

   1. True

2. _____ Loss of one-half of the visual field is possible because of the branching of the optic nerve fibers at the chiasm.

   2. True

Frame 24

Increased ICP also can cause papilledema, the engorgement and swelling of the optic disc at the back of the eye that is visible through an opthalmoscope. The sheath of the optic nerve is continuous with the subarachnoid space, and a rise in ICP is transmitted through it to the disc. Papilledema is often accompanied by distension of retinal veins, and it is a sign of dangerously high ICP. Body fluid imbalances resulting in edema may also cause papilledema.

True or False:

1. _____ The appearance of papilledema is an early sign of ↑ICP.

   1. False

2. _____ Papilledema is a serious sign.

   2. True

Frame 25

Summary:

Sympathetic fibers cause pupil dilation (mydriasis)

Pressure or lesions in pons and hypothalamus → constriction of pupils

Parasympathetic fibers cause pupil constriction (miosis)

Pressure or lesions on CN III (especially uncal herniation) →dilation of pupils on the same side.

Dangerously high ICP → dilated and fixed pupils bilaterally.

Drugs affect pupil size

Constriction—heroin, morphine

Dilation—cyclopegic eye drops, atropine, amphetamines

Assessment: size, equality, reaction to light

Eye movements are controlled by CN III, IV, VI

Nystagmus—involuntary eye movements in horizontal, vertical, rotary, and mixed directions.

Visual field defects are caused by damage to CNII optic nerve.

Papilledema is swelling of the optic disc at the back of the eye due to ↑ICP and/or venous engorgement due to body fluid imbalance.

Level of Consciousness

Frame 26

The next part of the assessment describes levels of consciousness. There are two distinct components of consciousness:

Arousal or alertness—function of reticular activating system (RAS) in the brain stem.

Content of consciousness or orientation, a function of the cerebral cortex particularly the frontal lobe.

1. A patient thinks that he is now a prisoner in a second world war zone. This is due to damage to the (RAS/cortex).

    1. cortex

2. A patient's only response to stimulation is moaning. This is a defect in (arousal/content) of consciousness.

    2. arousal

3. Arousal is dependent on the (cortex/RAS).

    3. RAS

Frame 27

The ARAS (ascending reticular activating system) in the brain stem is the center where impulses from the sensory modalities, the cerebrum, and the cerebellum enter and interact. Any one neuron may have synaptic input from over 4000 other neurons and interactions with about 25,000 neurons.

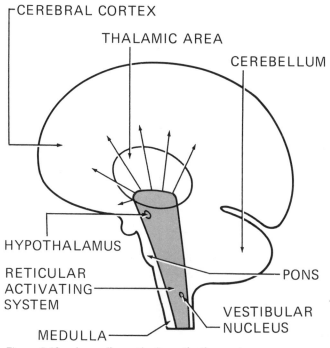

Figure 5.18. *Ascending reticular activating system*

Integration is a vital function of this area of the brain stem. When there is interference with blood circulation to this area either by direct pressure or blockage within blood vessels themselves, the level of consciousness is decreased.

Supratentorial lesions and/or edema are a common cause for decrease in level of consciousness. Look again at Figure 5.10, Frame 14, to see that downward pressure not only puts direct pressure on the brain stem but also causes pressure on the posterior cerebral artery which supplies the brain stem. The neurons in the brain stem do not receive the needed O_2 and glucose for normal functioning.

1. The ARAS integrates input from the
_____, _____, and
_____ _____.

1. cerebrum, cerebellum, sensory modalities

2. An expanding supratentorial lesion pushes the uncus of the temporal lobe through the tentorial opening, putting pressure on the _____ artery which supplies the brain stem.

3. Interference with the supply of _____ and _____ affect the functioning of the ARAS.

2. posterior cerebral

3. oxygen
   glucose

With minimal uncal herniation, some pressure is placed on the ARAS causing slowed responsiveness in the patient. More pressure further reduces the ability of the neurons to integrate incoming stimuli. Therefore, detection of decreasing consciousness is an indication for interventions to halt the progression of increasing pressure. The intervention used depends on the suspected etiology.

Frame 28

When Mr. Evans assessed the level of consciousness (LOC) of Ms. Olson, he stood by the bedside and greeted the patient in his normal manner. This did not elicit a response, so he used a louder tone of voice and gently shook Ms. Olson's arm. She then opened her eyes and said, "Who are you?"

If a stronger stimulus had been needed to arouse the patient, Mr. Evans could try slightly painful stimuli such as

a gentle thump on her sternum
application of pressure on the nailbeds or joints

These procedures should not break skin integrity or cause tissue damage.

Number the following assessment procedures in order of use.

_____ a. pressure on nailbeds
_____ b. shake patient gently
_____ c. normal greeting
_____ d. louder tone of voice

a. 4
b. 3
c. 1
d. 2

Frame 29

Other observations Mr. Evans needs to make are

154

—whether Ms. Olson *remains* responsive, and the pattern of her alertness

—other factors which may affect arousal such as sensory deficits, administration of sedatives, narcotics, and sleep deprivation.

1. Choose the patients who may be slow to respond.

    a. Mr. C. had 100 mg Demerol (IM) 30 minutes before

    b. Ms. Z. has damage to the ARAS

    c. Mr. P. is partially deaf in both ears

    d. Ms. R. has a field cut involving the left half of the visual field

    3. Mr. B. was in an accident at the end of a full night of driving his truck.

1. all

Frame 30

In recording LOC, terms or numbers may be used. Terms used to describe LOC are:

alert — responds immediately to minimal external stimulation

lethargic — state of drowsiness or inaction in which the person needs an increased stimulus to be awakened

obtunded — a duller indifference to external stimuli exists and response is minimally maintained

stuporous — person can be aroused only by vigorous and continuous external stimulation

comatose — stimulation fails to produce voluntary neural response in the patient

These terms, if they are used, should be carefully defined on the neuro sheet so all interpret them in the same manner. The parameters for numbers should be clear and careful noting of the assessment should be made. Mr. Evans wrote: "I had to shake Jenny to awaken her. She mumbled when asked questions and fell back to sleep immediately."

Match the word in Column B to the LOC described in Column A

Column A	Column B	
1. Requires vigorous shaking to arouse and then just opens eyes and groans	a. alert b. lethargic c. stuporous d. comatose	1. c
2. Does not respond to painful stimuli		2. d
3. Opens eyes and gives name when spoken to		3. a

Frame 31

Orientation to one's environment includes recognition of self, others, place, and time. Confusion first occurs regarding *time,* then *place* and lastly loss of recognition of *self*. Trauma often interferes with the normal transmission and storage of incoming stimuli resulting in the person being termed "disoriented" or "confused."

1. The doctor states that Ms. Olson is slightly confused. You would expect this to mean she had difficulty with:

   1. b

   a. the place where she was
   b. the time and/or date
   c. who was talking to her

2. The person who does not correctly identify himself is:

   2. c

   a. slightly confused
   b. moderately confused
   c. severely confused

Frame 32

Intact sensory modalities are essential for orientation. If incoming stimuli are blocked or distorted, the patient's perception of them and response to them is altered.

In determining orientation, assess the integrity of the senses. Lack of ability to see, hear, and touch may contribute to confusion. Also consider the quality of stimuli coming to the patient: meaningless noises, snatches of conversation, constant boring noise of machines, ability to see only ceiling and white walls.

True or False:

1. _____ If incoming stimuli are blocked, confusion is likely.

2. _____ Confusion due to sensory deprivation and sensory overload is unusual in ICU.

1. True

2. False

Frame 33

The prefrontal area in the cerebral hemisphere is thought to be the main association area for memory. Confusion after cerebral trauma occurs due to interference with transmission of neural impulses.

Amnesia, inability to remember, occurs when lesions or trauma affect the frontal and/or temporal lobes. There are several kinds of amnesia:

Circumscribed —for a certain time period
Anterograde —from the stress point forward
Retrograde —for events prior to the stress period

1. The primary memory association area is in the _____ part of the brain.

2. Mr. J. was found wandering in the street, unable to recall any of his past life. This is _____ amnesia.

3. Ms. Olson recalls the events before her car accident, but not the accident itself. She remembers being admitted to the hospital. She has _____ amnesia.

1. prefrontal

2. retrograde

3. circumscribed

Frame 34

Appropriateness of motor response is also an indicator of level of consciousness. Mr. Evans asked Ms. Olson to touch her mouth, blink her eyes, and move her legs. She responded to these requests correctly.

If Ms. Olson had not been able to follow directions, the nurse would assess her response to painful stimuli (such as nailbed pressure).

A normal response is withdrawal, pulling her hand away.

The decorticate response indicates a lower level of consciousness, and interruption of voluntary motor tracts. The motor pathways through the brain stem are intact and the patient responds by flexion of large muscle groups.

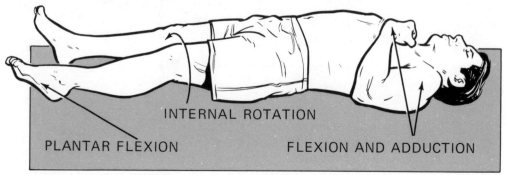

INTERNAL ROTATION

PLANTAR FLEXION   FLEXION AND ADDUCTION

Figure 5.19. *Decorticate response*

The decerebrate response indicates deeper brain damage. There is disruption of motor fibers in the midbrain and brain stem. The patient responds with stiffly extended arms and legs, hyperextended head, and clenched jaw. The opisthotonus position seen in meningeal irritation is similar, but the back is arched in opisthotonus.

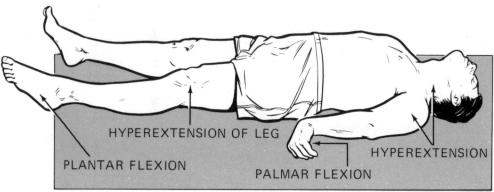

HYPEREXTENSION OF LEG

PLANTAR FLEXION   HYPEREXTENSION

PALMAR FLEXION

Figure 5.20. *Decerebrate response*

No response to pain indicates loss of both sensory and motor pathways.

Label the following responses to pain decerebrate, decorticate, or normal.

1. Flexion of arm and shoulder

2. Withdrawal of hand from pain

3. Extension of arm and neck

4. Internal rotation of hip

1. decorticate

2. normal

3. decerebrate

4. decorticate

Frame 35

Here is Mr. Evans' flow chart on Jenny Olson's level of consciousness the first two hours after admission.

NEUROLOGIC   CLINICAL FLOW SHEET

			1⁰⁰	1¹⁵	1³⁰	1⁴⁵	2⁰⁰	2¹⁵	2³⁰	2⁴⁵	3⁰⁰			
PATIENT'S NAME: *Jenny Olson*														
DATE: 4/25														
TIME:														
LEVEL OF CONSCIOUSNESS	EYES OPEN LID MOVEMENT	SPONTANEOUSLY												
		TO SPEECH												
		TO TOUCH	✓	✓	✓	✓	✓	✓	✓	✓	✓			
		NONE												
	BEST VERBAL RESPONSE	ORIENTED												
		CONFUSED (TIME, PLACE)	✓	✓	✓	✓	✓	✓	✓					
		INAPPROPRIATE WORDS												
		GARBLED								✓	✓			
		NONE												
	BEST MOTOR RESPONSE USUALLY BEST ARM	OBEY COMMANDS	✓	✓										
		APPROPRIATE RESP. TO PAIN			✓	✓	✓	✓	✓	✓	✓			
		FLEXION TO PAIN (DECORTICATE)												
		EXTENSION TO PAIN (DECEREBRATE)												
		NONE												

Figure 5.21. *Level of consciousness*

True or False:

1. _____ The flow chart shows that Ms. Olson's alertness would be described as lethargic.

2. _____ Motor response shows a decreased level of consciousness but no interference with cortical motor pathways.

3. _____ Ms. Olson's verbal response is within normal limits.

1. True

2. True

3. False

Frame 36

Summary:

Level of consciousness includes
  alertness—ARAS activity in brain stem and
    midbrain
  orientation—cortical function, especially
    prefrontal lobe

Levels in descending order: alert, lethargic, obtunded, stuporous, comatose.

Disorientation occurs in this order: loss of

recognition of time, place, people, self. Sensory defects, deprivation, and overload can contribute to disorientation.

Amnesia (memory loss) occurs with frontal lobe damage, and can be circumscribed, anterograde, or retrograde.

Motor response levels: obey commands, withdrawal from pain, flexion to pain (decorticate), extension to pain (decerebrate).

Motor and Sensory Function

Frame 37

A third major area of assessment is the functioning of the motor-sensory units. While the two units are represented in different areas of the brain, they are closely related and so are checked together.

Before advancing to the assessment of function, recall some terms related to motor-sensory dysfunction.

Monoplegia: paralysis of one limb, e.g., right arm

Hemiplegia: paralysis of one side of the body

Paraplegia: paralysis of the lower extremities

Quadriplegia: paralysis of all four extremities

Spasticity: abnormal increase in muscle tone, with rigidity and/or jerking contractions of the muscles.

Paresis: weakness of motor function in an extremity

Paralysis: complete absence of ability to voluntarily move an extremity.

Match the word in Column II to the phrase describing it in Column I

Column I	*Column II*	
1. Inability to voluntarily move left and right legs	a. monoplegia b. paresis c. decerebrate rigidity	1. f
2. Weakened grasp with right hand	d. decorticate rigidity	2. b
3. Arms and legs stiffly extended and teeth clenched	e. quadriplegia f. paraplegia	3. c
4. Inability to voluntarily move all four extremities		4. e
5. Arms flexed, legs internally rotated with plantar flexion		5. d

Frame 38

Mr. Evans checked Ms. Olson's ability to move all extremities as well as the strength and appropriateness of the movements.

Arms: He asked Ms. Olson to hold her arms straight out for a few moments and watched for a downward drift that indicates lack of strength. Mr. Evans then grasped both of Ms. Olson's hands, and asked her to squeeze his hands, to test the strength and equality of her grasp.

Legs: Ms. Olson was able to hold both legs off the bed. A weakened leg will flop to the bed. The nurse put his hands against the soles of Ms. Olson's feet and asked her to press down as hard as possible, to test strength and equality of motor function of the legs.

1. Why did Mr. Evans have the patient squeeze with both hands simultaneously?

1. To determine equality of grasp

2. Mr. J. has no ability to grasp on the left, and cannot lift his left leg off the bed. What is this called?

2. left hemiplegia

Frame 39

The Babinski reflex is determined by stroking the lateral margin of the sole. The normal response is plantar flexion of the toes. Dorsiflexion of the great toe with a fanning of the other toes is called a positive Babinski.

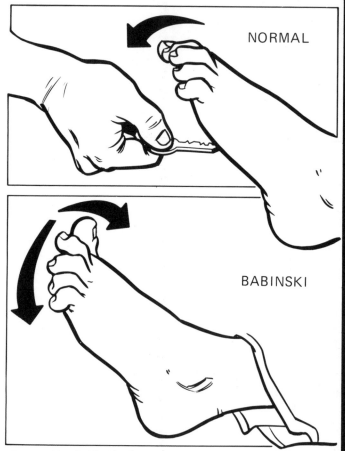

NORMAL

BABINSKI

Figure 5.22. *Babinski reflex*

The presence of the Babinski reflex is indicative of dysfunction in the voluntary motor system (corticospinal tract or motor area of the cerebrum).

Another reflex is the corneal reflex. When something touches the cornea, a person automatically blinks to remove it. Pressure on or dysfunction of the CN V eliminates the sensory portion of the reflex; similarly, dysfunction of the CN VII will eliminate the motor portion of the corneal reflex. Gentle blowing on the eye can be done to elicit the presence or absence of this reflex.

1. Which of the following describes a positive Babinski?

   a. great toe flexed up, toes fanned out
   b. all toes flexed down

2. A positive Babinski indicates dysfunction in:

   a. the sensory tracts
   b. the voluntary motor tracts
   c. the extra-pyramidal tracts

3. A person with an impaired corneal reflex will be unable to:

   a. blink his eyes
   b. produce tears
   c. turn his eyes

1. a

2. b

3. a

Frame 40

Alterations in the motor-sensory status may be related to dysfunction at many levels of the nervous system. The exact level may often be determined by the findings in all four extremities—hemiplegia indicates cerebral hemisphere or internal capsule involvement while paraplegia usually means dysfunction in the spinal cord. Inability to move an arm could mean a localized lesion affecting a small area in the motor strip.

Expanding intracranial lesions and/or edema, causing downward pressure, put increasing pressure on the corticospinal (motor) tract and the sensory tracts as they pass through the tentorial notch. Thus, decreased response to pain and decreased ability to move are found. Weakness and paralysis are first noted on one side of the body. As the lesion continues to expand, both sides may be involved.

1. Downward pressure through the tentorial notch initially causes weakness or paralysis on the (contralateral/ipsilateral) side.

2. Hemiplegia is due to damage in a (cerebral/cerebellar) hemisphere.

3. In monoplegia (one limb/one side of the body) is paralyzed.

1. contralateral

2. cerebral

3. one limb

Frame 41

Figure 5.23 shows the charting of Jenny Olson's motor abilities. Mr. Evans noted in the narrative section that her sensation was normal in all extremities. (See Chapter 14, Frame 3 for discussion of sensory assessment.)

NEUROLOGIC CLINICAL FLOW SHEET

				1:00	1:15	1:30	1:45	2:00	2:15	2:30	2:45	3:00			
PATIENT'S NAME: *Jenny Olson*															
DATE:							4/25								
TIME:															
L I M B M O V E M E N T	RECORD (R) AND (L) SEPARATELY IF THERE IS DIFFERENCE BETWEEN TWO SIDES R = RIGHT L = LEFT	A R M S	NORMAL POWER	✓	✓	✓	✓	✓	✓	✓	L	L			
			MILD WEAKNESS								R	R			
			SEVERE WEAKNESS												
			SPASTIC FLEXION (DECORTICATE)												
			EXTENSION (DECEREBRATE)												
			NO RESPONSE												
		L E G S	NORMAL POWER	✓	✓	✓	✓	✓	✓	✓	L	L			
			MILD WEAKNESS								R	R			
			SEVERE WEAKNESS												
			EXTENSION (DECEREBRATE)												
			NO RESPONSE												

Figure 5.23. *Motor response*

True or False:

1. _____ Ms. Olson's motor function remained normal.

2. _____ Weakness on one side of the body is called hemiparesis.

3. _____ The mild right hemiparesis noted at 2:45 is a sign of pressure or damage to motor tract pathways.

1. False

2. True

3. True

Frame 42

Summary:

Voluntary movement, strength, and sensation in the extremities are noted. Equality of motor and sensory function on both sides is also checked.

Terms:

-plegia, -paralysis: complete absence of voluntary motion; hemi-: one side; mono-: one; quadra-: four; para-: lower extremities

paresis: weakness

spasticity: abnormal increase in muscle tone

Reflexes:
   Babinski, normal: plantar flexion of all toes; positive: dorsiflexion of great toes, fanning of other toes. Indicates damage to motor pathways.
   Corneal: blink when cornea is touched. Loss indicates damage to CN V and CN VII.

Loss of sensory/motor function

   localized lesion in motor or sensory strip or ↑ICP with uncal herniation causes progressive loss of sensation and movement contralateral to the lesion. This gradually extends to both sides of the body if the lesion expands.

Homeostatic Balance

Frame 43

Assessment of the neurologic patient should also include monitoring of the homeostatic balance of the patient. The most important parameters in the critically ill patient are:

   body fluids
   electrolytes
   acid/base levels

Body fluid balance is indicated by:

   intake and output data
   changes in weight
   serum and urine osmolality (number of dissolved particles)
   signs of dehydration and edema

1. Retention of 500–600 ml of water is reflected by a weight gain of 1 lb or .5 kg. Mr. S. has an intake of 2,300 ml and an output of 1300 ml. You would expect him to gain about (1 kg/5 kg.) of body weight.

   1. 1 kg.

2. Mr. S. has papilledema, puffy eyelids, moist breath sounds, and dependent edema. These would indicate fluid (loss/retention).

   2. retention

3. Mr. S. also has ↑ICP. Body fluid retention would (help/hinder) the body's compensatory mechanisms.

   3. hinder

4. Mrs. J. is recovering from a craniotomy. Because of damage to her pituitary gland, she has diabetes insipidus with daily urinary outputs of 4–6,000 ml. Her urine is very dilute, and serum osmolality is high (many particles in low volume). You would expect her to tend toward (edema/dehydration).

4. dehydration

Body fluid balance disturbances can also cause neurologic effects:

Dehydration	*Fluid Retention*
weakness, dizziness, irritability, exhaustion	disorientation, headache, twitching, nausea, blurred vision

Frame 44

Blood electrolytes need to be within the correct range to ensure normal cell function. The electrolytes which most frequently cause problems in neuro patients are:

Sodium—changes also affect water balance
Potassium—functions in conduction of nerve impulses
Calcium—also affects nerve impulse conduction

True or False:

1. _____ Mr. L. has a serum potassium of 6.8 mEq (normal = 3.6–5.5). He has irritability, parethesias (tingling sensations), nausea, and changes in cardiac rhythm. These symptoms could be due to the electrolyte imbalance rather than neurologic disease.

1. True

2. _____ Signs and symptoms of electrolyte imbalance may distort the picture of neurologic status.

2. True

3. _____ Cell function continues normally within a wide range of electrolyte levels.

3. False

Frame 45

The acid-base balance (pH) of the body should also be monitored. Recall these facts:

Normal pH in arterial blood = 7.35–7.45, essential for normal cell function

Excess acid in blood = below 7.35
Excess alkali in blood = above 7.45

Acidosis is seen in shock as well as in respiratory, renal and certain metabolic diseases.

Physical signs include: deep respirations as the lungs blow off CO_2, and central nervous system depression with confusion, lethargy and ultimately coma.

Alkalosis may occur when the patient hyperventilates because of pathology affecting the respiratory center in the brain stem or excessive rates of mechanical ventilation.

Physical signs include: central nervous system excitation—paresthesia, muscle irritability and irregular heart rhythm—which progress to tetany, convulsions, coma.

1. Mr. L.'s serum pH is 7.31. He has (acidosis/ alkalosis).

2. You would expect Mr. L. to have signs of nervous system (stimulation/depression).

3. The range of pH within which cells can function normally is (narrow/wide).

4. Mr. T. has central neurogenic hyperventilation. He is at risk for (acidosis/alkalosis).

5. Mr. T. has twitching muscles and an irregular pulse. This (is/is not) a sign of alkalosis.

1. acidosis

2. depression

3. narrow

4. alkalosis

5. is

Frame 46

Summary:

Important parameters indicating homeostatic balance:
Body fluids: Intake and output data, weight changes, serum and urine osmolality, signs of dehydration and edema

Serum electrolytes: particularly sodium, potassium, calcium

Acid base balance: serum pH
acidosis—CNS depression
alkalosis—CNS stimulation

Use this method to assess your study habits . . .

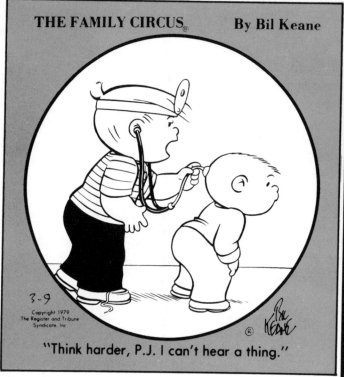

Figure 5.24.

PART II DETERMINING SIGNIFICANCE OF CHANGES

So far you have looked at *each component* of the nursing assessment: the underlying physiologic and pathologic factors, the technique, and significance of changes.

Now look at assessment findings as a whole and recognize the patterns that indicate deteriorating neurologic status.

Stage of Compensation

Frame 47

Figure 5.25 is Jenny Olson's whole clinical flow sheet. Use it to answer these questions.

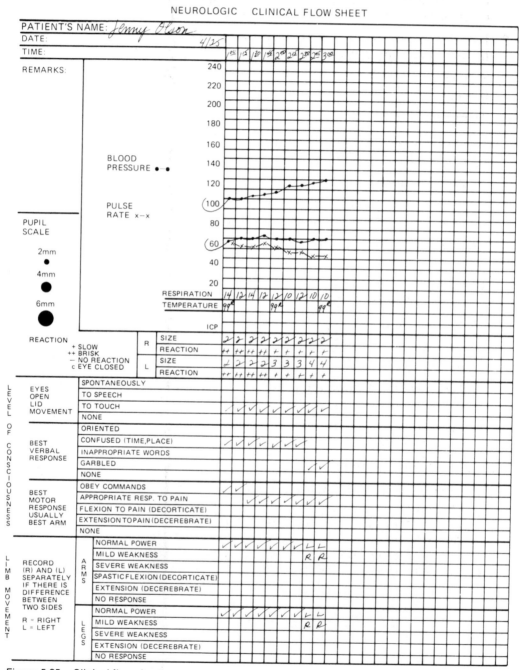

Figure 5.25. *Clinical flow sheet*

1. The pulse pressure (difference between the systolic and diastolic reading) is

   a. remaining the same
   b. narrowing (or decreasing)
   c. widening (or increasing)

2. The pulse rate is

   a. steady
   b. increasing
   c. slowing

3. Mr. Evans charted that the respirations are ataxic, deep, and stertorous. They are also

   a. faster
   b. slower

4. The pupils are becoming

   a. unequal and less reactive
   b. equal but reacting slowly

5. Dilation of the pupil indicates

   a. paralysis of CN III ipsilaterally
   b. stimulation of CN III contralaterally

6. Level of consciousness is

   a. slightly improved
   b. dramatically lower
   c. slowly deteriorating

7. Motor response is

   a. essentially the same
   b. weaker on the right

8. Motor weakness indicates damage to the motor pathways on the

   a. right side of the brain
   b. left side of the brain

9. Jenny Olson's clinical course indicates:

   a. beginning foramen magnum herniation on the right
   b. beginning uncal herniation on the left side of the brain
   c. brain stem paralysis
   d. right-sided trauma in the brain

1. c

2. c

3. b

4. a

5. a

6. c

7. b

8. b

9. b

Decompensation

Frame 48

The table in Figure 5.26 summarizes changes in consciousness, pupils and vital signs seen as neurologic status deteriorates.

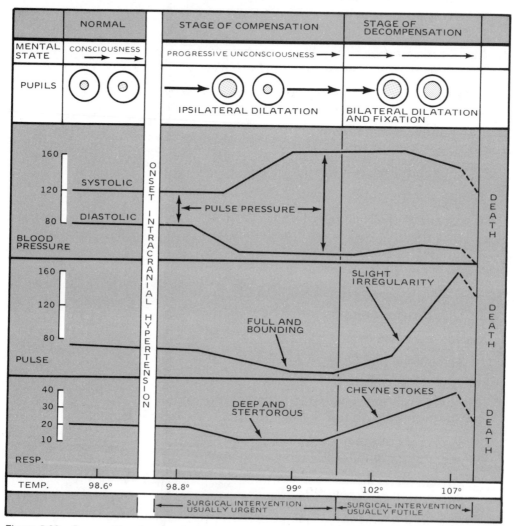

Figure 5.26. *Progression of neuro signs*

1. Use Jenny Olson's clinical flow sheet to determine what stage she is in.

   a. normal
   b. compensation
   c. decompensation

1. b

2. During the stage of compensation, which mechanisms are in operation due to ↑ICP?

   a. increased systolic pressure to overcome ↑ pressure on cerebral arteries
   b. pressure on the respiratory control center of the brain stem
   c. herniation of brain tissue out of the supratentorial space
   d. slower pulse as the heart beats more forcefully

2. all

3. What action(s) should be taken for Jenny Olson?

   a. continued close nursing observation
   b. use of mechanical ventilation
   c. immediate medical attention
   d. faster infusion of IV fluid

3. a and c

4. Which signs would show that Ms. Olson has moved into the stage of decompensation?

   a. hyperthermia
   b. pulse irregularity and increase in rate
   c. widening pulse pressure
   d. Cheyne Stokes respirations
   e. increased alertness

4. a, b, d

Frame 49

1. From this list of patients, choose the ones for whom the nurse should get immediate medical attention.

   a. Mr. L's pupil's were equal, but now the left one is slightly more dilated.
   b. Mr. P. has widely dilated pupils following a neurologic examination.
   c. Ms. Q's pulse pressure is wider, pulse is slower, and she is becoming more difficult to arouse.

1. a and c
   (b probably had cyclopegic eye drops.)

2. John Parks, a 15 year old, was admitted to ICU following an auto accident. On admission he did not respond to verbal stimuli but responded purposefully to pain. Two hours later his right pupil was dilated and nonreactive. He responded to pain by flexing his left arm and extending his left leg. His breathing was deep, regular and 26/min. His blood pressure and pulse remained stable. The nurse should

a. tell the family that John's condition is improving
b. call the physician to report the changes
c. observe John's condition for another hour before calling the physician

2. b

Cerebral Death

Panel 2

Brain Death

Continuous advancement in techniques of artificial life support have led to incidence of a clinical state in which patients have spontaneous cardiac function, but no apparent cerebral function or ability to breathe unaided. With mechanical respiration and supportive therapy vital functions can be maintained. These patients are alive in the traditional sense, but have no hope of recovery. They are sometimes potential organ donors for transplant procedures. Therefore, much research is being conducted to delineate the clinical entity of brain death as a determinant of the legal definition of death.

Various sets of criteria for brain death have been defined and are in use. Here are some common criteria:

A. Cause of coma—factors that result in permanent brain damage.

B. Physical examination of cortical and brain stem function
   —unresponsive
   —no spontaneous respirations (the respirator is detached for 3 or 4 minutes to see if the respiratory center can be stimulated by CO_2)
   —absence of brain stem reflexes: ciliospinal (dilation of the pupil when the cheek below the eye is pinched), oculocephalic (doll's eyes), oculovestibular (cold caloric), corneal, pupillary

C. *Other tests which may be helpful*
   —*EEG—isoelectric for 10–30 minutes*
   —*Arteriography—non-filling of cerebral vessels due to edema*
   —*Radioisotopes to measure cerebral flow*

D. *Timing of repeated tests: at least 12 hours are allowed to intervene before retesting to be sure changes are permanent.*

At this time, brain death is not yet a completely defined entity. More clinical study is needed to clarify the parameters of total irreversible cerebral damage.

Frame 50

Jason Pettis, age 23, was in ICU following an industrial accident causing severe cerebral trauma. His neurologic status steadily declined until there was total absence of responsiveness, spontaneous respirations, and brain stem reflexes. The physician explained the irreversibility of Jason's condition to the Pettis family and discussed the options open to them: continuation of treatment, or discontinuation of treatment with or without organ donation. The Pettis family decided that Jason would want to donate whatever organs he could for transplant procedures.

The next 24 hours were to be used to fulfill all the tests the hospital had adopted to define brain death.

1. The nurse tested Jason's neurologic status at frequent intervals. She (should/should not) explain the neuro assessment to the family.

   1. should

2. The nurse disconnected the respirator for four minutes and watched for signs of spontaneous respirations. She (should/should not) allow the family to be present during such tests.

   2. should

3. Mr. Pettis repeatedly told the nurse of his belief that Jason would want to be an organ donor. The nurse responded, "You are very concerned that you are making the right choice for Jason . . . ." This (is/is not) a response which will encourage Mr. Pettis to express his thoughts more fully.

   3. is

Frame 51

Summary:

Seriously increased ICP is recognized by: progressive loss of consciousness, single pupil dilation and loss of reactivity to light, widening of pulse pressure, slowing of pulse rate, changed respiratory patterns, loss of purposeful motor responses. Medical intervention is urgent.

Decompensated neuro status is indicated by: bilateral pupil dilation and fixation, narrowing of pulse pressure, rapid and irregular pulse, Cheyne Stokes respirations, hyperthermia. Medical intervention is often not successful at this stage.

Brain death is characterized by total absence of responsiveness, spontaneous respirations and brain stem reflexes for a period of at least 12 hours.

PART III
MONITORING
INTRACRANIAL
PRESSURE

Purposes

Frame 52

You are probably familiar with the monitoring of central venous pressure. The same idea has been applied to the measurement of intracranial pressure.

Recall that CSF, formed in the ventricles, circulates slowly into the subarachnoid space. The monitoring device called the subarachnoid screw is hollow, and its tip can be placed in the subarachnoid space to monitor ICP. Monitoring devices can also be placed in the epidural or subdural spaces and the ventricles of the brain.

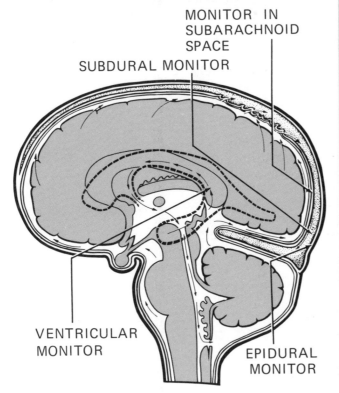

MONITOR IN SUBARACHNOID SPACE

SUBDURAL MONITOR

VENTRICULAR MONITOR

EPIDURAL MONITOR

Figure 5.27. *Location of CSF*

The screw provides *direct* recording of ICP, while observation of neurologic status provides *indirect* evidence of changes in ICP. Neuro changes are observed only after some pathologic changes have occurred.

1. Direct monitoring of ICP would result in (earlier/later) detection of changes.

2. Neurologic assessment provides (direct/indirect) evidence of changes in ICP.

1. earlier

2. indirect

Intracranial monitoring is most frequently used for patients with head trauma, posterior fossa lesions, hydrocephalus, and subarachnoid hemorrhage.

If ICP is dangerously high, treatment may include administering hyperosmolar solutions, surgery to relieve pressure, or draining CSF from the brain.

Equipment

Frame 53

Insertion of the subarachnoid screw

After the scalp is anesthetized, an opening is made in the skin. A small drill is used to make a hole through the skull bone. When the hole is drilled, the patient hears the noise but doesn't feel pain.

The screw is positioned to rest in the subarachnoid space. It picks up the variations in pressure of the cerebrospinal fluid.

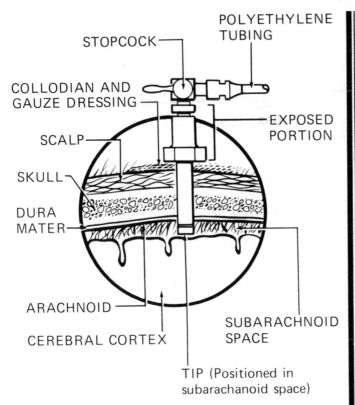

POLYETHYLENE
TUBING

STOPCOCK

COLLODIAN AND
GAUZE DRESSING

EXPOSED
PORTION

SCALP

SKULL

DURA
MATER

ARACHNOID

CEREBRAL CORTEX

SUBARACHNOID
SPACE

TIP (Positioned in
subarachanoid space)

Figure 5.28. *Subarachnoid screw placement*

True or False:

1. _____ The subarachnoid screw is placed
while the patient is under general
anesthesia.

      1. False

2. _____ Because an opening is made in the
dura, there would be a risk of meningitis in intracranial monitoring.

      2. True

3. _____ If intracranial pressure rises, the screw
tip would sense an increase in cerebrospinal fluid pressure.

      3. True

Frame 54

A stopcock and tubing is attached to the screw.
The tubing leads to a transducer that converts the
pressure waves into electrical current. This is
transmitted to the oscilloscope where it is displayed. The syringe is used to flush the screw
periodically. The flushing is always directed away
from the patient. Flushing is done if waves are flat
and obstruction in the screw is suspected.

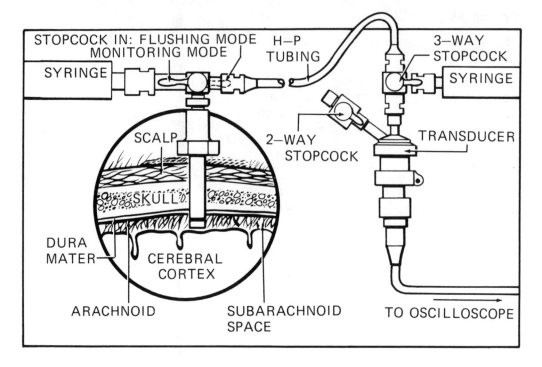

Figure 5.29. *Pressure monitoring equipment*

Match each component with its function.

1. screw tip
2. syringe
3. transducer
4. oscilloscope

a. displays CSF pressure waves
b. drills a small hole in the skull
c. changes CSF pressure waves to electrical current
d. flushes system to prevent obstruction
e. senses changes in CSF pressure

1. e
2. d
3. c
4. a

Frame 55

The monitoring equipment is calibrated to measure the pressure of the waves.

The range of readings reported as normal varies because of the variety of equipment and methods used. Clinical studies are needed to correlate findings from various techniques.

Normal range: 50–200 mm H_2O
4–15   mm Hg

The shape of waves is influenced by cardiac pulsations and the respiratory cycle. Figure 5.30 shows three waves encountered in intracranial pressure monitoring.

1. A or plateau waves

   A or plateau waves are pronounced when the cranial contents are increased. They may be greatly elevated for 5–20 minutes.

2. B waves

   B waves also are present with ↑ICP and may indicate pressure increases to 50 mm Hg. They are present for shorter periods of time than the A waves and last only ½ to 2½ minutes.

3. C waves

   The significance of C waves has not been definitely established.

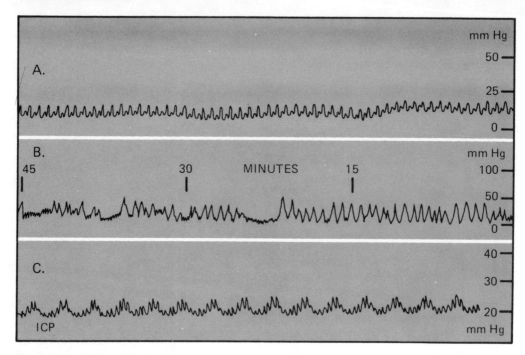

Figure 5.30. *ICP monitor waves*

1. Which tracing of ICP waves is within normal pressure limits (A/B/C)?

    1. A

2. A patient has dilated pupils and Cheyne Stokes respirations. You would expect his ICP reading to be closer to (15/50 mm Hg).

    2. 50

Frame 56

When a reading is done, the following items should be noted to assure as accurate a reading as possible:

—the subarachnoid screw and the transducer are at the same level
—patient is quiet: no coughing, restlessness, straining
—no leaks are present in the system
—if wave is flattened, flush system
—no kinks in tubing

True or False:

1. _____ Leaks will cause an inaccurate reading.

    1. True

2. _____ A flat wave is a normal finding.

    2. False

3. _____ The transducer should be higher than the head when taking a reading.

    3. False

4. _____ Wait for several minutes after the patient has had a bowel movement before taking a reading.

4. True

Nursing Care

Frame 57

Because the screw is a direct route to the subarachnoid space, care must be taken to avoid introducing infections. This includes

—routinely checking the tubing for any leaks as organisms can enter through these sites
—cleansing around the insertion site with hydrogen peroxide every day
—using sterile technique when flushing the line, flushing away from the patient.

1. List three ways organisms can be introduced into the subarachnoid space.

1. leaks in tubing, entry around the screw, in solution for flushing

Frame 58

The tubing should be long enough to allow the patient to move in bed and be turned, but lengths beyond 14 ft. may cause inaccurate readings. Care must be taken so that the tubing does not get caught or kinked.

1. Mary Lind is having a subarachnoid screw placed. The best way to determine the length of tubing to use is to:

   a. measure the length from the transducer to Mary and get that length of tubing
   b. have Mary turn to her side and measure this distance for the tubing
   c. have the tube long enough so she can get up into the chair freely

1. b

2. Before taking a reading you would:

   a. roll the head of the bed up to 90°
   b. make sure the transducer and screw are at the same level
   c. place her in trendelenburg position
   d. have the transducer one foot higher than the screw

2. b

3. Ms. Lind's ICP is gradually moving above 15 mm Hg. The nurse should:

    a. increase Ms. Lind's activity
    b. flush the tubing
    c. notify the physician

3. c

Frame 59

Summary:

Direct recordings of ICP are provided by placing a monitoring device in the epidural, subdural, or subarachnoid spaces or in the ventricles.

Components of the equipment are:
    screw (or sensing device) placed through a burr hole in the skull
    stopcock and flushing line to prevent obstruction
    tubing of sufficient length to allow for movement
    transducer to change pressure waves to electrical current
    oscilloscope to display waves

Normal range of ICP   50–200 mm H_2O
                        4–15   mm Hg

Inaccurate readings can be caused by:
    leaks
    obstruction of screw
    difference in height of screw and transducer
    kinks in tubing
    Valsalva maneuver
Careful sterile technique must be used to prevent infection.

CHAPTER 6

DISUSE PHENOMENA

Immobilization of the body due to bedrest or lack of nerve innervation produces a sequence of events called the disuse phenomena. One of the key features of neurologic nursing care is the prevention of these complications.

At the conclusion of this chapter you will be able to:

1. Explain the effects of immobility on the following structures: muscles, bones, joints, cardiovascular system, skin, lungs, kidneys, and GI tract
2. Suggest preventive measures for each of the disuse phenomena
3. Recognize the psychologic problems caused by immobility
4. Identify patients at risk for complications of immobility

Chapter outline

Effects of immobility and preventive measures
    Musculoskeletal system
    Skin
    Cardiovascular system
    Lungs
    Kidneys
    GI tract

Psychologic effects of immobility

PART I
EFFECTS OF IMMOBILITY
AND PREVENTIVE
MEASURES

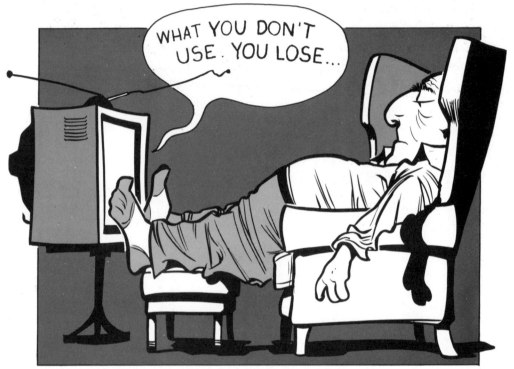

Figure 6.1.

Musculoskeletal System

Frame 1

Physical restriction of motion occurs in critical illness when there is extensive motor paralysis or when casts, splints, and traction are in use.

Where there is loss of nerve stimulation to muscles and/or little voluntary movement, the muscles atrophy (decrease in size). They become stiff and fibrotic and lose elasticity. In the unaffected parts of the body, the muscles loose strength and endurance due to lack of physical activity.

1. Mr. Kim has had left hemiplegia following a cerebral vascular hemorrhage two years ago. He is physically inactive now. You would expect:

    a. Right leg muscles swollen and hypertrophied
    b. Left arm and leg thin with reduced muscle mass
    c. No change in size of muscles
    d. Generalized muscular weakness

    1. b and d

2. Mr. Kim cries out with pain when his left arm is fully extended. This is because:

    a. Paralysis increases the sensation of pain
    b. Fibrotic muscles have lost capacity to stretch
    c. He is afraid to move his affected arm

    2. b

Frame 2

Mobility of the musculoskeletal system is dependent upon the formation of loose connective tissue wherever motion should occur. Study Figure 6.2 to appreciate the importance of connective tissue surrounding the joints: muscles, tendons, ligaments and joint capsule.

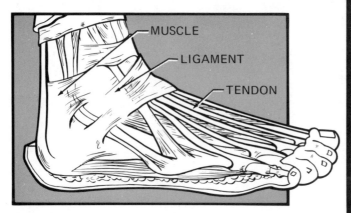

Figure 6.2. *Connective tissue on ankle*

This connective tissue is constantly being repaired and reorganized by the body's normal maintenance system.

Where there is frequent motion, the connective tissue developed is loose with widely spread points of attachment.

In areas where little or no motion occurs, the connective tissue becomes dense, stiff and closely attached. The progressive shortening of connective tissue occurs during a period of days following immobilization. This process is called *contracture* of the joint.

Normal motion in joints and soft tissues can be maintained only by normal movement and stretch through the full range of motion many times each day.

Frame 3

Normally, constant nerve stimulation to opposing flexor and extensor muscle groups allow the body to remain upright and resist the force of gravity. This also allows finely graded movements.

When nerve innervation is lost, the force of gravity and the strongest muscle groups (usually the flexors) take precedence, and the affected part is held in a characteristic position.

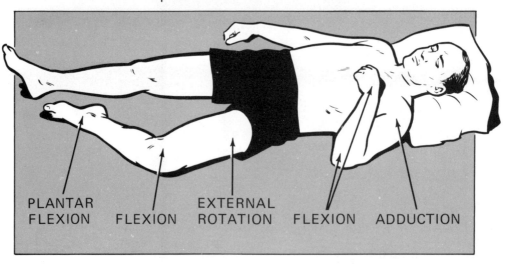

PLANTAR FLEXION   FLEXION   EXTERNAL ROTATION   FLEXION   ADDUCTION

Figure 6.3.   *Hemiplegic posturing*

If this nonfunctional position is maintained for long periods, the connective tissue becomes fibrotic and contractures occur. The most common and most disabling contractures are hip and knee flexion and shoulder adduction.

Mr. Kim has a severe adduction contracture in his left shoulder and flexion contractures of his elbow, wrist, and hand. This causes:

> pain when his arm is moved
> difficulty with hygiene in axilla, elbow, palmar areas
> difficulty in dressing.

Mr. Wells has a plantar flexion (foot drop) deformity of his right foot following cranial surgery. He had right hemiparesis which gradually subsided. When he was able to walk again, the flexion deformity prevented normal gait.

Agree or disagree?

1. Both Mr. Kim and Mr. Wells have serious limitations because of contractures.

   1. agree

2. Nursing care should have been planned to prevent these complications.

   2. agree

3. Extremities should be kept in positions of function.

   3. agree

Frame 4

The hallmarks of correct nursing intervention to prevent contractures and deformities are:

> maintaining the extremities in a functional position
> range of motion exercises.

1. These interventions should be initiated:

   1. c

   a. when the patient is able to be out of bed
   b. by the physical therapist
   c. on admission

2. The patient's hand should be positioned with:

   2. b and c
   This is the position of function.

   a. the fingers spread flat
   b. the fingers slightly flexed
   c. the thumb and index finger in a "pincer" position

Frame 5

Pillows and splints are used to position extremities. The splinted areas are frequently inspected for pressure spots, and position changes are done often.

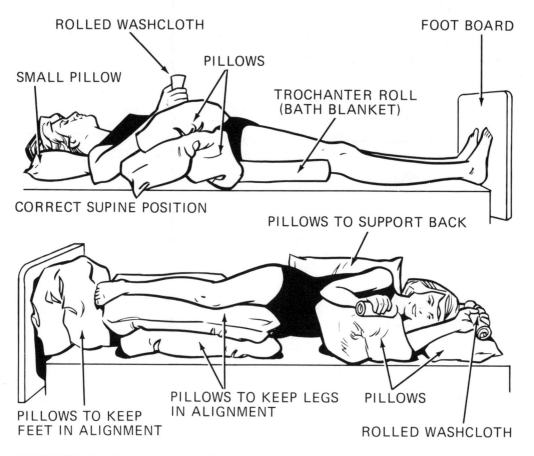

ROLLED WASHCLOTH

FOOT BOARD

PILLOWS

SMALL PILLOW

TROCHANTER ROLL
(BATH BLANKET)

CORRECT SUPINE POSITION

PILLOWS TO SUPPORT BACK

PILLOWS TO KEEP
FEET IN ALIGNMENT

PILLOWS TO KEEP LEGS
IN ALIGNMENT

PILLOWS

ROLLED WASHCLOTH

CORRECT SIDE-LYING POSITION

Figure 6.4.   *Correct positioning*

1. Larry Cole has paralysis of both legs. When he lies in bed, his toes point toward the foot of the bed. The nurse puts high-topped sneakers on his feet, to keep them at right angles to his legs. Is this a good intervention?

2. What observations are important for the nurse to make when removing the shoes?

1. yes; maintains position of function

2. observe for pressure areas

Most neuro patients are positioned with the head of the bed elevated 30°. This assists blood return from the cerebral vessels. Ventilation is improved in this position because abdominal contents are not pressing on the diaphragm. If the physician approves, the patient's bed should be rolled flat for 30–60 minutes each shift to prevent hip flexion contractures.

Panel 1

Range of Motion Exercises

Ms. Eggers cares for critically ill neurologic patients. While giving nursing care to her patients she spends a few moments putting each extremity through its range of motion. She assesses her patient's sensory integrity and motor strength at the same time.

Here is a review of the movements to be included in range of motion exercises. Put yourself through these range of motion exercises as you study Figure 6.5.

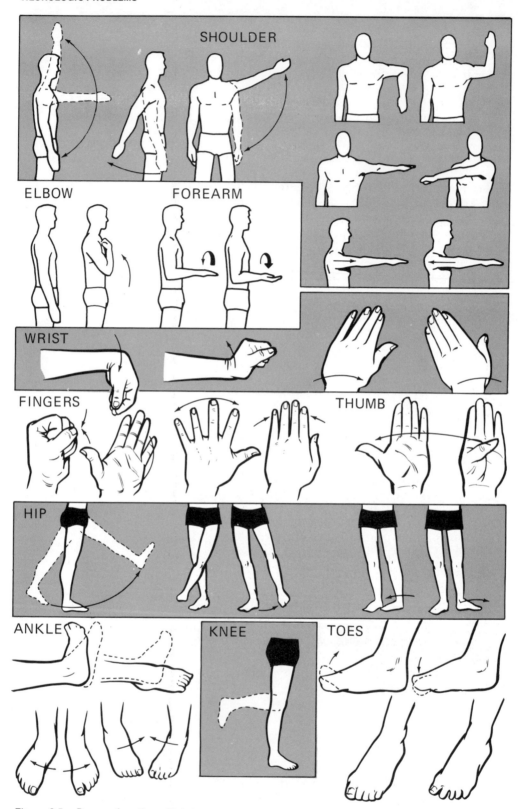

Figure 6.5. *Range of motion of joints*

Frame 6

Prolonged immobility causes the long bones in the body to lose calcium. As calcium is removed from bone, the structure becomes "honeycombed" rather than solid and hard. Lack of muscular pull and weight-bearing on the bones is the cause of this phenomenon.

Active exercise against resistance with the non-involved extremities, and early ambulation, can prevent this effect. Completely paralyzed patients may periodically use a standing (or tilt) table for this purpose. Figure 6.6 shows a patient positioned on a tilt table. This position also promotes optimal ventilation and psychologic well-being.

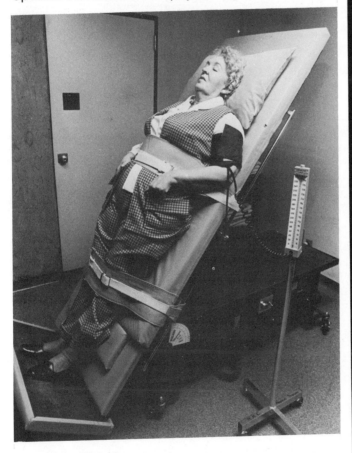

Figure 6.6. *Tilt table*

True or False:

1. _____ Passive exercise will prevent osteoporosis.

2. _____ Weight-bearing is related to deposit of calcium in the long bones.

1. False

2. True

Frame 7

The calcium ions removed from bone increase the serum calcium level. This often leads to formation of calcium-type kidney stones. Restriction of dietary calcium (especially milk products) and high fluid intake are methods to prevent renal calculi. Sometimes foods that result in acidic urine are encouraged as a preventive measure.

1. Choose interventions which are important for patients with calcium imbalances.

    a. diet high in calcium
    b. resistive exercises of non-involved extremities
    c. monitor serum calcium
    d. high fluid intake to prevent kidney stone formation

1. b, c, d

Research is in progress to find methods of stimulating deposit of calcium in bone and inhibiting calcium removal. Various combinations of hormones, vitamins, and ions such as fluoride and phosphate are being tested.

Frame 8

Summary

Lack of voluntary movement and/or loss of nerve innervation causes muscle atrophy, weakness and loss of endurance, and shortening of connective tissue around joints.

Lack of balance of opposing muscle groups results in shortening and fibrosis of connective tissue, contractures and deformity of joints.

Nursing interventions:

maintain extremities in position of function
range of motion exercises.

Prolonged immobility causes osteoporosis, hypercalcemia and kidney stones. Lack of muscle pull and weight bearing on the long bones contributes to this process.

Nursing interventions:
    active exercise of noninvolved extremities
    early ambulation
    restriction of dietary calcium
    high fluid intake
    monitor serum calcium.

Skin

Frame 9

Immobility adversely affects skin integrity. Briefly review the mechanisms causing decubitus ulcers (skin breakdown due to immobility).

Blood pressure in skin capillaries is 30 mm Hg. If pressure greater than this is applied, the capillaries close, depriving cells of nourishment and preventing removal of metabolic wastes.

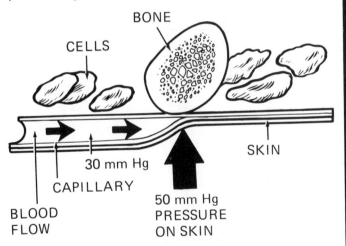

Figure 6.7. *Pressure closing skin capillaries*

If the weight of a patient in bed were evenly distributed over his whole body surface, the pressure over any one area would be about 10 mm Hg. This amount of pressure does not close capillaries.

But when a person is lying down, most of his weight is borne over the bony prominences. Pressure in these areas is much greater than 30 mm Hg. Figure 6.8 shows bony prominences which bear high pressure in the back and side-lying positions.

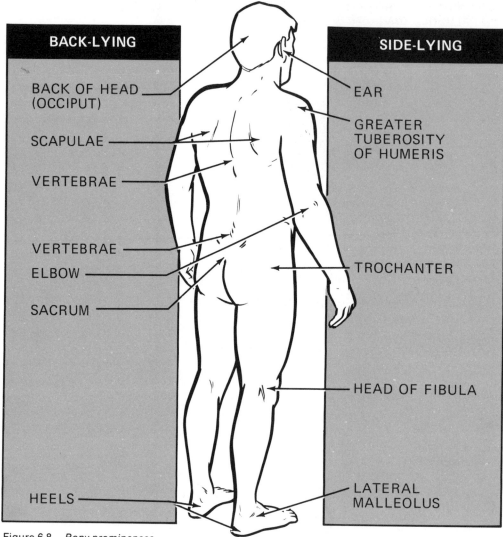

BACK-LYING

BACK OF HEAD (OCCIPUT)

SCAPULAE

VERTEBRAE

VERTEBRAE

ELBOW

SACRUM

HEELS

SIDE-LYING

EAR

GREATER TUBEROSITY OF HUMERIS

TROCHANTER

HEAD OF FIBULA

LATERAL MALLEOLUS

Figure 6.8. *Bony prominences*

1. Pressure on the skin greater than (10/30/150) mm Hg will close the capillaries.

    1. 30

2. Obstruction of capillary flow causes (increased/decreased) amounts of metabolic wastes in the interstitial spaces.

    2. increased

3. The bony prominences are areas of (high/low) pressure during bedrest.

    3. high

Frame 10

Figure 6.9 shows the effect of pressure on the bony prominences when the patient is lying in bed. The hard bed surface and the bone press the tissue as in a vise. If pressure is not relieved in 60–90 minutes, cell damage can occur.

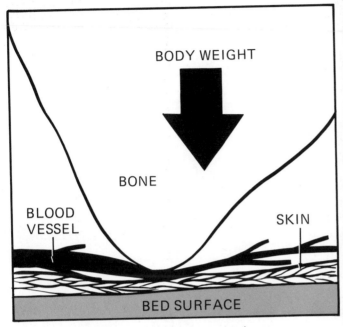

BODY WEIGHT

BONE

BLOOD VESSEL

SKIN

BED SURFACE

Figure 6.9. *Effect of pressure over bony prominences*

1. How could this pressure be alleviated?

   a. Make the surface of the bed softer
   b. Turn the patient often
   c. Massage the area to stimulate blood flow

2. Mrs. Parker is comatose following a basilar skull fracture. When Mr. Evans turns her, he notices that the skin over her bony prominences is reddened. This is due to:

   a. elevated temperature
   b. build-up of metabolic wastes due to pressure on the capillaries
   c. lack of neural stimulation to the area
   d. none of the above

3. Mr. Evans consults the central supply manual to find a special mattress to reduce pressure. All have been tested by the manufacturer. Which should he choose?

   a. an air mattress which reduces skin pressure to 30 mm Hg half of the time
   b. a gel-type mattress producing skin pressure of 15 mm Hg
   c. a foam mattress which is easy to keep clean but specifies no skin pressure

1. a, b, c

2. b, patient should not lie on the area until redness is gone

3. b

4. Mr. Evans knows that a decubitus ulcer can begin after several hours of unrelieved pressure. He should plan to:

   a. change Mrs. Parker's position every two hours

   b. rotate Mrs. Parker through a series of "quarter turns" at half hour intervals

   c. not disturb the patient because the mattress relieves pressure

Methods are continually being invented to decrease pressure on bony prominences. The use of water flotation mattresses of various types is an effective and practical method in common use for immobilized patients. However, body alignment is difficult to maintain when using water flotation mattresses.

4. b

Frame 11

Shearing force is another cause of decubitus ulcers. To get an idea of this, put your elbow firmly on the table and move the bone back and forth as your skin adheres to the table. Now look at Figure 6.10. The patient has slipped down in bed and his skin is rumpled above the coccyx. The force of the bone moving one way and skin pulling the opposite direction tears ("shear") the blood vessels as they go through the fascia to the skin. A triangular and widely undermined area of tissue necrosis results.

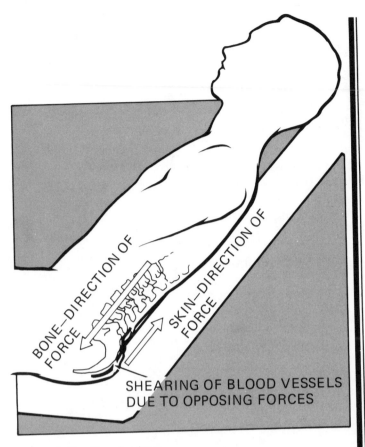

BONE—DIRECTION OF FORCE

SKIN—DIRECTION OF FORCE

SHEARING OF BLOOD VESSELS DUE TO OPPOSING FORCES

Figure 6.10. *Shearing force*

1. What are some other ways that shearing force occurs?

2. How can this be prevented?

1. Slipping down in a chair, being pulled across the bed, and lifted improperly

2. Use of "lifting sheets" under patient, seat belts in chair, careful positioning, enough persons to help with lifting

Frame 12

Patients who run a high risk of decubitus ulcers are those who:

A. are unable to move about freely in bed and shift position frequently (as everyone does during normal sleep)
B. are thin and lack natural cushioning over the bony prominences
C. are malnourished and have inadequate protein and vitamin intake to keep tissues healthy
D. are incontinent, causing chemical irritation to skin
E. have cardiovascular problems causing hypotension, diminished peripheral circulation, or edema
F. have sensory deficits in parts of the body.

Match the causes just listed to the conditions described here.

1. _____ Mr. L. is comatose.

2. _____ Mrs. T. is heavily sedated.

3. _____ Mr. J. has congestive heart failure.

4. _____ Mrs. R's serum albumin is 1.5 (normal = 3.2–5.6).

5. _____ Mrs. Q. is 5'8" tall and weighs 120 lbs.

6. _____ Mr. O. is quadriplegic.

7. _____ Ms. S. has had no oral intake and is maintained only on IV solutions for one week.

8. _____ Mr. M. is confused and often incontinent.

1. A

2. A

3. E

4. C

5. B

6. A (also D and F)

7. C

8. D

Frame 13

The development of a decubitus ulcer is painful and places stress on the patient's healing capacity. The additional cost of care for one pressure sore averages $5,000. Once tissue breakdown has started, it is most difficult to heal.

Prevention is the watchword.

Remember the types of high risk patients and begin preventive measures on admission. Test yourself by making a list of all the preventive measures you can use:

Make sure you include: frequent position changes, modify the mattress, inspect bony prominences for redness, massage areas, maintain adequate protein intake, keep skin clean, prevent shearing by using lifting sheet, care in positioning.

Frame 14

Summary:

Pressure greater than 30 mm Hg on the skin over the bony prominences causes capillary obstruction and tissue damage if pressure is prolonged.

Areas of increased pressure are occiput, scapula, elbows, coccyx, heels in back-lying position; ears, shoulders, elbows, iliac crest, knees, ankles in side-lying position.

Shearing force causes capillary disruption and deeply undermined areas of skin necrosis.

Patients at high risk: immobilized, ↓ physical activity, lack of adipose cushion, malnourished, incontinent, poor peripheral circulation.

Prevention: modify bed surface, change position frequently, inspect and massage areas, good protein intake, skin cleanliness, prevent shearing.

Cardiovascular System

Frame 15

When a normal, healthy person shifts from a recumbent (lying-down) position to standing, does all his blood rush to his feet because of gravity?

No

The body has special reflexes to prevent this from happening. However, when healthy people are kept flat in bed for only two weeks, this reflex may be lost. The effect is *orthostatic hypotension,* a drop in blood pressure and cerebral circulation due to change from recumbent to upright posture. Symptoms include weakness, pallor, dizziness, ↑pulse, nausea. Tests have shown that it can take five weeks to regain the ability to tolerate upright posture.

True or False:

1. _____ Prolonged recumbency can affect vasomotor reflexes which adjust the cardiovascular system to changes in posture.

2. _____ Mr. P. has been lying flat in bed for three weeks in skeletal traction. He now has a cast, and is able to sit up. He is not at risk for orthostatic hypotension.

3. _____ Signs of orthostatic hypotension include: pallor, dizziness, buzzing in ears, feeling faint, diaphoresis, ↑pulse rate, dyspnea.

1. True

2. False

3. True

Frame 16

When a patient has orthostatic hypotension, the blood vessels in the abdomen and legs have lost their power of reflex contraction.

1. This would cause blood to (pool in/leave) the abdomen and legs.

2. Use of elastic hose and an abdominal binder (would/would not) help to prevent pooling of blood in the lower part of the body.

3. The nurse is caring for a patient who has been recumbent for a week. The patient can now sit up. Adaptation to upright posture should be done (quickly/gradually).

1. pool in

2. would

3. gradually

Patients with spinal cord injury and lumbar sympathectomy have added physiologic problems, which will be explained in Section 2. Very gradual postural changes are planned using a tilt table or CircOlectric bed. Sometimes anti-gravity pressure suits (space-flight suits) are used to support circulation.

Frame 17

The heart works 30% harder when the patient is in a recumbent rather than a sitting position. Signs of increased cardiac work seen during immobility are increased pulse rate, lower systolic and diastolic blood pressure, and cardiac dysrhythmias.

In addition, there is a decreased volume of circulating blood and much pooling of blood in the venous system. Cardiac insufficiency and failure may result.

True or False:

1. _____ Blood is forced through the venous system by contraction of muscles.

2. _____ A recumbent and inactive patient would have less blood volume, that flows quickly in the venous system.

3. _____ Edema can result from venous stasis.

Pressure on the calf muscles from recumbency can cause endothelial damage in the blood vessels.

4. _____ This would predispose the patient to blood clotting around the damaged surfaces.

5. _____ Think of all the ways you know to prevent cardiovascular complications:

1. True

2. False

3. True

4. True

5. Did you include: use of elastic hose, frequent change of position, exercise, early ambulation, and close observation of cardiovascular status?

Frame 18

Summary

Orthostatic hypotension—loss of vasomotor reflexes which adjust for postural shifts.

Signs: pallor, dyspnea, diaphoresis, ↑pulse rate, dizziness when patient assumes upright position

Prevention: Elastic stockings, abdominal binder, gradual adaptation to upright position

> *Cardiovascular changes*—↑ pulse, ↓ BP and circulating blood volume, dysrhythmias, venous stasis and thrombosis, edema.
>
> Prevention: Elastic hose, frequent change of position, exercise, early ambulation, close observation of cardiovascular status.

Lungs

Frame 19

Adequacy of ventilation depends on free movement of the chest. When a patient is recumbent, the part of the chest lying against the bed is restricted in movement.

1. This would (increase/decrease) ventilation.

1. decrease

Neurologic patients may have paralysis of chest muscles which also limits ventilatory movement. The force of gravity causes lung secretions to pool in the dependent lobes of the lung and block air passages and alveoli. Gravity also affects distribution of blood supply to lobes of the lungs. Blood pools in dependent areas of the lung, reducing the exchange of O_2 and CO_2.

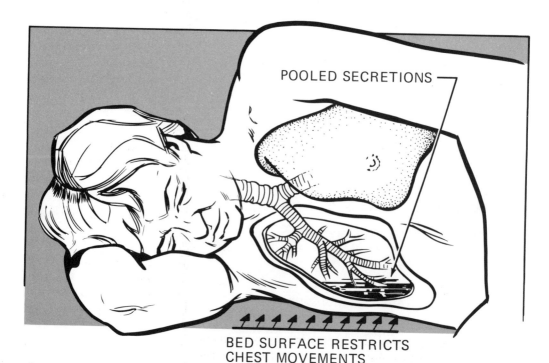

POOLED SECRETIONS

BED SURFACE RESTRICTS CHEST MOVEMENTS

Figure 6.11. *Effects of immobility on respiratory adequacy*

2. The effects of recumbency on respiratory function are:

   a. interference with chest movement
   b. clogging of small airways with secretions
   c. better distribution of blood supply
   d. more blood available where secretions block oxygen supply

2. a, b, d

3. Which disease processes occur in the lungs when secretions and blood are pooled?

   a. allergic reactions
   b. lung infection (hypostatic pneumonia) from pooled secretions
   c. pulmonary thrombosis or embolus due to circulatory problems

3. b and c

Frame 20

Mr. W. has been unconscious for three days following a head injury. He is unable to cough and needs frequent suctioning. The nurse's plan to prevent the development of pneumonia includes:

Positioning: when lying on side, position to allow expansion of upper chest wall
change position frequently

Airway
Hygiene: maintain unobstructed airway, chest physical therapy and intermittent positive pressure breathing treatments (IPPB)

1. Are these interventions appropriate?

1. yes (the physician may also order prophylactic antibiotics)

2. Mrs. A. is conscious but very lethargic. What should be added to this plan for her?

2. Cough and hyperventilation exercises.

3. What are some signs of hypostatic pneumonia?

3. fever, change in amount and character of secretions, changes in breath sounds over affected lobes

Hypostatic pneumonia is a critical development, as it is a frequent cause of death in neurologic patients.

Frame 21

Summary:

Immobility causes:

Restriction of chest movements with ↓ ventilation

Pooling of secretions in dependent parts of the lung

Pooling of blood in dependent parts of the lung.

Prevention of pneumonia: clear airway, frequent change of position, position to allow free movement of chest, chest physiotherapy, cough and hyperventilation exercises, IPPB, prophylactic antibiotics

Hypostatic pneumonia is a frequent cause of death in neurologic patients.

Kidneys

Frame 22

Gravity helps the flow of urine out of the kidneys into the urinary tract when a person is in the upright position. The recumbent position, however, slows the flow of urine through the kidneys and causes pooling of urine in the ureters and bladder.

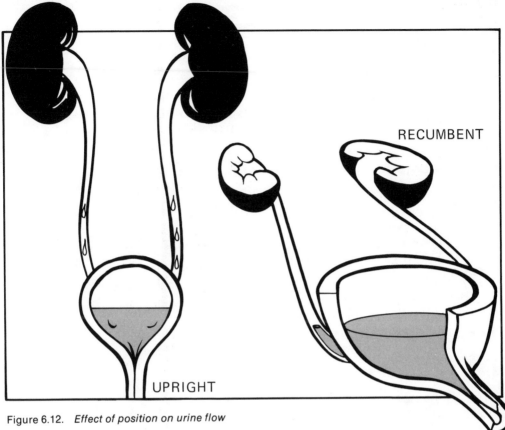

RECUMBENT

UPRIGHT

Figure 6.12. *Effect of position on urine flow*

The effects of pooled urine in the system are:

risk of infection
precipitation of calcium salts to form stones.

1. An effect of immobility on bones is (more/less) calcium deposited in bone tissue.

2. This results in (higher/lower) blood calcium levels, and (more/less) calcium excretion by the kidney.

3. There is greater risk of urinary tract infection when urine is (concentrated and pooled/dilute and rapidly excreted).

1. less

2. higher, more

3. concentrated and pooled

Some neurologic patients have lost nerve innervation to the bladder requiring the use of an indwelling catheter. This increases the chances for infection.

Frame 23

Here are the symptoms of common urologic complications.

	Renal Calculi	Bladder Infection
Pain	sharp	dull, burning on urination
Location	lumbar area	lower abdominal area
Temperature	normal	fever
Output	decreased	foul smelling urine frequency of urination

1. Mr. R. has been on bedrest for several weeks. He began to complain of sharp, colicy pain in the small of his back on the right. He has tenderness over the right kidney. Urinary output has decreased by almost half. He has signs of:

   a. urinary tract infection (UTI)
   b. kidney stone blocking the right ureter
   c. back pain from immobility

2. Which interventions are helpful in preventing urinary complications?

   a. high fluid intake to keep urine dilute and "flush" the system
   b. ↓ dietary intake of calcium
   c. frequent position change and early activation
   d. attention to perineal hygiene
   e. prophylactic antibiotics

1. b (UTI usually causes fever)

2. a, b, c, d, e

GI Tract

Frame 24

Lack of activity decreases peristalsis, the smooth muscle movements which propel food through the GI tract. Some neurologic patients lack nerve innervation of the GI tract. Sedative drugs can depress the vagal system and slow peristalsis.

Immobility may result in malabsorption of nutrients from the small intestine.

1. Choose the GI problems most likely in immobilized patients:

   a. diarrhea
   b. gastric dilatation
   c. malnutrition
   d. constipation

2. Choose interventions to alleviate these effects:

   a. intake of roughage, prune juice, etc.
   b. regular time and routine for bowel movement
   c. use of suppositories
   d. high intake of fluids
   e. early activation

1. b, c, d

2. a, b, d, e,

Frame 25

Summary:

Urinary stasis in the bladder and ureters → infection and precipitation of stones (particularly calcium).

Prevention: high fluid intake, ↓ dietary calcium, frequent position change, early activation, perineal hygiene, prophylactic antibiotics.

Decreased peristalsis causes gastric dilatation and constipation

Prevention: high fluid and fiber intake, use of bulk laxatives, stool softeners and suppositories may be included in the regimen. Establish regular time and routine for elimination.

Malabsorption → malnutrition

PART II
PSYCHOLOGIC EFFECTS
OF IMMOBILITY

During the 3 P.M. shift report Dan O'Brien's nurse mentioned that Dan seemed withdrawn and depressed. Linda Zeller, R.N., had cared for Dan O'Brien from the beginning of his hospitalization for treatment of a head injury and multiple fractures. He had been comatose for several days, but was now awake and alert. His neurologic signs had stabilized, but he had much pain and discomfort from his other injuries and immobilization by traction apparatus. While Ms. Zeller was caring for Dan O'Brien, he began to tell her how he felt.

I'm going crazy here. There's nothing to do, and nothing to think about except what will happen to me now. I'm no good—can't even turn over in bed by myself, feed myself or go to the bathroom. I'm like a baby.

Every day is the same. I can't look at that ceiling another minute. There are only the 'White Coats' to talk to and they have given up on me, too. Sometimes I think that the only part of the real me left is my head, and I wish I could turn that off, and wake up 10 years from now.

Frame 26

1. Choose the feelings Dan O'Brien seems to be expressing:

   a. isolation
   b. depression
   c. low self-esteem
   d. boredom
   e. withdrawal

2. Which of these feelings is related to being immobilized?

3. Which of these responses would be appropriate?
   a. Come on, Mr. O'Brien, you're just feeling sorry for yourself. You're getting better every day.

1. all

2. all

b. I thought you were pretty brave about all of this, before.

c. You are feeling so isolated, bored and miserable that you'd like to escape somehow, is that right?

d. Maybe you should ask to see a psychiatrist so you can get some help for your mind as well as your body.

3. c
(The other responses imply that his disgust with himself is justified.)

Frame 27

Confinement to bed with restricted environmental interactions can cause severe disruption of body image. Any change in normal body posture and activity can disturb a person's self-image. Loss of control of one's body is a frightening experience.

1. Choose the statements that Dan O'Brien made which indicate some problems with body image.

1. "I'm like a baby," "The only part of the real me is my head."

2. What usual elements of body image feedback are changed for Mr. O'Brien?

a. posture
b. clothing
c. activities, schedules, routines
d. appearance
e. reaction of other people

2. all

Frame 28

Immobilized patients often experience distortion of their perceptions.

Sensory overload can be caused by the unending strange sounds, sights, smells, and people in the unit. The patient may become hypersensitive and fearful.

Sensory deprivation can occur simultaneously with sensory overload. All familiar cues are lost. The patient is isolated from the familiar people in his life. There is unending monotony of the room, a loss of the sense of time and no pleasant sensations.

1. Mr. O'Brien seemed to be suffering from sensory (deprivation/overload).

1. deprivation

2. Deprivation and overload (can/cannot) occur together.

2. can

Frame 29

Because of noise and activity in the unit, Dan also suffered from sleep deprivation.

One cycle of sleep takes about 90–100 minutes and consists of several levels. Loss of the following levels can cause adverse effects:

—REM (rapid eye movement) stage in which the brain is active and dreaming takes place
—Deep sleep with profound muscle relaxation

Frequent awakening interrupts progression to REM and deep sleep and causes symptoms of irritability, anxiety, and fatigue, as well as disruption of the body's rhythmic production of adrenal hormones.

True or False:

1. _____ Sleep deprivation causes psychologic effects rather than physiologic harm.

2. _____ Dan should be allowed 40 minute periods of uninterrupted sleep.

3. _____ Nurses should minimize sounds, light and activity during nighttime hours in ICU.

4. _____ Sleeping pills which suppress the REM stage are indicated for Dan O'Brien.

1. False

2. False, 2 hour periods are better, as a whole cycle can take 1½ hours.

3. True

4. False, loss of the REM stage is harmful

Frame 30

All of these factors: immobility, body-image problems, sensory overload and deprivation can combine to cause delirium. This can range from a slight clouding of consciousness to hallucinations. Illusions are common; paranoid delusions and visual hallucinations are sometimes present. Often patients try to cover up these symptoms because they are afraid of "going crazy." It is helpful to encourage the patient to discuss these feelings and experiences and to provide reassurance that this is a temporary phenomenon.

1. The day after Dan O'Brien talked about his feelings, he again told Ms. Zeller he was afraid

of "being nuts." Which response would be most helpful?

a. Of course you aren't nuts. This is a tough situation but you're getting better.
b. Tell me about what's happening that makes you feel "nuts."
c. We'll move you to a place where you'll feel more protected.

2. He said that he sometimes saw "things" climbing on the traction ropes and heard people calling him when no one was around. What should Ms. Zeller do?

a. Explain that these symptoms frequently occur when people are immobilized in an unfamiliar environment, that they are not signs of mental illness, they eventually go away, but that it's perfectly OK to talk about it with her.
b. Arrange for referral to a psychiatrist.
c. Increase reality orientation and meaningful stimuli.

1. b

2. a, c

Frame 31

From this list, choose interventions which would help immobilized patients like Dan O'Brien to cope with psychologic effects.

1. Move him into a private room.

2. Increase visiting hours for family and friends.

3. Find self-help devices he can use for personal activities.

4. Establish a strict routine and schedule with few deviations.

5. Try to find a task the patient can do to help you such as watching another patient's IV, keeping track of his own intake and output, watching for a doctor's arrival.

6. Use posters, pictures, maps, greeting cards for visual stimuli.

7. Expect television to keep the person occupied.

8. Arrange for tapes or "talking books" on topics of interest.

9. Keep sleep disruption to a minimum.

2, 3, 5, 6, 8, 9

Frame 32

Summary:

Psychologic effects of immobility are:
Feelings: isolation, depression, low self-esteem, boredom, withdrawal, despair

Body image disturbances

Sensory deprivation and overload

Delirium with illusions, delusions and hallucinations

Prevention: Encourage patient to talk about his feelings and symptoms, increase meaningful sensory input, increase independence and control over self and environment.

CHAPTER 7

ALTERATIONS IN TEMPERATURE REGULATION

Fever is a frequent complication in neurologic patients which requires nursing intervention and monitoring. It is important to maintain body temperature within a normal range. During fever the metabolic demands of the body are greatly increased and compete with the brain for available oxygen and nutrients.

At the conclusion of this chapter you will be able to:

1. State common causes of fever in the neurologic patient
2. Identify indications for the use of the hypothermia blanket
3. Describe the major components of a hypothermia blanket and machine
4. Recognize parameters for monitoring patients on hypothermia blankets
5. Select nursing interventions to be used for patients receiving this therapy.

Chapter outline

Causes of fever
   Intracranial
   Extracranial

Hypothermia units
   Components
   Induction phase

Nursing care
   Observation and assessment
   Interventions

PART I
CAUSES OF FEVER

Intracranial Causes

Frame 1

Damage to the hypothalamus frequently leads to elevated temperatures. The anterior portion of the hypothalamus normally initiates mechanisms for *cooling the body.*

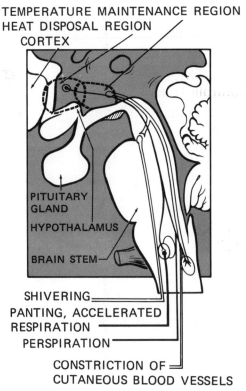

TEMPERATURE MAINTENANCE REGION
HEAT DISPOSAL REGION
CORTEX

PITUITARY GLAND
HYPOTHALAMUS
BRAIN STEM

SHIVERING
PANTING, ACCELERATED RESPIRATION
PERSPIRATION
CONSTRICTION OF CUTANEOUS BLOOD VESSELS

Figure 7.1. *Hypothalamic areas controlling body temperature*

The cells in the anterior lobe detect higher than normal blood temperature. They then initiate compensatory mechanisms:

vasodilation	—sends more blood to the peripheral vessels, with resultant heat loss through the skin
sweating	—evaporation with cooling of the body surface.

The cells in the posterior hypothalamus regulate *conservation of body heat* by these mechanisms:

vasoconstriction—keeps blood in the core areas

shivering, increased muscle tone—uses heat from muscular contraction to warm the body.

1. Damage to the anterior hypothalamus causes:

   a. hyperthermia
   b. hypothermia

1. a

2. Choose problems which could cause damage to the hypothalamus:

   a. surgery in the pituitary area
   b. head injury
   c. interruption of the blood supply
   d. edema causing pressure

2. a, b, c, d

3. Match the compensatory mechanism and the lobe of the hypothalamus controlling it.

   a. ___vasoconstriction   A = anterior lobe
   b. ___vasodilation   P = posterior lobe
   c. ___shivering
   d. ___sweating

3. a. P
   b. A
   c. P
   d. A

Frame 2

Hyperosmolar IV solutions are frequently used to reduce ICP. Removal of fluid may result in hypernatremia and fever.

Patients who have elevated serum sodium levels (hypernatremia) may have a fever because high sodium concentrations i ritate the hypothalamus.

True or False:

1. _____ Hypokalemia causes the hypothalamus to initiate vasoconstriction.

1. False

2. _____ Edema in the area of the pituitary can affect function of the hypothalamus.

2. True

3. _____ Patients with brain stem injuries frequently have elevated temperatures as the hypothalamus is involved.

3. True

4. _____ Fever decreases the metabolic oxygen needs of the body cells.

4. False

5. _____ Increased cerebral oxygen demand is dangerous for patients with ↑ ICP.

5. True

Frame 3

Fevers caused by hypothalamic dysfunction are usually very high—above 102° (39.5C). They are also characterized by lack of diurnal variations; that is, they remain high constantly around the clock. The compensatory mechanism of sweating is absent.

An exception to this is a low-grade fever resulting from blood or foreign elements circulating in the subarachnoid space. A low-grade fever is found. Subarachnoid hemorrhage or a traumatic spinal tap could cause a low-grade fever.

1. Cerebrally caused fevers are characterized by (high/low) grade fevers.

2. A subarachnoid hemorrhage causes a (high/low) fever.

3. Cerebrally caused fevers (remain high/fluctuate greatly) during a 24 hour period.

1. high

2. low

3. remain high

Extracranial Causes

Frame 4

Extracranial causes of elevated temperatures are more common. Urinary tract infections and infectious processes in the lungs are two of the most common causes of fever. Immobility and decreased levels of consciousness may lead to atelectasis and pneumonia unless vigorous preventive efforts are made. Likewise, decreased levels of consciousness and/or neurologic damage often necessitate an indwelling catheter which increases the likelihood of urinary tract infections.

Other extracranial causes of elevated temperature in the neurologic patient include dehydration from administration of hyperosmolar solutions, wound infections, and drug reactions.

Frame 5

Mr. L. has a fever of 104° following a brain stem injury. His medical orders include:

    A. prophylactic antibiotics

B. antipyretics (aspirin)
C. sponge baths and ice bags
D. use of the hypothermia blanket
E. chest physiotherapy

Fill in the blank with the letter(s) of the treatment listed above.

1. _____ Which treatment(s) act directly upon the heat control center in the hypothalamus?

1. B

2. _____ Which treatment(s) cool the body surface and peripheral blood supply?

2. C, D

3. _____ Which treatment(s) prevent or eliminate infectious causes of fever?

3. A, E

Frame 6

Summary:

Intracranial cause:
Elevated temperatures are caused by damage to the body heat-control mechanism of the hypothalamus.
anterior lobe controls cooling of the body by vasodilation and sweating
posterior lobe conserves body heat by vasoconstriction and shivering

Intracranial fevers are usually above 102°F and do not vary diurnally. (Fevers due to subarachnoid space problems are an exception.)

Extracranial causes:
pulmonary and urinary tract infections, dehydration, wound infection, drug fevers.

Fever is treated with antipyretics, sponge baths and ice bags, and hypothermia blankets.

PART II
HYPOTHERMIA UNITS

Components

Frame 7

Now review the general principles of operation for these units. All types of hypothermia units include a machine and a blanket.

The blanket consists of tubes running within the surfaces of the rubberized material. Cooled distilled water enters the blanket via one hose and is removed through the second hose. It is important that the patient's skin is in close contact with the blanket so that heat exchange can take place. Only one layer of sheet or bath blanket should be used between the patient and the hypothermia blanket.

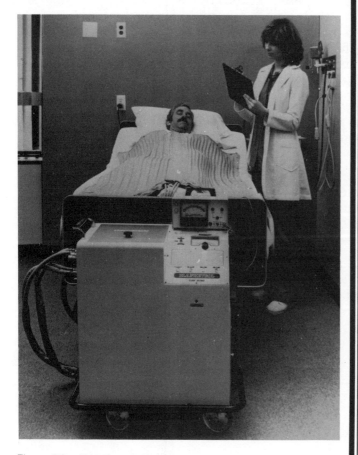

Figure 7.2.   *Hypothermia blanket*

A second hypothermia blanket may be placed on top of the patient for increased cooling. Some companies manufacture one large blanket that wraps around the patient.

1. List three common ways used to lower elevated temperatures in neuro patients.

    1. antipyretics, sponge baths, hypothermia blanket

2. The fluid circulating in the hypothermia blanket is _____.

    2. distilled water

3. To obtain good heat exchange only a _____ should be between the patient and the cooling blanket.

    3. single sheet

Induction Phase

Panel 1

Induction of Hypothermia

Karl Evans was placing Mrs. Lanz on a hypothermia blanket.

First he obtained baseline information: vital signs, neurologic assessment, assessment of respiratory, cardiovascular and skin condition. He made sure the IV was patent, as it would be difficult to restart because of vasoconstriction caused by cooling.

Mr. Evans inserted a rectal thermometer probe at an anterior angle for 3–5 inches. (Esophogeal and/or skin probes are sometimes used.) He frequently rechecked placement and accuracy of the probe.

Automatic setting: *Mr. Evans set the dial to the desired patient temperature. The unit automatically turns cooling on and off to maintain desired body temperature. The rectal probe relays the patient's temperature to the machine. The dial registers the patient's body temperature.*

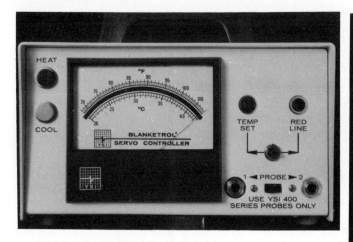

Figure 7.3 *Hypothermia blanket controls*

Mr. Evans was careful not to set the blanket temperatures too low. Rapid cooling of Mrs. Lanz's body could cause dysrhythmias and cardiac arrest. Mr. Evans closely monitored her vital signs every five minutes during the cooling phase. Because of vasoconstriction, Mrs. Lanz's blood pressure and pulse rate increased, but she had no cardiac dysrhythmias. Mr. Evans also observed for cyanosis of nailbeds indicating inadequate peripheral blood flow. Decrease in renal output can also occur due to vasoconstriction.

The nurse had an airway and suction tube close at hand since hypothermia can decrease the seizure threshold.

Manual Setting: *The patient's temperature is shown on the dial but does not cause the machine to cool and heat automatically.*

The nurse sets the desired blanket temperature, monitors the patient's temperature, and turns the cooling unit off when the desired body temperature is reached.

Maintenance of correct temperature—Manual Setting

The machine is turned off when the patient's temperature reaches 99°–100°F. The body temperature will drift down a degree or two after the cooling is discontinued. This is because the probe measures warmer blood at the core of the body. The peripheral blood is cooler and will continue to lower the core temperature.

Frame 8

Answer the following questions about use of the hypothermia blanket.

1. Induction of the cooling phase should be (rapid/slow).

   1. slow

2. When the machine is on the automatic setting, cooling is cycled by the (nurse/patient's temperature).

   2. patient's temperature

3. In the manual mode, the (blanket's/patient's) temperature is set by the nurse.

   3. blanket's

4. The rectal probe should be inserted at a (anterior/posterior) angle for (1/3/9) inches.

   4. anterior 3

5. The core temperature measured by the probe (is/is not) higher than peripheral blood temperature.

   5. is

PART III
NURSING CARE

Frame 9

1. Application of cold to the skin causes (vaso-dilation/vasoconstriction).

2. Vasoconstriction (increases/decreases) blood supply to the skin.

3. Use of hypothermia would (increase/decrease) risk of skin breakdown due to poor circulation.

4. Mrs. F. is lying on a cooling blanket. When the nurse turns her, she notes reddened areas on the scapula and coccyx. She does not massage the areas because this would warm the skin. Do you (agree/disagree)?

1. vasoconstriction

2. decreases

3. increase

4. disagree, meticulous skin care is necessary to prevent a worse complication—decubitus ulcer

Observation and Interventions

Moisture increases the conduction of heat and causes increased vasoconstriction. Attention should be paid to the presence of fluids from feedings, IV's, and urine. Wet bedding should be promptly removed.

Frostbite, while infrequent, must also be kept in mind. Turning—at least every 1–2 hours—and massage are important preventive measures.

Frame 10

Shivering may occur when the patient is being cooled. It is less frequent when elevated temperatures are being lowered than when hypothermia is used as therapy to decrease metabolism and cellular oxygen demand. An example of this is cooling of the patient during surgery.

Shivering increases basal metabolic rate (BMR) and thus causes a greater demand for O_2 and nutrients. Remember, shivering is a compensatory mechanism of the posterior hypothalamus to maintain body temperature, therefore it negates the desired effect of hypothermia. Medications such as chlorpromazine (Thorazine) may be administered to relieve shivering. Shivering is very uncomfortable for the patient. Prolonged shivering and anxiety may elevate blood pressure and increase intracranial pressure and cause discomfort to the patient.

1. Shivering _____ the BMR.

2. A medication which will reduce shivering is _____.

3. Shivering may _____ blood pressure and ICP.

1. increases

2. chlorpromazine

3. increase

Frame 11

Other items to note when using the hypothermia blanket include:

Watching the level of distilled water in the machine and adding water if needed. A gauge displays the level.

Using grounded electrical receptacles.

Keeping pins and other sharp objects away as they can puncture the blanket resulting in leakage of the distilled water.

Providing adequate explanation of the blanket and machine to the patient and the family.

True or False:

1. _____ A catheter tube should be secured to the sheet over a hypothermia blanket with tape.

2. _____ Tap water is added when the fluid level is low.

1. True

2. False

Frame 12

When a patient is on a hypothermia blanket, caution should be used in the administration of subcutaneous and intramuscular medications. Vasoconstriction reduces the rate at which the medication is absorbed. Thus the effects of medications such as sedatives and narcotics may be delayed. When cooling is discontinued, vasodilation results in rapid absorption. Overdosage may occur if several doses are given while the patient is being cooled.

1. When the patient is cooling, absorption time of intramuscular medications is (lengthened/shortened).

    1. lengthened

2. The absorption of IM drugs (would/would not) be enhanced by massage of the site.

    2. would

3. During hypothermia the best route for drug administration is (IM/IV).

    3. IV

Frame 13

Summary:

Nursing care involves:

Correct assembly and setting of controls:
automatic—set desired body temperature, machine cycles according to rectal probe temperature
manual—set desired blanket temperature, turn off cooling when correct body temperature is reached

Monitoring vital signs, general condition and adequacy of peripheral circulation

Careful skin care to prevent breakdown

Watching for shivering and giving medication to control it

Prevention of leaks, electrical hazards, and a low water level in the machine

Explanation of the blanket and course of treatment to patient and family

Care in administering medications—IV is the preferred route because cumulative effects of IM medications may occur with warming and vasodilation.

CHAPTER 8

NURSING MANAGEMENT OF PATIENTS WITH ALTERED BEHAVIOR AND COMMUNICATION

Interaction with others is an important aspect of human life. Many patients on neurologic units have difficulties interacting due to disorientation, memory loss, decreased levels of consciousness, lessened attention span, aphasia, dysarthria, and sensory deficits. Nurses increase a patient's interactive patterns by thorough assessment and specific nursing actions.

At the conclusion of this chapter you will be able to:

1. Identify the anatomic area related to memory, judgment, receptive aphasia, expressive aphasia, and dysarthria
2. Select causes of confusion and/or disorientation
3. Choose nursing actions which will lessen confusion
4. Describe safety considerations for confused patients and those with deficits in memory and judgment
5. Differentiate fluent (receptive) and nonfluent (expressive) aphasia
6. Select nursing actions that assist the aphasic patient
7. Identify interventions to promote communication with the dysarthric patient
8. Describe nursing actions for patients experiencing the post-concussion syndrome
9. Relate techniques to stimulate patients with altered levels of consciousness

Chapter outline

Perceptual Problems
    Confusion
    Loss of memory
    Judgment deficits
    Post-concussion syndrome
    Decreased alertness

Communication problems
    Types of aphasia
    Dysarthria

PART I
PERCEPTUAL PROBLEMS

Confusion

Frame 1

Perception is the process of acquiring knowledge of the environment. It involves

- —focusing selectively on stimuli
- —maintaining attention, and
- —placing the new information into the framework of past learning.

Confusion results when the quality of sensory input is changed, when all stimuli are not perceived simultaneously, and/or when there is interference with integration of information with past experience.

For the following situations, choose the probable cause for confusion from this list.

- A. change in quality of sensory input
- B. damage to association areas of the brain
- C. damage to some of the tracts bringing information to the brain

1. Mrs. P. had surgery in the pituitary area and her vision is diminished. She is confused and gets lost when walking in her room and the hall.

   1. A

2. Mrs. P. often calls the staff, her friends and family members by the wrong names as she tries to identify them by their voices and the sound of their footsteps.

   2. A and C

3. Mr. I. was transferred to a different room on the unit. Although this change has been explained often, he is confused about where he is, and talks about being moved to "the poorhouse."

   3. B

Frame 2

Any of the causes of cerebral dysfunction presented in Chapter 3 can result in confusion. However, lesions in the pre-frontal area are the most frequent cause. Drugs, electrolyte imbalance, and sensory overload are also common causes of confusion. Careful assessment of the total patient situation helps to identify the source and suggests treatment methods.

True or False:

1. _____ Lesions in the parietal area are the most frequent cause of confusion.

2. _____ Detection of electrolyte imbalance and its correction may clear up confusion.

1. False

2. True

Loss of Memory

Frame 3

Two needed components for accurate perception and action are memory and judgment. The auditory and visual association areas are located in the superior temporal gyrus of the temporal lobe. Characteristically, memory for recent events is lost first while knowledge of earlier occurring events is retained longer.

1. Loss of memory is associated with a lesion in which of the following areas?

   a. frontal lobe
   b. temporal lobe
   c. occipital lobe
   d. parietal lobe

1. a and b

2. Mrs. James has memory problems. Which of the following would be most difficult for her to remember?

   a. her sister's name
   b. what she wore on her wedding day
   c. what she had for lunch
   d. the name of the president of the U.S.A.

2. c and d

Judgment Deficits

Frame 4

Eric Smith suffered a gunshot wound in the anterior frontal lobe of his brain. As a result, he has severe difficulties in making correct judgments. He often overestimates his abilities and makes boastful claims. Family members seem embarrassed by his behavior. Defects in judgment are sometimes difficult to detect as the patient may talk quite normally. Careful analysis of conversation is needed to recognize problems with judgment.

1. Mr. Smith states that he knows how to make a million dollars in one day. Such a statement is probably a consequence of damage to his _____ lobe.

   1. frontal

2. It may be _____ to ascertain if a patient has problems with judgment.

   2. difficult

Frame 5

Nursing care for patients with faulty perception focuses on providing a safe environment. Restraining neurologic patients may be harmful as fighting against restraints can precipitate intracranial bleeding and/or an increase of intracranial pressure. Siderails are essential and the bed should be kept in low position for safety. Providing a stable, uncluttered environment may help decrease confusion. Familiar personal items and visits by the family often decrease anxiety and calm the patient.

1. Which of the following nursing actions should be used with confused patients?

   1. a, c, e

   a. Allow the patient to have a pillow from home
   b. Place the patient in four point restraints
   c. Have the same nurses provide care
   d. Restrict visits from family members
   e. Obtain full-bed siderails

Frame 6

Orient the patient to the environment. Directions should be simple, focusing on one item at a time. Constant reminders are needed. Providing these is taxing to both the patient and the staff. Conversation should be about concrete items. Discussing abstract ideas adds to the confusional state.

1. Which of the following statements would be best to use with a confused patient?

    a. "Would you like to brush your own teeth or should I do it for you? It's good to do things for yourself."

    b. "Here is your toothbrush for brushing your teeth."

    c. "What would you like to do first—brush your teeth or take your bath?"

1. b

Post-Concussion Syndrome

Frame 7

The post-concussion syndrome is the behavioral state exhibited by some persons who have suffered head trauma. It is characterized by a short attention span, inability to concentrate, poor memory, tiring quickly, irritability, and mood shifts. The exact cause of the symptoms and why they occur in some persons and not others is not known.

Time required for the processing of stimuli is increased and the patient expends more energy on this, and tires more quickly. Irritability is related to increased fatigue.

True or False:

1. _____ Post-concussion syndrome is characterized by inability to concentrate.

2. _____ Fatigue increases irritability.

3. _____ All persons who have had a concussion exhibit poor memory.

4. _____ Time for processing stimuli is shortened after a person has suffered a concussion.

1. True

2. True

3. False

4. False

Frame 8

Nursing care of patients following head trauma should include:

    avoid placing overwhelming demands on the patient

231

keep the environment as simple as possible

give simple directions

provide for ample sleep.

The family needs to be aware of the problems and ways to help, as the post-trauma patient may appear strong and healthy and able to do everything. However, return to work or school may result in failure. The patient cannot give the necessary attention to these added demands. Time, up to several years, is needed for complete recovery.

1. Mrs. Smith is concerned about her 18-year-old son who suffered a concussion from a fall. "I'm afraid he won't graduate as he just won't study." What nursing response would be best?

   a. "Make sure he gets enough sleep. Try to have him study for very short periods of time."
   b. "He's in school? Don't you think you're expecting too much of him?"
   c. "Make him study instead of watching TV. He can do it if he wants to."

1. a

Frame 9

Summary:

Confusion is caused by: sensory disturbances, damage to association tracts or areas, drugs, electrolyte imbalance and sensory deprivation and overload.

Memory loss—temporal lobe damage, recent memory lost first

Judgment problems—frontal lobe damage

Nursing implications: safe, stable, uncluttered and predictable environment, familiar people and personal items

Orient frequently using simple concrete words and one idea at a time

Post-concussion syndrome: short attention span, inability to concentrate, poor memory, fatigability, irritability, mood swings. Gradually clears up over time

Management: ↓ demands, simple directions, ample rest, coach family to meet patient's needs.

Decreased Alertness

Frame 10

The comatose state, which may accompany or follow cerebral lesions, may be transient or permanent. Removing the lesion or decreasing intracranial pressure often results in improvement in the level of alertness. Recall that the ARAS in the brain stem is responsible for alertness.

1. The ARAS in the ___ ___ is primarily responsible for the level of consciousness.

2. Not responding to stimuli is termed ___.

1. brain stem

2. coma

Frame 11

Sensory input helps in increasing alertness and orientation. The amount of input should be regulated to avoid overwhelming the patient. Stimuli should be varied and altered because monotonous input is ignored. Auditory stimuli are frequently used (talking, radio, records or tapes) but stimuli for other senses should also be included.

Textures and touching are tactile stimulants. Visual stimuli include bright colors, TV, family pictures, other scenes of personal interests. Olfactory stimultants used are coffee, mint, vinegar, and perfumes. Vary flavors of food when the patient is able to drink and eat.

Mr. Tam is just beginning to respond. Look at the following lists and select the strongest stimulus.

1. Tactile stimulation

   a. vigorous pressure when drying after bath
   b. cooling blanket
   c. use prop pillows with varying textures of materials

2. Visual stimulation

   a. black and white TV
   b. colored TV

3. Olfactory stimulation

   a. scented after-shave lotion
   b. unscented lotions

1. a

2. b

3. a

4. Auditory stimulation

   a. tape of family members talking for ten minutes

   b. continuous background music

   c. entire baseball game

4. a

PART II
COMMUNICATION
PROBLEMS

Types of Aphasia

Frame 12

This diagram illustrates the many areas of the brain involved in communication.

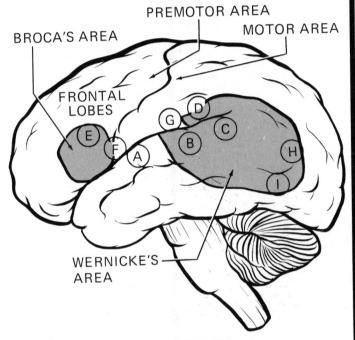

PREMOTOR AREA

MOTOR AREA

BROCA'S AREA

FRONTAL LOBES

WERNICKE'S AREA

A. WORDS HEARD IN PRIMARY
   AUDITORY AREA

B. WORDS RECOGNIZED IN AUDITORY
   ASSOCIATION AREA

C. MEANINGS OF WORDS INTERPRETED
   IN COMMON INTEGRATIVE AREA

D. ORIGIN OF VOCAL RESPONSE TO
   INCOMING THOUGHT IN
   IDEOMOTOR AREA

E. PATTERN OF WORDS IN BROCA'S AREA

F. COORDINATE CONTROL OF RESPIRATION

G. CONTROL OF LARYNGEAL MUSCLES

H. WORDS SEEN IN PRIMARY
   VISUAL AREA

I. WORDS RECOGNIZED IN VISUAL
   ASSOCIATION AREA

Figure 8.1. *Pathways for communication in cerebrum*

The middle cerebral artery supplies blood to many of the communication areas. Damage to this artery and/or interference with blood flow will interfere with normal cell function in these areas.

Match the communication problems listed here with the associated area of the brain in Figure 8.1, labeled A through I.

1. inability to understand written material		1. I
2. unable to comprehend simple directions		2. B, C
3. cannot form words to speak intelligibly		3. G
4. cannot hear		4. A
5. lacks ability to coordinate breathing and speaking		5. F
6. takes a long time to formulate a simple verbal response		6. D
7. loss of visual fields		7. H

Frame 13

Varying degrees of impairment are found in the ability to process symbols and respond appropriately. There may be problems with:

speaking—expressive aphasia
interpreting speech and/or writing—receptive aphasia.

Global aphasia is the inability to interpret incoming symbols as well as to communicate thoughts.

Match the items:

1. Wernicke's area	a. receptive aphasia	1. a
2. Broca's area	b. expressive aphasia	2. b
3. difficulty understanding others		3. a
4. difficulty in speaking		4. b
5. global aphasia		5. a, b

Frame 14

Another system for classification of aphasia is fluent and nonfluent. Fluent aphasia results from lesions in the temporal or parietal lobes or interruption of the blood supply to the area. It is equivalent to receptive aphasia. The area around the auditory association area is damaged. The person has clear articulation, normal rhythm, and uses phrases or sentences. However, the content is nonsensical and is characterized by circumlocution and substitution of words. Spontaneous speech is present but often unintelligible.

True or False:

1. _____ Fluent aphasia is similar to expressive aphasia.

2. _____ Lesions in the temporal lobe result in fluent aphasia.

3. _____ The message in fluent aphasia lacks meaning.

4. _____ There is no rhythm in the speech of a person with fluent aphasia.

1. False

2. True

3. True

4. False

Frame 15

Nonfluent or expressive aphasia results when the motor strip in the frontal lobe is damaged or the anterior branch of the middle cerebral artery is disrupted. No speech, little speech, or poor articulation are evidence of this type of aphasia. Since Broca's area is in the motor area, persons with nonfluent aphasia usually have hemiplegia. The language that persists in nonfluent aphasia is often automatic or stereotypic in nature. Profanity, "Oh, yes", "O.K." and days of the week are examples of automatic speech. Nouns and verbs may be used without connecting words.

True or False:

1. _____ Interruption of the posterior cerebral artery causes nonfluent aphasia.

2. _____ Hemiplegics often have nonfluent aphasia.

3. _____ "Me sleep" is characteristic of sentences in nonfluent aphasia.

4. _____ Profanity is an example of automatic speech.

1. False

2. True

3. True

4. True

Frame 16

Assessment of the patient's language ability is necessary. The nurse must differentiate between sensory deficits in hearing and seeing and aphasia. Sometimes hearing aids and glasses are needed for accurate sensory input.

Patients with fluent aphasia may seem to be normal as they respond when they are addressed. The content of the message needs to be analyzed to differentiate between confusion and fluent aphasia.

A brief, simple assessment:

Is the content relevant to the question asked?
Does the person have the ability to name an object shown?
Can the person follow spoken simple requests?
Can the person follow written directions?
Are there any sensory deficits?

1. What group of patients may speak as if they also have fluent aphasia?

1. confused

2. What factors other than aphasia may contribute to a person's difficulty in communicating?

2. hearing or visual problems

Frame 17

Persons with aphasia often show behavioral or personality changes. These changes are caused by damage to cerebral areas which control emotional responses. Frustration results from the inability to communicate with others. Crying and withdrawal, anger, hitting objects or people, and profanity are common behaviors. Patience and understanding are required. Interventions include sitting with the patient, giving objects such as a piece of sponge to use for hitting siderails to disperse frustrations, and frequent visits. Personal items should be placed close to the patient, but a stable, noncluttered environment is helpful.

1. Emotional outbursts in persons with aphasia are due to:

1. a, b

a. frustration because no one understands them
b. damage to the brain center that controls emotions
c. decreased level of consciousness

2. Which of the following would be good items for the patient to use in releasing frustrations?

2. b, c, d

a. a bell to ring
b. a piece of foam
c. a pillow or bag to punch
d. Play-dough

Frame 18

Aphasic persons take longer to respond to questions and directions. The nurse should allow sufficient time for activities and avoid rushing the patient. Eliminate extraneous noise such as TVs, radios, and noisy halls. The patient has difficulty processing stimuli and added stimuli such as noise from TV increases the processing problems.

The nurse gives simple directions: requests to do *one* thing, or questions asking for one item. Activities to help the patient communicate should be instituted when he is rested, because this requires much energy.

1. The best time to practice speech with Mrs. Thompson who is aphasic is (before/after) her nap.

2. Soft music should be turned (on/off) when trying to communicate with the patient.

3. Processing time for sensory input is (increased/decreased) in aphasic patients.

1. after

2. off

3. increased

Frame 19

Remember, most aphasic patients are not deaf! Slow speech in a normal tone of voice is most easily understood. Talk to the patient and not about him. If assessment reveals the patient understands written communication better than spoken words, use that modality. When the patient is groping for a word, wait for him to think of the word, but don't let him become frustrated. Frustration interferes with his ability to communicate.

1. What would be the best initial approach with the aphasic who states, "I want a _____" and stops?

   a. Wait for the patient to tell you the missing word.
   b. Immediately show nearby objects such as water glass and tissues.
   c. Give a list of objects.
   d. State that you'll be back later.

1. a

Dysarthria

Frame 20

Clyde Freeman had a thrombosis in the medullary area which interfered with the nuclei of CN IX, X, and XII. One result was difficulty in articulating words or dysarthria. Mr. Freeman comprehends all that is spoken to him, but innervation of the muscles for speech has been lost.

1. In dysarthria, the person has difficulty with _____.

1. articulation

2. One would also expect Mr. Freeman to have difficulty _____ if CN IX, X and XII are damaged. (Refer to Chapter 1, Frame 16.)

2. swallowing

3. CN IX, X, and XII originate in the _____.

3. medulla

Frame 21

Therapy in dysarthria is aimed at strengthening the muscles to improve articulation. While Mr. Freeman is expressing himself, listen attentively. He can write on a slate if his speech is incomprehensible. Teach him to tilt his head slightly forward while speaking. This pulls the tongue forward by gravity and lifts the palate, which helps in articulation. Because of his garbled speech, other people may think that Mr. Freeman is confused or intoxicated. Family and visitors may need reminders that his mental ability is not affected.

1. Which of the following nursing actions would help in dysarthria?

   a. Get an alphabet board
   b. Face him when he is talking
   c. Do therapy after lunch
   d. Exercise the jaw muscles
   e. Have him in a reclining position while speaking

1. a, b, and d

Frame 22

Summary:

Aphasia—
   Receptive or fluent—problem understanding verbal stimuli, damage to

temporal or parietal lobes. Speech clear and sounds normal but content lacks meaning.

Expressive or non-fluent—unable to express ideas verbally, poor articulation, damage to Broca's area. Often associated with hemiplegia.

Global—both receptive and expressive aphasia

Assessment
rule out sensory deficits, confusion
observe: relevance of content, ability to follow verbal and written requests

Associated behavior—uncontrolled emotional responses, frustration: crying, withdrawal, anger.

Communication:
eliminate extraneous noise
simple words
simple directions, one at a time
adequate rest
slow pace, wait for patient to find words
try written communication

Dysarthria—loss of innervation to muscles of speech. Mental ability is normal. Slow pace, use written communication, tilt head forward.

CHAPTER 9

SEIZURES

Seizures occur frequently in neuro patients. Nursing care involves assessing the seizure pattern, preventing injury and allaying the fears of the patient and his family.

At the conclusion of this chapter you will be able to:

1. Identify the characteristics of common types of seizures
2. Specify the underlying mechanisms of seizure activity
3. Select safe care for tonic-clonic seizures
4. Describe care needed in status epilepticus.

Chapter outline

Causes

Partial Seizures
   Jacksonian
   Psychomotor

Generalized Seizures
   Absence
   Tonic-clonic
   Status Epilepticus

Nursing care

PART I
CAUSES

Frame 1

Seizure activity is indicative of underlying cranial pathology. This pathology causes certain nerve cells to depolarize often and rapidly. Cells in the *epileptic focus area* differ from the other neurons in that they:

—have increased electrical excitability (more sensitivity to stimuli)
—possess a longer period of electrical negativity
—exhibit an intense, high-frequency impulse caused by sudden depolarization.

It is not fully understood why some persons have seizures while others with similar pathology do not. Cellular and biochemical differences may account for this variability.

True or False:

1. _____ The presence of cerebral pathology (tumors, vascular problems, head injury) increases the likelihood that seizure activity will occur.   1. True

2. _____ Seizures occur because nerve cells are abnormally sensitive to stimuli and depolarize suddenly.   2. True

Frame 2

The new international classification of seizures:

Partial (focal)	involve a circumscribed area of the brain
	consciousness may or may not be lost
	may progress to involve other areas
Generalized	bilaterally symmetrical
	no local onset
	loss of consciousness

Choose the classification in Column II that fits the description in Column I:

Column I

1. _____ jerking muscle contractions in all four extremities
2. _____ twitching of muscles on one side of face
3. _____ uncontrollable movements of one arm progressing to the leg
4. _____ loss of consciousness for several minutes

Column II

a. partial
b. generalized

1. b

2. a

3. a

4. b

PART II
PARTIAL SEIZURES

Jacksonian

Frame 3

Jill Smith, R.N., is doing Mr. Hill's neuro check. Mr. Hill had a left frontal tumor removed the previous day. While making the assessment, she notes Mr. Hill's right cheek twitching. As the facial twitching continues, alternating movements begin in Mr. Hill's right arm. The arm movement and twitching subside in about 45 seconds. Ms. Smith notifies the physician. Phenytoin (Dilantin) 100 mg. t.i.d. is begun.

This is an example of a jacksonian (partial) seizure, seen in patients who have pathology involving the motor strip or a nearby area. Seizure activity may remain localized or progress to involve one entire side of the body and then both sides. Consciousness may or may not be lost when the seizure is focal. Because of the proximity of the parietal lobe, the patient may also have sensory disturbances.

1. A jacksonian seizure would be more common in a person with a (occipital/frontal) tumor.

2. Jacksonian seizures (sometimes/never) spread to involve an entire side of the body.

1. frontal

2. sometimes

Psychomotor

Frame 4

A second type of partial seizure is the psychomotor (temporal lobe) seizure. This type has gained notoriety because aggressive or bizarre behavior may occur. The temporal lobe is closely associated with the limbic system and these two areas are the seat for much of man's elementary and emotional behavior.

Psychomotor seizures usually involve some impairment of consciousness. Other symptoms vary widely but may include problems with thinking and emotional control, automatic behavior, or psychosensory disturbances. The person may look alert but does not respond to questions. A safe environment needs to be provided so that the person does not injure himself. The family needs to understand the reason for behavioral changes and the person's lack of control over behavior during the seizure.

Medications—phenytoin, primidone (Mysoline), mephenytoin (Mesantoin), and carbamazepine (Tegretol) are used in controlling psychomotor seizures. Surgery may be done to remove scar tissue if it is believed to be the cause of the seizure.

True or False

1. _____ Psychomotor and temporal lobe seizures are synonymous terms.

2. _____ Bizarre behavior during the seizure is beyond the patient's voluntary control.

3. _____ The close connection of the temporal lobe and cerebellum account for the behavior changes.

4. _____ Scar tissue in the temporal lobe may cause psychomotor seizures.

1. True

2. True

3. False

4. True

PART III
GENERALIZED SEIZURES

Absence

Frame 5

Absence (petit mal) seizures have unknown causes and occur most frequently in children. Behavior resembles day-dreaming but is actually a brief loss of consciousness. The person momentarily stops an activity and appears to be staring into space. The episode may last only seconds but may occur many times a day. Medications are used to control these seizures, primarily ethosuximide (Zarontin) and trimethadione (Tridione). Patients may have absence seizures along with other kinds of seizure activity.

True or False:

1. _____ Absence seizures are most common in children.

2. _____ Consciousness is lost in absence seizures.

3. _____ Absence and other kinds of seizures do not occur in the same person.

1. True

2. True

3. False

Tonic-clonic

Frame 6

Tonic-clonic (grand mal) seizures progress in two phases.

Phase 1—tonic

—loss of consciousness
—stiffening of body (heightened tonicity of muscles) lasting 30–45 seconds
—depressed respirations, cyanosis
—heightened autonomic activity with increased salivation

Phase 2—clonic

—jerking and shaking of body as muscles contract spasmodically
—incontinence of urine and/or feces
—frothing at the mouth

The seizure lasts about 3–5 minutes. Afterwards the patient is exhausted and sinks into a deep sleep.

Phenytoin and phenobarbital are drugs often used to control tonic-clonic seizures.

1. What two medications are used most frequently to control tonic-clonic seizures?

2. Why does increased salivation occur?

3. During which phase of the seizure is breathing depressed?

1. Phenytoin and phenobarbital

2. ↑ autonomic activity

3. Phase 1—tonic

Status Epilepticus

Frame 7

Status epilepticus demands immediate medical attention. In status, the patient proceeds from one tonic-clonic seizure to another. Not only is the energy drain on the patient exhausting, but the oxygen supply to the brain is severely decreased. Because suctioning the patient is often impossible, aspiration of saliva and blood occur.

Diazepam (Valium) and phenytoin (Dilantin) are two medications administered intravenously to stop the seizure activity.

1. The most critical problem in status epilepticus is decreased cerebral _____ supply.

2. _____ and _____ are two medications used to stop status epilepticus.

3. ____ ____ may occur following status epilepticus because of difficulties encountered in suctioning the patient.

1. oxygen

2. Diazepam phenytoin

3. Aspiration pneumonia

Frame 8

Summary:

Seizures are caused by increased irritability of neurons due to underlying cranial pathology. They are common in patients with head injury, craniotomy, brain tumor.

Partial seizures: circumscribed brain area, may not lose consciousness, symptoms may progress from one area of the body to another.

jacksonian—localized motor symptoms due to pathology of motor strip.

psychomotor—impairment of consciousness, thinking, behavior control due to pathology of temporal lobe and limbic areas.

Generalized seizures: bilaterally symmetrical, no focal onset, loss of consciousness.

absence—momentary loss of consciousness

tonic-clonic—rigidity and contraction of muscles, loss of consciousness

status epilepticus—continuous tonic-clonic seizures, a medical emergency due to $\downarrow O_2$ to brain.

PART IV
NURSING CARE

Panel 1
Nursing Mangement

Mrs. Lutz had a frontal craniotomy two days ago. Her nurse, Mr. Evans, anticipated the possibility of seizures, so he padded the siderails and had suction equipment available.

When he came to give the 12 P.M. medications, Mr. Evans found the patient in a tonic-clonic seizure. Because her jaw was clenched, he did not try to insert a tongue blade or airway. He stayed with Mrs. Lutz to protect her from injury, to prevent dislodgment of the IV and monitoring lines, and to carefully observe the progress of the seizure.

When Mrs. Lutz's jaw relaxed, he suctioned her airway and turned her on her side. He did a neuro assessment and compared it to pre-seizure data. Mrs. Lutz was more difficult to awaken after the seizure but demonstrated no new deficits.

Mr. Evans' charting is as follows:

12:05 Tonic-clonic seizure lasting 2–3 minutes. Onset not observed. Clonic contractions of all four extremities. No incontinence. Neuro signs stable after seizure (see flow sheet), patient hard to arouse.

Mrs. Lutz's sister was at the bedside during the seizure and looked wide-eyed and frightened. Mr. Evans explained that sometimes after surgery the nerve cells in the brain are irritable and seizures occur. He added that the physician would order medication to control the seizures. He explained that Mrs. Lutz would sleep for a while and awaken with no remembrance of the episode.

Because the seizure could have precipitated intracranial bleeding, Mr. Evans did a neuro assessment every 15 minutes.

Frame 9

Evaluate the care Mr. Evans gave during his patient's seizure.

True or False:

1. _____ His first action should have been to insert a padded tongue blade.

   1. False, her jaw was clenched

2. _____ He lowered the siderail nearest himself to prevent bumping of the patient's arm and IV site. This is acceptable.

   2. True, he was in position to prevent a fall

3. _____ He should have waited until all seizure movements subsided before suctioning Mrs. Lutz.

   3. False, should be done as soon as the jaw relaxes

4. _____ A decreased level of alertness could be expected after the seizure.

   4. True

5. _____ Frequency of neuro checks did not have to be increased.

   5. False

Frame 10

1. Choose patients who are likely to have seizures and need seizure precautions.

   a. head injury
   b. previous history of seizures
   c. craniotomy
   d. brain tumor

   1. all

2. What should the nurse do during a seizure?

   a. try to suction the patient's throat
   b. call the physician
   c. protect the patient from injury and dislodgment of tubes
   d. observe progress of seizure

   2. c, d
   (a as soon as possible after the jaw relaxes)

3. What is the optimum position following a seizure?

   a. back-lying
   b. side-lying

   3. b—prevents aspiration

4. List the factors to be included in good charting following a seizure.

4. events at onset, time, parts of body involved, progression, types of movement, incontinence, neuro and vital signs afterward

Frame 11

An explanation of reasons for the seizure helps reduce anxiety of the patient and the family. The stigma attached to seizures still exists. Most persons want to know, "Will it happen again?" and "What will they do for it?" Medications are helpful in controlling seizure activity in about 80% of persons with seizures. Anticonvulsant medications are often prescribed prophylactically for patients with head injuries. Families need to be taught what to do if a seizure occurs.

Frame 12

Summary:

Nursing Care:

Protect patients susceptible to seizures—pad siderails, have suction equipment available

Insert padded tongue blade or airway before tonic phase

Protect from injury and dislodgment of IV and monitoring lines

Observe: onset, progression, kinds of movements, parts of body affected, time, incontinence, neuro and vital signs.

After seizure: turn to side, suction, assess frequently, explain situation to family and patient.

INTRODUCTION TO CASE STUDIES

In order to simulate the clinical situation more closely in the case studies, we will use another method of programming in this section. It will allow you to confront a large amount of information and select the appropriate factors, to explore the relationships between the factors, and to use your creativity and decision-making ability. This method is called "structural communication," and here is a brief example.

It is the year 1992. You are working in a computerized critical care unit. You have continuous access to a large amount of information about each of your patients. The response indicator below lists some of the available information. Use it to construct solutions to the following problems.

Problem 1

What information would you request to monitor the patient's intracranial pressure? Squares numbered: _____

Problem 2

If your patient's ICP was rising, which of these values would progressively *increase*? Squares numbered: _____

Response Indicator			
Respiratory rate and pattern 1	Motor response to pain 2	ECG pattern 3	Hourly urine output 4
Systolic blood pressure 5	Pupil size 6	Level of consciousness 7	Body temperature 8
Body weight 9	Pressure of arterial O_2 (PaO_2) 10	Readings of pressure from Richmond screw 11	Pulse rate 12

Next you will compare your answers with the suggested responses. Explanations are then given about the most important factors which must be included and those which are clearly wrong. This is the system for alerting you to these key factors:

Problem 1 Increased intracranial pressure

Suggested responses: 1, 2, 5, 6, 7, 8, 11, 12

O   5, 12 ▷   *(Means: If you OMITTED 5 or 12, read this comment to see why these parameters are important)*

The vital signs change to reflect the body's attempt to compensate for ↑ICP. Blood pressure and pulse rise to pump blood into the brain against higher resistance.

I   3, 4, 9, 10⟩   *(Means if you INCLUDED 3, 4, 9 or 10 read this comment.)*

While these parameters are important in assessing the general condition of the patient, they do not directly reflect changes in ICP.

O   1, 8⟩

These parameters change as increased pressure is transmitted to their respective regulatory centers in the brain stem.

O   2, 7, 11⟩

The Richmond screw is a direct reading of ICP. Motor response and the level of consciousness change due to the effect of ↑ICP on the reticular activating system and motor tracts in the brain.

O   6⟩

If increased pressure forces brain tissue into the tentorial opening, CN III is compressed causing pupil dilation.

Problem 2   Values which increase
Suggested responses: 5, 6, 8, 11

O   5, 6, 8, 11⟩

Re-read the explanations above to recall why systolic blood pressure rises, pupil size increases, and temperature may rise. Elevated temperature may also be caused by extracranial infection, particularly in the lungs and urinary tract. As ICP increases, the Richmond screw readings will also rise unless there is an equipment failure.

I   2, 7⟩

Motor responses and level of consciousness will *decrease* as ICP rises dangerously.

I   1, 10⟩

The respiratory rate may increase or decrease, and the pattern will also change with pressure on the brain stem. Pneumonia, obstructed airways and loss of adequate chest expansion can cause changes in respiratory rate and pattern and Pao_2.

In the comment section the most troublesome wrong answers will be discussed, as well as the most important correct answers. You may come up with some combinations that did not occur to us, or that show a broad understanding of the relationships between factors. This also reflects the reality of clinical practice. There are many ways to identify relevant information and to solve problems.

CHAPTER 10

CASE STUDY: BRAIN TUMOR, CRANIOTOMY

The symptoms of a brain tumor are related more to anatomic location than to its tumor type. Malignant tumors grow rapidly and do not allow the cranial components to compensate for the increased content. This causes increased intracranial pressure. Diagnostic tests and neurologic assessment are used to pinpoint the location of the tumor before a craniotomy is done. The patient, Jim Douglas, has a malignant tumor in the parietal area. The nursing care planned for him is typical of patient care after a craniotomy.

At the conclusion of this chapter you will be able to:

1. Describe the clinical course of a person with a malignant brain tumor
2. Describe medical therapies and the related nursing interventions
3. Determine the key patient parameters to assess both pre-operatively and post-operatively
4. Develop a nursing care plan based on these assessments.

Chapter outline

Pre-operative period
   Condition on admission
   Nursing assessment
   Nursing care plan

Craniotomy

Post-operative period
   Medical regimen
   Nursing interventions
   Clinical course
   Post-discharge plans

PART I
PRE-OPERATIVE PERIOD

Case Presentation

Condition on Admission

Jim Douglas, age 64, was admitted to the emergency room on September 1 via ambulance. Mr. Douglas' son had found him lying on the bathroom floor unable to use his left arm and leg. The son stated that he had to shake his father to get him to open his eyes, and when he tried to speak, the words were garbled and difficult to understand. On admission Mr. Douglas moaned occasionally. When aroused, he nodded in response to questions rather than answering verbally. No signs of trauma were evident.

Mr. Douglas' son was stunned by his father's condition—"He's always been healthy. He saw the doctor a little over a year ago and was okay." When questioned about any recent problems his father may have experienced, the son related that his father had complained of some clumsiness: "I've dropped a few things," "The left leg feels like it's sometimes asleep." Mr. Douglas did not have a history of hypertension or heart disease.

Mr. Douglas had lived alone since his wife died three and a half years ago. He was retired from his work as a postal employee. He kept house, loved yardwork, and played with his grandchildren. The son related that his father prided himself on his independence and "being young for his age."

The neurologic exam on admission revealed the following:

Fundi and discs flat

CN III, IV, and VI OK. Intact to horizontal movement. No ptosis or nystagmus

Corneal reflex ↓ on L

Pupils small and react to light

Gag reflex intact but some weakness noted

Left sided weakness. Upper extremity weaker than lower extremity. Strength and movement ↓

Vital signs: BP   150/82
           P   68
           R   24
           T   100°F (R)

Skin warm and dry

Mr. Douglas was admitted to the intensive care unit for observation and possible diagnostic tests. The physicians suspected either a right intracerebral hematoma or a tumor.

Discussion

Nursing Assessment

Frame 1

1. In addition to the information in the preceding history, what information should be secured from the family while assessing Mr. Douglas?

   a. difficulty in hearing and/or use of hearing aid
   b. food likes and dislikes
   c. hobbies and interests
   d. facial symmetry
   e. visual acuity

2. Assessment of Mr. Douglas' status for signs of ↑ ICP is an important nursing activity. Which of the following would indicate that ICP is increased?

   a. T 100° (R)
   b. difficulty arousing
   c. skin warm and dry
   d. no sign of papilledema
   e. abrupt onset of symptoms
   f. moans

Frame 2

1. On-going nursing assessment of Mr. Douglas would center on which parameters?

   a. vital signs
   b. pupillary size and response to light
   c. x-rays of the skull
   d. level of consciousness
   e. motor response

2. Neuro checks should be done and charted

   a. every 15–30 minutes
   b. every hour
   c. every two hours

1. a, d, e
   (b and c are not essential at this time)

2. b

1. a, b, d, e

2. a

Nursing Care Plan

Frame 3

1. Which of the following would you do in positioning Mr. Douglas?

   a. elevate head of bed 90°
   b. elevate head of bed 30°
   c. turn Mr. Douglas to his side
   d. keep left arm and leg fully extended
   e. supply support for weakened extremities
   f. give skin care q2h but keep Mr. Douglas on his back

1. b, c, e

Frame 4

Mr. Douglas was moaning. The family requested that he be given "something for pain."

Sedatives and narcotics are used cautiously in neurologic patients because it is difficult to accurately determine the level of consciousness after sedatives or narcotics have been administered. Morphine sulfate is contraindicated because it:

   lowers the level of consciousness
   decreases respirations
   affects pupil size.

Codeine sulfate is a medication often prescribed for pain in patients with suspected intracranial lesions.

1. Which parts of the neuro assessment would be affected by morphine?

1. LOC
   pupil size
   respirations

2. If a patient with increased intracranial pressure requires analgesia, the medication most likely to be prescribed would be _____.

2. codeine

The physician's orders for Mr. Douglas were:

   Neuro checks q 30 minutes
   5% Dextrose in .2 Normal Saline at 75ml an hour
   Acetaminophen q4h for temperature above 101°F (R)
   Bedrest
   Indwelling catheter with straight drainage

Frame 5

Because Mr. Douglas displayed signs of increased intracranial pressure, it was decided to monitor intracranial pressure. A Richmond screw was placed in the subarachnoid space. The procedure was done in the intensive care unit.

1. What would you include in your explanation to the family concerning the pressure monitoring equipment?

    a. It is used to regulate intracranial pressure.
    b. It allows for early detection of changes in pressure.
    c. It is one of several ways we are monitoring your father.
    d. It's perfectly safe, so don't worry.
    e. We don't have to arouse your father as often for checks when he's monitored.

2. Which of the following readings would indicate clogging of the monitoring line?

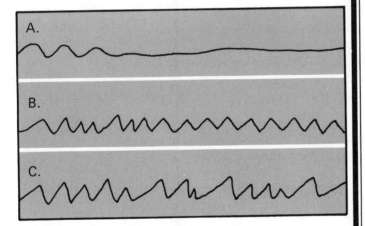

Figure 10.1. *ICP monitoring waves*

3. Before taking readings the nurse would make certain that

    a. the transducer is level with the screw
    b. Mr. Douglas isn't restless or straining
    c. the saline is flowing into the screw
    d. Mr. Douglas is rolled up to a 90° angle

The intracranial pressure readings varied between 25 and 32 mm Hg. This indicated a significant elevation of pressure.

1. b, c

2. A

3. a, b

Frame 6

Mr. Douglas' lab work included the following findings:

Hemoglobin 15.5 (n = 14–18 Gm)
11,600 (n = 5–10,000 per cu. mm)

Arterial blood gases (ABG)

pH	7.30	(7.35–7.45)
PCO_2	45	(35–45 mm Hg)
PO_2	65	(80–100 mm Hg)

1. Which of the findings in the lab work would contribute to increasing intracranial pressure?

1. low PO_2, high PCO_2 pH acid (See Chapter 2, Frame 14)

2. Why would it?

2. ↓O_2 supply to brain causes vasodilation

3. What nursing action would be instituted to help decrease the effect?

3. O_2 administration, patent airway, position for effective ventilation

Frame 7

Mr. Douglas' corneal reflex was decreased on the right so normal moistening of the eye by tears will not occur. Nursing care focuses on keeping the cornea moist and preventing injury. Foreign bodies may remain in the eye, scratching the cornea. An eye pad may be used to prevent such injury.

1. Which of the following nursing actions is indicated?

   a. stand on right side of patient
   b. instill methylcellulose drops q4h
   c. keep the room darkened

1. b

The Response Indicator contains information found in the nursing care plan for Mr. Douglas.

Problem 1

What nursing care actions are aimed at reducing intracranial pressure? Squares _____.

Problem 2

Which actions would promote adequate respiration? Squares _____.

Problem 3

Nursing actions which will prevent complications related to the disuse phenomena include squares _____.

Response Indicator

Elevate head of bed 30 degrees 1	Suction via nasopharynx PRN 2	Reposition q2h and give skin care 3	Check skin over bony prominences every two hours for redness 4
Stand on right side of the patient when talking to him 5	Orient patient to time and place frequently 6	Regulate fluids to prevent over-hydration (75 ml/hr) 7	Provide eye care methylcellulose drops q4h 8
Passive and active range of motion 9	Talk to Mr. Douglas when giving care 10	Administer stool softener 11	Monitor arterial blood gases 12
Go with family to bedside and stay with them for a few minutes 13	Catheter care each shift 14	Deep breathing exercises q2h 15	Place articles on right side of bed 16

Comments

Problem 1   Reduce intracranial pressure

Suggested responses 1, 7, 11, 12

Remember: O means if you omitted *these*
I means if you included *these*

O [1⟩

Elevating the head of the bed improves venous return from the brain and also flow of CSF, through force of gravity. Elevating the head of the bed is done for many reasons, but ↑ICP is an important one.

O [7⟩

Overhydration is a big contributor to increasing ICP. Restriction of fluids is a medical order but nurses are responsible for the regulation and monitoring of fluid balance. One needs to be alert to both signs of overhydration and dehydration.

O [11, 12⟩

Stool softeners will help prevent straining for bowel movements. Noting arterial blood gas results and initiating action if the PO_2 is low will help prevent vasodilation and increased pressure.

I [2, 3, 15⟩

Suctioning and deep breathing will help promote oxygenation of the lungs and thus maintain normal O_2 levels. Re-positioning may also loosen lung secretions and promote oxygenation. However, the discomfort and stimulation of these procedures may contribute to ↑ICP.

I [6, 13⟩

If you chose these because they decrease anxiety, you're correct. Anxiety may increase blood pressure sending more blood to the brain. These actions probably don't have any great effect on ↑ICP, however.

I [4, 5, 8, 14⟩

There seems to be little relationship of these items to ↑ICP

I [9⟩

One study has shown that hip flexion, a part of range of motion, may increase ICP.

I [10⟩

Conversation *about* the patient, whether he is comatose or awake can ↑ICP, but talking *to* the patient in a calm manner is thought to be beneficial.

Problem 2   Promote adequate respiration

Suggested Responses   1, 2, 3, 9, 12, 15

O [9⟩

Exercise and movement promote circulation and aid ventilation.

O [1, 3⟩

The bed limits chest expansion so turning the patient onto his side promotes fuller expansion of the chest. The pooling of secretions in the lung is lessened as the cough reflex may be stimulated. Elevating the head of the bed allows for more effective diaphragm movement. Aspiration of secretions is prevented. Preferably, patients with decreased levels of consciousness should be placed in side-lying position.

O | 2, 15 >

Deep breathing exercises help decrease pooling of secretions. Mr. Douglas may not be able to cooperate so intermittent positive pressure breathing may be needed. Suctioning may be necessary to remove secretions. Careful assessment of the patient, noting secretions, and listening for sounds of congestion, will tell you if suctioning is needed.

O | 12 >

Arterial blood gases give valuable information about the respiratory status of the patient. A PO_2 below 80 mm Hg is indicative of hypoxia. This may be due to accumulated lung secretions, restricted ventilatory movement, or disturbances in cerebral regulation of respiratory rate and depth.

I | 6, 10 >

Orienting the patient is important, but it has little reference to respiration. However, you may have thought that anxiety affects respiration and hence included these two items.

I | 7 >

Adequate hydration is needed to keep secretions moist and easy to expectorate. However, fluid intake is closely monitored to prevent ↑ICP. The use of mist inhalations helps to keep secretions moist and loose.

I | 4, 5, 11, 13, 14, 16 >

None of these relate to promotion of respiration.

Problem 3   Prevent disuse phenomena

Suggested Responses 3, 4, 6, 8, 9, 10, 11, 14

O | 3, 9 >

Exercise promotes circulation and lessens chances of skin breakdown. This kinesthetic stimulation also arouses the patient and orients him to his environment.

O | 11 >

Stool softeners alleviate constipation, one of the complications of immobility.

O | 6, 10 >

You may have thought of complications in terms of the physical ones, but remember the psychological factors also. Hearing one's name and having information provided helps the patient to be oriented and cooperative.

O | 4, 8 >

A right parietal lesion decreases sensory awareness of the left side increasing the need to monitor skin condition. Early detection prevents decubitus, but regular good skin care keeps adequate circulation to the area. Eye care prevents corneal drying and ulceration.

O | 14 >

A catheter was probably inserted because of Mr. Douglas' decreased level of consciousness. Prevention of infection and adequate drainage are important.

Case Presentation

Two days after admission, a CAT scan (computerized axial tomography) was done on Mr. Douglas. It showed a large shift of the cerebral contents to the left. The location of the lesion was determined to be in the right temporal-parietal area.

To further verify the location of the lesion and the possible type of lesion, an angiogram was done. The femoral artery was utilized for inserting the catheter. Angiogram films showed the lesion to be highly vascular. The x-rays demonstrated that the internal cerebral vein was shifted and the anterior choroidal vein widened. Uncal herniation was believed to be imminent. Following the angiogram the femoral site showed no signs of a hematoma.

Discussion

Frame 8

1. Which of the following nursing actions should be done following Mr. Douglas' angiogram?

   a. check breathing because hematoma formation in neck may occur
   b. keep flat in bed for eight hours
   c. observe for possible reactions to the dye
   d. check femoral site for hematoma or bleeding

1. d only

a—appropriate for carotid site
b—head should be raised 30°
c—occurs during test

Frame 9

Dexamethasone (Decadron) was given to Mr. Douglas to decrease cerebral edema. He received 10 mg. of dexamethasone IV at 2 p.m. followed by 4 mg IV q6h

The exact mechanism of corticosteroids in reducing cerebral and spinal cord edema is uncertain. Three possible actions are:

Corticosteroids may exert an effect on the permeability of blood vessels, thereby reducing the transudate that moves from the blood into cranial tissue.

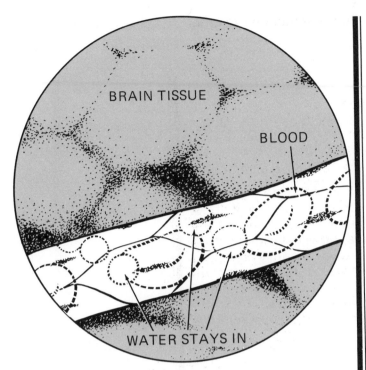

Figure 10.2. *Effect of corticosteroids on capillary membrane*

Corticosteroids may also stimulate metabolic mechanisms which increase the removal of edema fluid from the tissues.

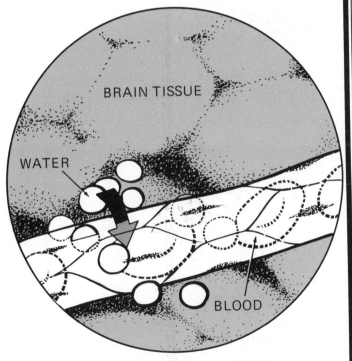

Figure 10.3. *Effect of corticosteroids on metabolism*

Steroids may promote the integrity of cerebral cells thus decreasing the escape of intracellular fluid. This is supported by the fact that steroids impede or restrict the spread of cerebral edema. Steroids stabilize the cell wall.

True or False:

1 _____ Steroids increase the permeability of the vascular wall allowing fluid to escape out of the vessels.

1. False

2 _____ After steroid therapy is begun, the spread of cerebral edema is reduced.

2. True

3 _____ Steroids may enhance metabolic processes to increase removal of fluid from tissues.

3. True

4 _____ Steroids are only effective on lessening cerebral edema and not spinal cord edema.

4. False

Frame 10

Corticosteroids may cause GI irritation and bleeding. Because of this, antacids are often given q2h. These may be administered orally or via nasogastric (NG) tube. An associated nursing action includes guiac tests of stools to detect any blood. If the patient has an NG tube, aspirated contents can likewise be tested for presence of blood.

1. One of the nurses is reading Mr. Douglas' care plan and asks, "Why do we guiac his stools? He doesn't have a history of ulcers." Which of the following statements would be best?

1. b

   a. steroids interfere with clotting mechanisms
   b. steroids irritate the GI system
   c. steroids stimulate production of hydrochloric acid.

2. Antacids should be administered

2. b

   a. every hour
   b. every two hours
   c. every four hours

Frame 11

The length of time steroids are administered varies with the situation. The patient's condition dictates when corticosteroids should be discontinued. If cranial surgery is planned, steroids are often continued until after surgery. Before discontinuing the dexamethasone, the dosage is tapered. This is done to allow the adrenal cortex to gradually resume its normal function. Tapering also helps avoid rebound cerebral edema. When this occurs, fluid again escapes into the tissues because the mechanisms for edema are still present. When tapering dexamethasone, the dosage is reduced and the time between administrations is lengthened.

1. Which factors are altered when tapering steroids?

2. What could happen if steroids were stopped abruptly?

1. time, dose

2. rebound cerebral edema and adrenal insufficiency

Frame 12

One complication of corticosteroid therapy is gastric bleeding from stress ulcers. Cimetidine (Tagamet) is a medication administered to prevent or reduce GI bleeding. Cimetidine blocks histamine from stimulating the production of hydrochloric acid in the stomach. It specifically blocks the H_2 receptor sites on the parietal cells of the gastric mucosa. Gastric secretion is reduced by 90% to 100% for up to four hours. Few side effects have so far been demonstrated.

True or False:

1 _____ Cimetidine neutralizes hydrochloric acid.

2 _____ Cimetidine has few known adverse effects.

3 _____ Corticosteroids can cause stress ulcers.

1. False

2. True

3. True

Frame 13

Mannitol was administered intravenously to Mr. Douglas to give prompt reduction of increased intracranial pressure and/or cerebral bulk. Mannitol withdraws water from cerebral tissue by an osmotic gradient. It is a hyperosmolar solution and causes water to move from the tissue spaces into the blood stream. If a urinary catheter is not in place, close observation of urinary output is needed. Severe bladder distention can quickly occur in patients with decreased levels of consciousness.

True or False:

1. _____ Mannitol draws fluid into the intracellular space.

    1. False

2. _____ All patients receiving Mannitol require a urinary catheter.

    2. False

3. _____ Mannitol quickly reduces cerebral edema.

    3. True

Frame 14

Because Mannitol rapidly removes fluid from the tissue spaces into the vascular system, transient systemic hypertension may occur. Slower administration of Mannitol is warranted in patients with cardiac problems. The usual length of time for administering Mannitol is 60 to 90 minutes. The usual dosage is 2.5–3 gm/kg of body weight.

1. The length of time over which to run the Mannitol for Mr. Douglas is _____ minutes.

    1. 60–90

2. Mr. Douglas weighs 180 pounds (2.2 lb = 1 kg). He should receive _____ gm of Mannitol.

    2. about 200 gm

Frame 15

Rebound edema may occur following administration of hyperosmolar solutions. The possible causes of rebound edema are:

> The hyperosmolar solution may eventually enter the lesion because of changes in the blood-brain barrier and thus draw fluid from the circulation into the brain.

> The lowering of intracranial pressure may stimulate production of CSF.

The phenomenon of rebound edema is decreased when corticosteroids are administered simultaneously.

1. Which of the following could account for rebound edema following administration of
   Mannitol?

   a. increased CSF is produced
   b. tissue irritation is caused by the Mannitol
   c. Mannitol enters the lesion site
   d. systemic hypertension decreases the blood
      flow to the brain

2. In rebound edema, the nurse would note which
   of the following in the patient?

   a. increased alertness
   b. decreased level of consciousness
   c. hyperactivity

1. a, c

2. b

PART II
CRANIOTOMY

Case Presentation

Surgery was scheduled for 8 A.M. on 9/6. Mannitol and dexamethasone had decreased cerebral edema somewhat and Mr. Douglas was less lethargic. The Douglas family asked numerous questions including:

"Will they have to shave Dad's head?"
"How will they get through the bone?"
"Will he be able to use his left side after surgery?"
"Why is his left side weak when the tumor is on the right side?"
"How long will the surgery take?"

These are common questions asked by the family or the patient. Even though the physician explains the surgical procedure, the nurse frequently has to clarify the explanations and answer questions.

Pre-operative orders for Mr. Douglas included:

Shampoo hair

Mannitol 250 gm—to be in by 7 A.M. on 9/6

Atropine 0.4 mg (h)

Promethazine (Phenergan) 50 mg (IM)} 1 hour pre op

Elastic hose from toes to groin

Foley catheter

The Richmond screw was removed prior to surgery, and Mr. Douglas' head was shaved after he was anesthetized. A right parietal craniotomy was performed. Drawing A of Figure 10.4 shows the site of the skin incision.

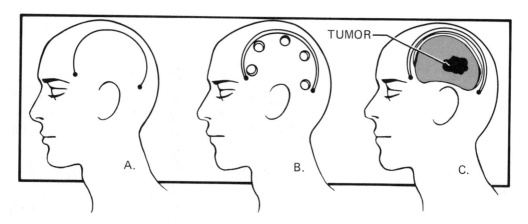

Figure 10.4. *Craniotomy*

Since the skin and scalp muscle are highly vascular, special clamps were used to compress the incision to reduce bleeding. Five holes were placed in the bone with a drill, as shown on drawing B. A Gigli saw was used for sawing between the holes to free the flap of bone. The dura was incised and opened The tumor mass was not visible on the surface of the brain so a cannula was used to probe the brain. The surgeon felt an area of softened tissue in the parietal-temporal area. The grey matter was cut and coagulated, exposing the tumor. Drawing C shows the tumor site. A specimen was sent to the laboratory and it was identified as a glioblastoma multiforme, a rapidly growing tumor. The tumor was not circumscribed or encapsulated, no strict differentiation existed between the tumor cells and the surrounding tissue. A large segment of the tumor (4 × 6 × 5 cm.) was removed. Meticulous care was used in stopping any bleeding in the tumor site and dura. The bone flap was wired in place and the muscle and skin closed. A large pressure dressing was applied to reduce bleeding in the muscle and skin. The surgical procedure took three and a half hours. Mr. Douglas was in the recovery room for one hour before returning to the ICU.

PART III
POST-OPERATIVE PERIOD

Medical Regimen

Post-operative orders included:

Neuro check q 15 min × 8
                   q 30 min until 8 A.M. then
                   q 1 hour unless condition is unstable

Dexamethasone   4 mg q6h × 8 doses
                    3 mg q6h × 4 doses
                    2 mg q6h × 4 doses
                    1 mg q6h × 4 doses
              0.5 mg q12h × 2 doses

Cefazolin (Ancef) 1 gm IV q6h

5% Dextrose in .2 Normal saline with 30 mEq KC1, 1500 ml/q24h

Magaldrate (Riopan) via N.G. tube q2h

Codeine 30 mg q3–4h PRN

Acetaminophen (Tylenol) q4h for temp ↑101°F (R)

Heated mist with O_2 40%

In addition, a CVP line had been inserted. Hourly readings were ordered.

Discussion

Nursing Interventions

Frame 16

Initial assessment on return to the ICU was:

alert
confused as to time and place
speech thick
grasp with right hand strong and holds right
   leg off of bed
weakened grasp on left and unable to hold left
   leg off of bed—moves foot slightly

VS: BP 130/76 P94 R20 T100.6°(R)
      CVP 7mm H_2O

1. A priority nursing goal for Mr. Douglas at this
time would be:

   a. Prevent increased intracranial pressure
   b. Promote use of left side
   c. Decrease anxiety

2. His family asks if the strength will return on his
left side. A correct response would be:

1. a

a. once movement is lost it never returns
b. cerebral edema is present so it is difficult to know at this time
c. the tumor was removed so he should be able to use his left side

2. b

3. A glioblastoma arises from which of the following tissues?

a. connective tissue
b. meningeal tissue
c. dendrites

3. a (Review Chapter 3, Frame 13.)

Clinical Course

Frame 17

On the day following surgery some twitching on the left side of Mr. Douglas' face was noted. After about 15 seconds the twitching stopped. Mr. Douglas did not respond during this time. Several checks later the nurse again noted twitching and notified the physician.

1. The twitching is probably:

1. b

a. a sign that function is returning on the left side
b. seizure activity of a focal nature
c. a sign of increasing intracranial pressure
d. a sign of hypokalemia

Frame 18

On the third post-operative day Mr. Douglas was transferred out of ICU. His neuro checks showed:

Weakness—left side
Pupils equal and react to light (PERL)
Responds to name, confused about place and time, speech is slow but does talk intelligibly
BP 130/78   P80   T100.8° (R)

Frame 19

Mr. Douglas complained of a slight headache and codeine was given. He was allowed out of bed. The CVP line, NG tube, and foley catheter were discontinued. A liquid diet was ordered.

1. Which of the following nursing actions would be useful in relation to Mr. Douglas' confusion?

   a. keep the shades in the room drawn
   b. have the family bring his watch and several other personal objects
   c. introduce yourself each time you enter the room
   d. keep the TV on all of the time
   e. try to arrange for a roommate who is oriented

1. b, c, e

2. In helping Mr. Douglas to walk, the nurse should place a safety belt around his waist and:

   a. provide support on his left side
   b. provide support on his right side
   c. put a sling on his left arm
   d. use a Hoyer lift

2. a, c

3. Mr. Douglas' temperature was 100.8° (R). The *best* nursing action would be:

   a. push fluids to 3000 ml
   b. have him deep breathe q1h, move about in bed and be up several times each day
   c. ask the doctor to increase the antibiotic dosage
   d. send a urine culture to the lab

3. b

4. The tumor was in the right parietal area. Because of the location the nurse should:

   a. give special attention to skin care as Mr. Douglas will have decreased sensation
   b. talk louder as hearing is decreased
   c. make sure all items are placed in his right hand
   d. stand on his right side when speaking to him to be sure he sees you

4. a
   (c—the nurse should encourage Mr. Douglas to use his left hand for some activities)

Frame 20

On the day Mr. Douglas was transferred to the surgical floor a nursing care conference was held. The following problems were identified:

Decreased strength and movement on left side
Malignant tumor, possible depression due to prognosis
Seizure activity
Risk of post-operative hematoma and/or edema
Risk of GI bleeding

On the fourth post operative day the IV was discontinued as Mr. Douglas was taking fluids well. A regular diet was ordered. Dioctyl (Colace) 100 mg bid. was used to retain fluid in the large bowel and thus prevent constipation.

1. Dioctyl promotes (retention/secretion) of fluid in the large bowel.

    1. retention

Frame 21

Post-operatively, the assessment for signs of increasing intracranial pressure have the same importance as pre-operatively. Post-operative hematomas and edema from trauma to the brain during surgery are two possible causes for ↑ pressure. In addition, such activities as straining, Valsalva maneuver, and vomiting can increase pressure and initiate intracranial bleeding.

1. Cerebral edema post-operatively is related to
_____.

    1. trauma from surgery

2. Dioctyl was initiated to prevent _____.

    2. straining

Mr. Douglas progressed well following surgery. He noted itching of his scalp in the incisional area. After three days the large pressure dressing was changed to a smaller gauze dressing. The wound was healing well. Five days post-operatively the dressing was removed and Mr. Douglas wore a surgery cap. On the eighth day the stitches were removed.

Frame 22

Radiation therapy was begun ten days after surgery. When the doctor explained radiation treatment, Mr. Douglas asked, "But you removed the tumor. Why do I need radiation?"

1. Mr. Douglas' question probably indicates:

    1. b

   a. he is denying his condition
   b. he doesn't have an adequate understanding of the condition
   c. he's afraid of radiation

Frame 23

The glioblastoma multiforme is a highly malignant tumor. Radiation therapy will decrease the size of the remaining tumor and delay its growth. On the second day of radiation therapy, Mr. Douglas was drowsy and less responsive. Radiation therapy initially causes tissue edema.

1. Mr. Douglas' son is very concerned about his father because he keeps falling asleep. This is the second evening after radiation therapy has begun. Your explanation would include the concept that:

   a. his tumor is growing and causing pressure
   b. edema is transient with the beginning of radiation
   c. the radiation caused a vessel to rupture

1. b

Post-discharge Plans

Frame 24

Mr. Douglas remained in the hospital for the majority of the radiation therapy treatments. His left side was less weak but there was still some deficit. His speech was normal.

Mr. Douglas seemed quiet and withdrawn. When the nurse talked with him he said "What's the use. I can't do things for myself. I can't live alone. I'm a burden to my family."

1. Which would be the best response for the nurse to make?

   a. Life can be very hard. You seem to have had your share of knocks.
   b. It's sometimes hard to look to the future. I've noticed, though, that your left hand is stronger today than a week ago.
   c. Let's see what you can do. You just can't sit there feeling sorry for yourself.

1. b

The nursing staff participated with the other members of the rehabilitation team to plan Mr. Douglas' home care with his family. He went to his own home, and his widowed sister came to stay with him.

A home health care agency was contacted to assist Mr. Douglas with self care. The family spent time discussing other options which might be considered in the future, such as hospice and skilled nursing care.

CHAPTER 11

CASE STUDY: CLOSED HEAD INJURY

Coma may be caused by many factors. In this case study you will learn about the care of a patient with brain stem injury. This comatose patient is completely dependent on others, particularly the nursing staff, for her safety and well-being. Good care prevents complications and promotes recovery.

At the conclusion of this chapter you will be able to:

1. Select nursing actions for a comatose patient
2. Determine nursing actions based on findings in laboratory tests and the neurologic exam
3. Choose approaches which would be helpful in giving support to the family of a comatose patient
4. Identify nursing actions related to the medical plan of care for a patient with a brain stem contusion
5. Recognize rehabilitation techniques appropriate to the critical phase of illness.

Chapter outline

Critical Phase
    Medical regimen
    Nursing assessment
    Nursing care plan

Recovery Phase
    Medical plan of care
    Nursing goals and interventions

PART I
CRITICAL PHASE

Case Presentation

Ginny Dale, a 17-year-old, was unresponsive following a head-on car accident.

Skull x-rays showed a basilar skull fracture. The CAT scan and angiogram revealed no localized intracranial mass. The diagnosis was closed head trauma with brain stem contusion.

The following were noted on admission:

PO_2	80	(80–100 mm Hg
PCO_2	40	(35–45 mm Hg)
pH	7.29	(7.35–7.45)
Hgb	14	(12–16 Gm/100 ml)
WBC	4,500	(5–10,000)
BP	130/68	
P	64	
R	28	
T	99°F (R)	

Pupils—equal, 4 mm, react sluggishly
Responsiveness to pain: assumes decerebrate posturing

Medical Regimen

Richmond intracranial screw

Foley catheter to straight drainage

Dexamethasone (Decadron) 10 mg IV stat; 4 mg q6h

IV 5% Dextrose in .2 Normal Saline at 60 ml/hr.

Neuro checks q15 min

Acetaminophen (Tylenol) 600 mg for temperature above 101°F (R)

Hypothermia blanket for temperature above 102°F (R)

Blood gases q12h

Vitamins 1 ampul IV qd

Based on arterial blood gas findings and increasing respiratory difficulty, a tracheostomy was performed and a cuffed tube was inserted into the trachea. Ginny was placed on a volume-cycled mechanical ventilator. She required suctioning almost every hour to maintain a patent airway. A mist attachment to the tracheostomy tube kept secretions loose.

Initial readings from the Richmond screw were 20–24 mm Hg, which is higher than normal. Mannitol was administered to control rising ICP.

Discussion

Nursing Assessment

The Response Indicator displays the assessment parameters noted four hours after admission.

Problem 1

Choose the parameters that show respiratory problems with depressed cerebral O_2 tension. Squares numbered _____.

Problem 2

Which parameters indicate problems with fluid and electrolyte balance? Squares numbered _____.

Problem 3

The signs of Ginny's increased intracranial pressure have already been discussed. Now choose the signs which would specifically indicate *rebound edema* following Mannitol administration. Squares numbered _____.

Response Indicator			
Richmond screw reading 28 mm Hg 1	ABG PO$_2$ 60 PCO$_2$ 42 2	Decerebrate posturing 3	Serum sodium 156 (n = 135–145 mEq/L) 4
Slight cyanosis of lips and nail beds 5	Intake—250 ml past four hours 6	Temperature 103°F (R) 7	Respirations 30 8
BP 140/76 9	Pupils react sluggishly 10	Serum chloride 92 (n = 98–109 mEq/L) 11	Hgb 12.5 (n = 12–16 Gm) 12
Urine output 800 ml past four hours 13	Skin warm and dry 14	blood pH 7.32 (n = 7.35–7.45) 15	Serum Potassium 3.9 (n = 3.5–5.5 mEq/L) 16

Comments

Problem 1   Respiratory problems

Suggested responses: 2, 5, 8, 15

O ⎜ 2, 5, 8, 15 ⟩

Arterial blood levels of oxygen are low and carbon dioxide is building up in the blood. This makes blood pH more acidic. Respiratory rate and depth increase to blow off excess CO_2 and more O_2 is inspired. However, occluded airways or alveolar inflammation can prevent O_2 from reaching the blood. Low O_2 levels are reflected in cyanosis.

I   7 >

Fever could be investigated as a sign of pneumonia due to airway obstruction; retained, infected secretions; or collapse of a lobe of the lung. Lack of diaphoresis, however, would point to a fever caused by damage to the heat regulating center in the hypothalamus.

I   1, 3, 10 >

These are signs of ↑ICP. They will become worse as cerebral oxygen levels decline. But they are not specific signs of respiratory problems.

Problem 2   Fluid and Electrolyte Balance

Suggested Responses: 4, 6, 7, 11, 13, 14

O   6, 13 >

The output far exceeds the intake. Specific gravity of the urine should be tested as diabetes insipidus is a possibility. Intake and output comparisons are essential elements of assessment.

O   4, 11 >

Hypernatremia may occur following administration of hyperosmolar solutions. Corticosteroids also may add to retention of sodium. The chloride level is slightly decreased. IV solution components may have to be changed to reduce sodium.

O   7, 14 >

Don't forget that the body uses more water when the temperature is elevated. The nurse sometimes has to remind the physician of this and ask to increase the IV rate of flow.

I   8, 14 >

Moisture is lost through respirations. In Ginny's case, the mistogen nebulizer should prevent water loss through this source. Ginny is not diaphoretic, so she is not losing large amounts of water through the skin. You are correct in remembering to calculate fluid loss including all channels: urine, feces, skin and lungs.

I   1, 10 >

The increased intracranial pressure reading and ↓ pupil reaction point to ↑ ICP. You may have thought that pressure is transmitted to the hypothalamus causing interference in fluid regulation. Damage to the pituitary could interfere with the secretion of fluid-regulating hormones. Neither seems likely at this point.

I   2, 15 >

Disturbances in blood gases may affect fluid and electrolytes indirectly by increasing respirations and causing water loss through this source.

I $\boxed{3, 9}\!\!>$

Decerebrate posturing consumes more energy but does not seem to be directly related to fluid and electrolyte imbalance. The BP elevation is probably related to ↑ICP rather than ↑fluid loading.

I $\boxed{12, 16}\!\!>$

These are normal findings and do not contribute to changes.

Problem 3   Rebound Edema

Suggested Responses: 1, 9, 10

O $\boxed{1}\!\!>$

Note that the intracranial pressure has increased to 28 from the initial reading of 20–24. This indicates rebound edema and is usually noted 3–4 hours after Mannitol has been given.

O $\boxed{9, 10}\!\!>$

Increasing systolic pressure (from 130–140) and sluggish pupil response indicate that edema is probably causing ICP. Steroid doses are often administered to prevent this rebound edema after the use of hyperosmolar solutions.

I $\boxed{4, 13, 14}\!\!>$

These are frequently found after Mannitol is administered but are not signs of rebound edema.

I $\boxed{2, 8, 15}\!\!>$

Rebound edema would not affect the respiratory status directly, but extreme elevation of ICP causing downward herniation could affect the respiratory center in the brain stem.

I $\boxed{3, 7}\!\!>$

Again, increased pressure could cause these. However, the original pathology is the more likely cause, rather than rebound edema.

I $\boxed{11, 12, 16}\!\!>$

These parameters do not directly reflect rebound edema.

Case Presentation

Nursing Care Plan

Linda Zeller, R.N., was responsible for Ms. Dale's nursing care. She developed a nursing care plan which focused primarily on these goals:

Prevent ↑ICP
Actions: Administer mannitol and dexamethasone as ordered
Monitor ICP readings and physical signs of ICP
Elevate head of bed
Monitor intake and output balance
Minimize pain and discomfort by skillful performance of nursing procedures

Support respirations
Actions: Adjust respirator settings according to arterial blood gas levels
Maintain patent airway
Turn every hour
Auscultate breath sounds four times/shift

Maintain homeostatic balance
Actions: Administer IVs and electrolytes as ordered
Monitor electrolyte, pH, and fluid balance

Prevent disuse phenomena
Actions: Place body in functional alignment
Skin care: special mattress, turning schedule, massage
Passive range of motion to all extremities two times/shift

The Dales were at the hospital most of the time. Mr. Dale, an insurance salesman, and Mrs. Dale, a secretary at the elementary school, took vacation time. Ginny's older brother was away at college, and her two younger brothers, 15 and 13 years old, came occasionally. The extended family of grandparents, aunts, uncles and cousins mobilized to help the family.

The nurse encouraged the family members who were staying with Ginny to touch her and talk to her frequently. Ms. Zeller explained that comatose patients can sometimes hear and understand everything that is said, and appreciate knowing about the family activities, their friends, the weather, etc. Mr. Dale said, "I've noticed that you always talk to Ginny and explain everything you are going to do, just as if she were awake. I wondered why you bothered and now I understand."

PART II
RECOVERY PHASE

One week after the accident, Ginny Dale's status was improved. Her vital signs stabilized and intracranial pressure readings were improved. Decerebrate posturing persisted. Suctioning and other treatments increased the rigidity. The ventilator had been gradually discontinued and Ginny's arterial blood gases were maintained adequately by the administration of 40% oxygen through a tracheostomy hood equipped with a heated nebulizer.

The following clinical flow sheet describes Ginny's condition.

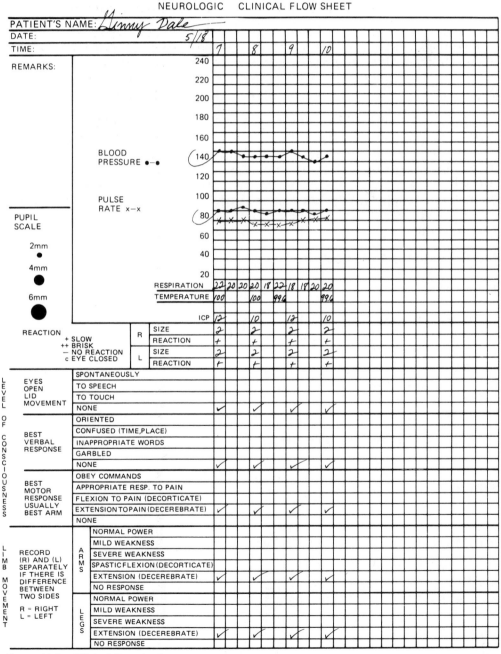

Figure 11.1. *Clinical flow sheet*

MEDICAL PLAN OF CARE

Current medical orders were:

> Nasogastric (NG) tube feeding with a preparation containing essential proteins, carbohydrates, fats, vitamins, and minerals; 100 ml q4h followed by 50 ml water
> Cefazolin sodium (Ancef) 500 mg q4h IV
> Acetaminophen (Tylenol) 600 mg q3–4h PRN for temperatures greater than 101°F
> Magnesium and aluminum hydroxide (Maalox) and aluminum hydroxide gel (Amphojel) alternate q2h via NG tube
> Dexamethasone (Decadron) 4 mg q6h IV
> Hypothermia blanket for temperatures above 102°F (R)

Linda Zeller had modified her care plan as the patient's condition changed. Here are the current goals:

Nursing goal	Patient outcome
1. Prevent contracture	Joints will maintain normal ROM
2. Promote adequate respirations	ABG's in normal range
3. Promote responsiveness	Level of alertness increased
4. Maintain skin integrity	Skin intact
5. Prevent infection	Temperature within normal limits
6. Maintain general hygiene	Overall appearance will be pleasing
7. Reduce demands on brain	No deterioration of neurologic function

Discussion

Nursing Goals and Interventions

Frame 1

1. Which of these goals would have highest priority?

1. 2—Respiratory. (If you chose Number 7, this also is very important and would include Number 2.)

2. Is Ginny's neurologic condition stable?

2. Yes

Frame 2

PROMOTE ADEQUATE RESPIRATION

In addition to noting the rate of respirations, it is particularly important in brain stem injuries to assess the rhythm of the respiratory pattern. After admission Ginny had central neurogenic hyperventilation.

1. Diagram the pattern you would see with CNH.

1.

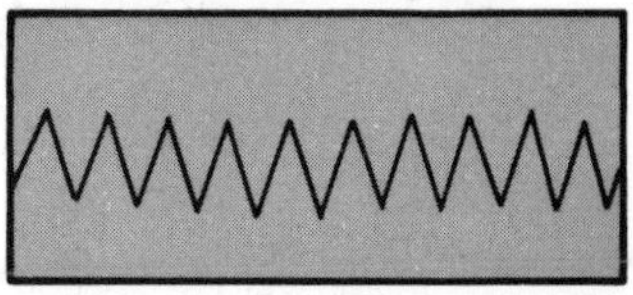

Figure 11.2. *CNH respirations*

2. The presence of this pattern indicates involvement of what area of the brain stem?

2. Lower midbrain, upper pons

Frame 3

1. Which of the following signs would indicate a significant change in respiratory status?

    a. rate—12/min.
    b. no breath sounds over one section of lung fields
    c. breath sounds that resemble the effervescence of a carbonated beverage
    d. cough producing thick greenish sputum
    e. fever of 102°F (R)

1. all
(a—much slower than baseline
b—atelectosis
c—presence of fluid in alveoli
d and e—possible infection)

Frame 4

Because the tracheostomy eliminates the functions of the nasal cavity, moistening and filtering air, these must be considered in providing care.

1. Which of the following would you include for Ginny because she has a tracheostomy?

    a. inform the family to stay away if they have colds
    b. humidify the air delivered to the trachea
    c. wear rubber gloves when caring for Ginny
    d. be careful when using powders, so they are not inspired
    e. use a heated nebulizer

1. a, b, d, e

Maintain Skin Integrity

Frame 5

Many nursing actions are needed to achieve this goal. Frequent position changes, at least q2h, are needed to promote circulation to tissue.

1. Since noxious stimulation initiates decerebrate posturing, which method(s) of turning and positioning would be least likely to cause this?

    a. have several persons to help turn Ginny
    b. do the turning quickly
    c. support limbs while turning
    d. use a turning sheet

1. a, c, d   (If you left out the turning sheet, you may also be including the fact that the patient is on the hypothermia blanket and shouldn't have an extra sheet in place.)

Frame 6

The frequent temperature spikes cause difficulty in achieving the goal of skin integrity. Elevated temperatures consume more body energy leaving less for maintenance of tissue. Perspiration results in damp skin surfaces. Rigidity keeps body limbs in tight proximity, trapping moisture.

1. Choose the therapeutic nursing actions.

    a. place face towels between upper arm and body
    b. bathe patient with hot water
    c. cover patient sparingly
    d. put talcum powder in areas where skin surfaces rub together
    e. refrain from using body lotion
    f. change bed linen when damp

1. a, c, d, f

Frame 7

Dexamethasone caused a rash on the upper part of Ginny's chest, as shown in Figure 11.3. Acetic acid compresses were helpful in clearing the rash.

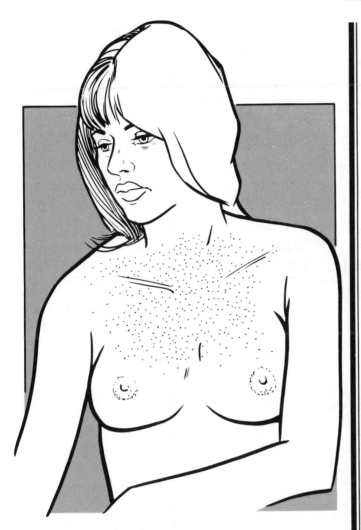

Figure 11.3. *Allergic rash*

Frame 8

Figure 11.4 shows Ginny in a side-lying position.
Evaluate the body alignment.

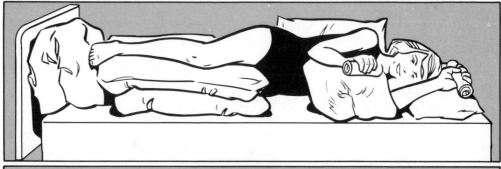
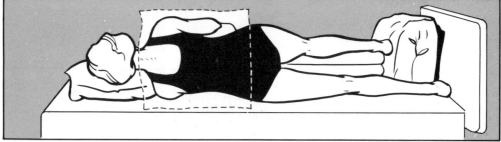

Figure 11.4. *Side-lying position*

1. Ginny's arm is supported by a pillow for what reason(s)?

   a. to promote chest expansion
   b. to prevent a flexion contracture of the elbow
   c. to prevent muscle wasting

   1. a, b
   (c—prevented only by active exercise)

2. The position of Ginny's leg and foot:

   a. prevents hip adduction
   b. prevents skin excoriation
   c. keeps hip, knee, and ankle joints in alignment

   2. a, b, c

3. The head of the bed is raised to:

   a. promote return of blood from the head
   b. flex the back
   c. prevent aspiration

   3. a, c

4. Which of Ginny's problems would make positioning and skin care more difficult?

   a. inability to respond to stimuli
   b. decerebrate rigidity
   c. fever
   d. incontinence

   4. all

5. Linda Zeller has trouble keeping Ginny's feet in alignment because her rigidity causes plantar flexion. Which of these would be a good solution?

   a. more pillows
   b. put high topped tennis shoes on Ginny
   c. wrap an elastic bandage around her ankle
   d. put her feet against a footboard

Promote Responsiveness

Frame 9

Injuries to the brain stem often interfere with the reticular activating system. Sensory input may promote the patient's responsiveness.

1. Which of the following nursing actions would be helpful in achieving this goal?

   a. talk to Ginny when giving care
   b. use a favorite cologne or perfume after bath
   c. tape voices of her family to play occasionally
   d. keep the lights on at night
   e. place bright colored posters in the room.

Prevent Infections

Frame 10

Good oral hygiene decreases the possibility of fungal infections of the mouth. Antibiotic therapy and poor nutrition predispose to fungal infections. Thrush, a common fungal infection, appears as white spots on the mucosal tissue. Nystatin (Mycostatin), an antibiotic mouth wash, or gentian violet swabs may be utilized to eradicate the infection.

1. List two factors which made Ginny susceptible to thrush.

2. Name an antibiotic mouth wash used in treating thrush.

5. b
(d—sometimes pressure of the footboard increases rigidity)

1. all but d would be helpful. (Continuous bright lights would most likely prevent any sleep-wake cycle Ginny may have.)

1. antibiotics, clenched jaw

2. Nystatin

Frame 11

Oral hygiene is a problem in the patient with decorticate or decerebrate rigidity. Stimulation increases the tightness with which the jaws are clenched. One approach is to place the patient on her side with the head elevated. While one nurse suctions, the second nurse sprays water or mouth wash against the teeth with a Water Pik or syringe and tubing.

When the patient is relaxed, a padded tongue blade dipped in mouthwash may be used to clean the tongue and inner mouth. Never force items between the teeth, pressure only increases rigidity. A tooth brush can be used on the outer surfaces of the teeth and gums.

1. How many nurses are needed when using a Water Pik for Ginny's oral hygiene?

2. In what position will you place Ginny for oral care?

3. What will increase the tightness of her clenched teeth?

1. two

2. on side with head of bed elevated

3. trying to force her mouth open

Frame 12

1. Mrs. Dale inquires why Ginny's temperature keeps spiking. "Is it an infection?" she asks. Which would be the best explanation to give her?

   a. it's common for persons with a tracheostomy to spike temperatures.
   b. the brain stem controls body temperature, and the area is damaged.
   c. the hypothalamus is located in the area of the brain that was damaged. It regulates temperature.
   d. there are so many ways that Ginny can be infected. We'll have to be more careful.

1. c

Provide Adequate Nutrition

Frame 13

After injury and stress to the body, its nutritional requirements increase to 2,000–3,000 calories, and the need for protein is four times normal. Intravenous feedings are not able to meet these needs on a long term basis. Therefore, nasogastric feedings are often given to comatose patients.

Many commercial preparations are available. The feedings are high in calories and protein. In addition, they contain the necessary amounts of other nutritional requirements. Feedings should be begun slowly because the richness of the formula may cause diarrhea. Occasionally medication is needed to control diarrhea.

When doing nasogastric feedings, it is necessary to:

—Roll the patient into a sitting position.
—Determine placement of the tube by injecting 10 ml of air and listening with a stethoscope immediately beneath the xiphoid process.
—Aspirate to determine if the previous feeding has been absorbed. This aspirate is returned through the tube and if it exceeds 60–75 ml, the feeding is not given.
—Administer the feeding over a 20–30 minute period.
—Follow the feeding with 50 ml water to cleanse the tubing and provide the patient with adequate hydration.
—Keep the patient in an upright position for 30–40 minutes following the feeding.
—If the patient has a tracheostomy with a cuff, be sure the cuff is inflated prior to the feeding.
—These measures are aimed at preventing aspiration; however, a suction machine should be available during the procedure.

True or False:

1. _____ The bed may be rolled to a 30° angle immediately after completing the tube feeding.

2. _____ To determine correct placement of the tube, listen below the xiphoid process with a stethoscope as you insert air.

1. False

2. True

3. _____ Aspirated contents should be discarded as they are contaminated.

3. False

4. _____ Water following the tube feeding helps prevent clogging of the tube.

4. True

Ginny continued to improve, but the gains seemed slight. By the third week the IV was discontinued. The tracheostomy was removed. Decerebrate posturing continued but was less frequent. The neuro check showed some weakness of her right arm and leg. Pupils were equal and reacted to light. Ginny still did not verbally respond, but she sometimes winced when painful stimuli were applied. She was transferred out of the acute neuro unit.

Frame 14

1. Mrs. Dale said, "I feel so helpless around Ginny. I wish there was something I could do for her." Which would be suitable activities the mother could do?

1. a, b, c, d

   a. assist in giving personal hygiene: bathing, combing hair, etc
   b. do range of motion exercises
   c. read to Ginny for 5-10 minutes each evening
   d. periodically supply smell and sound stimulation

Frame 15

At one point during her recovery Ginny became very hyperactive but was still not able to process incoming information. Her behavior was bizarre, non-purposeful, and sometimes aggressive. Ginny chewed everything in sight including her hands, sheets, and clothing. She seemed unaware of her surroundings and did not recognize family or staff. Occasionally she cried and moaned. Her family found this behavior very distressing.

1. What safety factors need to be included in her plan of care?

1. all but d—may be in chair restrained

   a. remove breakable items from surrounding area
   b. keep restrained unless someone is with her
   c. cut fingernails short
   d. keep in bed with siderails at all times

Sensory stimulation was important at this time to orient Ginny. This included

> repetitive motor contacts
> use of reflexes to facilitate and inhibit movement
> joint compression
> resistive exercises
> interaction with others

Careful assessment was needed to avoid over-stimulation and fatigue.

Ginny began eating soft foods and started saying occasional words and phrases. The grasp on her right side became stronger. Ginny's rehabilitation included physical and occupational therapy. By the time she was discharged, Ginny was eating independently and walking with assistance, but had difficulty communicating. Mrs. Dale took a leave of absence from her job to care for Ginny.

Five months after the accident Ginny returned to the nursing unit. She had regained complete use of her right side, had no difficulty eating or talking, and had returned to school.

SECTION II

Spinal Cord Problems

In this section you will study the nursing care of patients with dysfunction of the spinal cord. However, you will find occasional references to the anatomy of the cranial part of the central nervous system. Like the brain, the cord is a complex structure, and an extremely fascinating entity. Both physiologic and psychosocial aspects of nursing care are vital to the well-being of patients with spinal cord problems. Because spinal cord dysfunction frequently involves the peripheral and autonomic nervous systems, these divisions will also be considered.

CHAPTER 12

THE SPINAL CORD

You will begin by reviewing the anatomy of the spinal cord, the peripheral nervous system, and the autonomic nervous system. When alternate names are used for structures, both will be included. Your understanding of this chapter will assist your learning in the rest of the book.

At the conclusion of this chapter you will be able to:

1. Specify the segments of the spinal column
2. Label the components of the reflex arc
3. Identify the location and functions of the major ascending and descending tracts
4. Recognize the differences between vertebrae at different levels
5. Identify the segments of a vertebra
6. Differentiate the actions of the sympathetic and parasympathetic nervous systems
7. Describe the relationship of the peripheral nervous system and the central nervous system
8. Relate the major sources of blood supply to the cord
9. Recognize the differences in cord structure at the various levels.

Chapter outline

Protective structures
    Vertebral column
    Meninges

Blood supply

Nerve tracts
    Sensory
    Motor

Autonomic nervous system
    Sympathetic
    Parasympathetic

PART I
PROTECTIVE
STRUCTURES

Vertebral Column

Frame 1

The spinal column is composed of vertebrae which encase and protect the spinal cord. Because vertebrae play an important role in cord pathology, take a moment to examine the structure more closely.

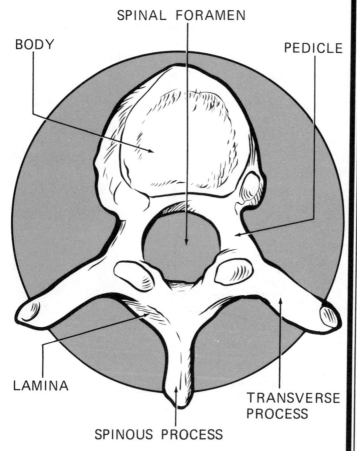

Figure 12.1. *Vertebral structure*

Use the words in Figure 12.1 to finish these sentences.

1. The spinal cord goes through the _____ _____.

1. spinal foramen

2. The most solid weight-bearing portion of the vertebrae is the _____.

2. body

3. There are two processes projecting laterally from the vertebrae, these are called _____ processes.

4. The _____ process lies opposite the body of the vertebrae.

5. The _____ connects the transverse and spinous processes.

6. The _____ form the sides of the wall of the foramen.

3. transverse

4. spinous

5. lamina

6. pedicles

Frame 2

The shape of the vertebrae varies according to function.

The first two cervical vertebrae are:

atlas—the skull rests on the superior articular facet
axis—articulates with the atlas and forms the axis of rotation of the skull

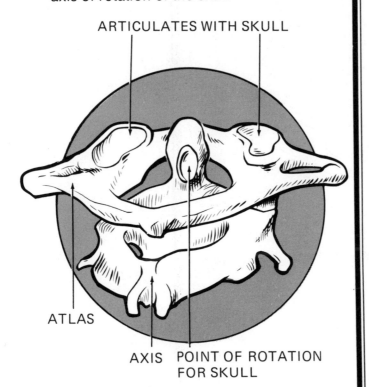

ARTICULATES WITH SKULL

ATLAS

AXIS POINT OF ROTATION FOR SKULL

Figure 12.2. *Atlas and axis*

These two vertebrae are built to support the weight of the skull and to allow the head to rotate.

The other cervical vertebrae have wide transverse processes for muscle attachments. These muscles hold the head erect and allow for a wide range of movements.

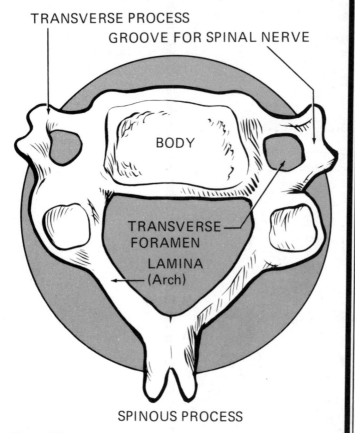

TRANSVERSE PROCESS

GROOVE FOR SPINAL NERVE

BODY

TRANSVERSE FORAMEN

LAMINA (Arch)

SPINOUS PROCESS

Figure 12.3. *Cervical vertebra*

1. The center of rotation of the skull is the (atlas/axis).

2. Muscles holding the head erect attach to the (transverse, spinous) processes of the cervical vertebrae.

1. axis

2. transverse

Frame 3

Note the difference in vertebral structure in thoracic, lumbar and sacral areas.

The thoracic vertebrae have points of attachment for the ribs on the transverse processes.

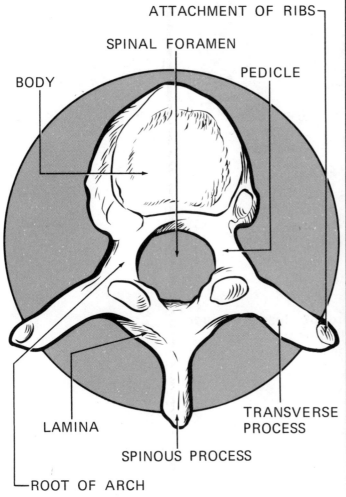

ATTACHMENT OF RIBS

SPINAL FORAMEN

PEDICLE

BODY

LAMINA

TRANSVERSE PROCESS

SPINOUS PROCESS

ROOT OF ARCH

Figure 12.4. *Thoracic vertebra*

The lumbar vertebrae have large bodies because they bear most of the body weight.

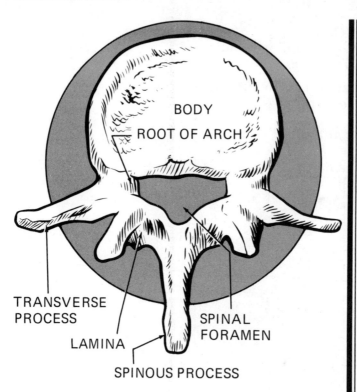

BODY

ROOT OF ARCH

TRANSVERSE
PROCESS

SPINAL
FORAMEN

LAMINA

SPINOUS PROCESS

Figure 12.5.   *Lumbar vertebra*

The sacrum and coccyx are large fused vertebrae.
Spinal nerves exit through the foramina.

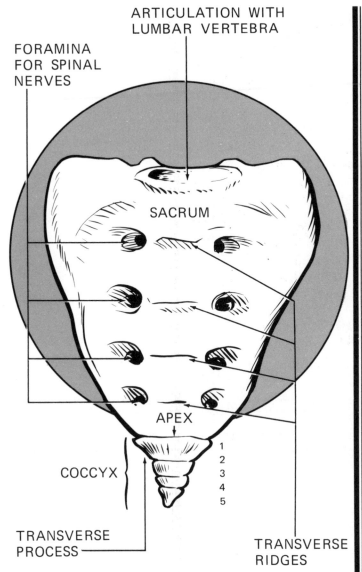

ARTICULATION WITH
LUMBAR VERTEBRA

FORAMINA
FOR SPINAL
NERVES

SACRUM

APEX

COCCYX

1
2
3
4
5

TRANSVERSE
PROCESS

TRANSVERSE
RIDGES

Figure 12.6. *Sacrum and coccyx*

Match the description with the type of vertebrae

1. _____	Point of rotation for skull	a. atlas	1.	c
2. _____	Fused vertebrae	b. cervical	2.	f
3. _____	Large bodies for weight bearing	c. axis	3.	e
4. _____	Rib attachment on transverse processes	d. thoracic	4.	d
5. _____	Supports the skull	e. lumbar	5.	a
6. _____	Wide transverse processes for muscle attachment	f. sacrum and coccyx	6.	b

Frame 4

In addition to protecting the cord, the spinal column has a major role in keeping the body upright
and giving it stability. There is limited movement
of the vertebrae except for C1 and C2. Several ligaments attach on each vertebrae and provide
stability to the spinal column. The two main ligaments are the anterior and posterior longitudinal
ligaments. Note their location on Figure 12.7.

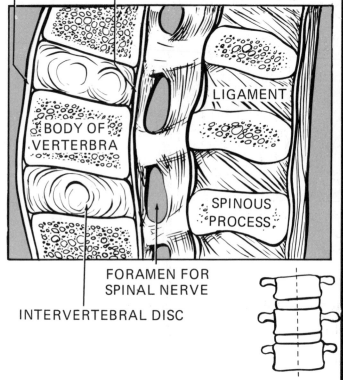

Figure 12.7. *Anterior and posterior longitudinal ligaments*

1. The two main functions of the spinal column
   are:

   1. protect cord
      stability to body

2. The major ligaments for stabilizing the spinal
   column are:

   2. anterior and
      posterior
      longitudinal
      ligaments

Frame 5

Located between the bodies of the vertebrae is a cushion of cartilage which is called the intervertebral disc. The disc absorbs shocks, force, and pull applied to the spinal column. The thicker outer layer of the disc is called the annulus while the inner part is the nucleus pulposus. Damage to the annulus results in the nucleus protruding out and applying pressure on the adjacent nerve root.

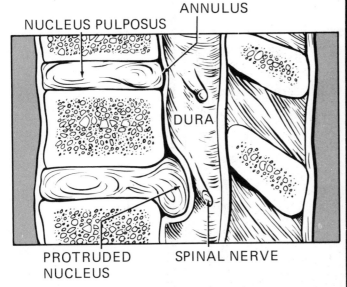

Figure 12.8. *Herniated intervertebral disc*

1. The function of the intervertebral disc is: 1. b

   a. motion of the vertebrae
   b. shock-absorber
   c. lubrication of joints

2. Which part of the disc herniates and presses on the nerve root?   2. b

   a. annulus
   b. nucleus pulposus

3. The disc is made of: 3. c

   a. bone
   b. muscle
   c. cartilage

Frame 6

This figure shows the alignment of the vertebrae and the spinal nerves which exit between them.

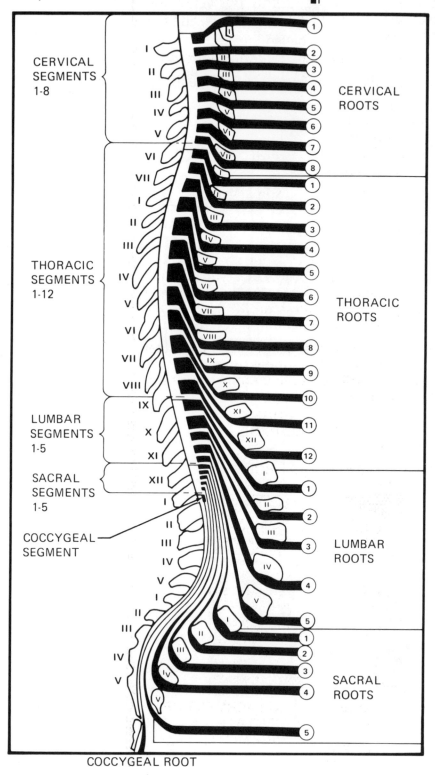

Figure 12.9. *Vertebrae and nerve roots*

Note that the spinal cord is divided into segments to correspond to adjacent vertebrae, and that the nerve roots are also numbered. (This figure shows nerves emerging on one side only. Recall that spinal nerves are paired and emerge on both sides of the vertebrae.)

Use the figure to answer the following questions.

1. How many paired spinal nerves emerge as

    a. cervical roots _____
    b. thoracic roots _____
    c. lumbar roots _____
    d. sacral roots _____
    e. coccygeal roots ____

2. There is a total of _____ spinal nerves.

1. a. 8
   b. 12
   c. 5
   d. 5
   e. 1

2. 31

Meninges

Frame 7

Ligaments attach the cord to the surrounding vertebral structures so that motion doesn't cause the cord to hit the bony structure with force. One of these is the dentate ligament.

Meningeal layers: dura, arachnoid and pia mater cover the cord and also supply protection. The membranes are a direct continuation of those surrounding the brain.

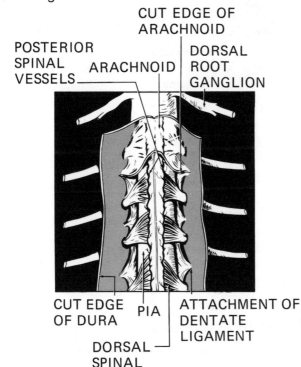

CUT EDGE OF ARACHNOID

POSTERIOR SPINAL VESSELS

ARACHNOID

DORSAL ROOT GANGLION

CUT EDGE OF DURA

PIA

ATTACHMENT OF DENTATE LIGAMENT

DORSAL SPINAL ROOT

Figure 12.10. *Support tissues for the cord*

True or False:

1. _____ The cord moves freely within the vertebral column.

2. _____ Cerebrospinal fluid flows in the subarachnoid space.

3. _____ The dura is the tough outer covering of the brain and cord.

1. False

2. True

3. True

Frame 8

The spinal cord extends to the level of about the second lumbar vertebra. The end of the cord is called the conus medullaris. Nerves from the cord descend down the column; they are called the cauda equina (horses tail). A segment of the pia meningeal layer continues to the coccyx. This is called the filum terminale.

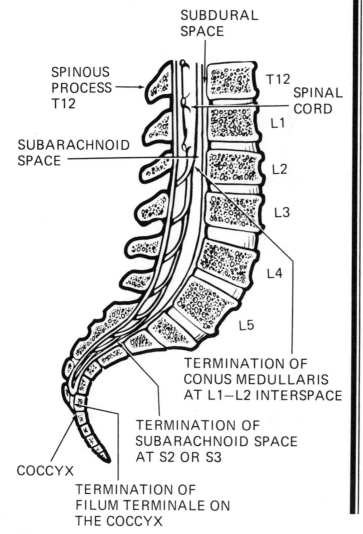

Figure 12.11. *Structures at the end of the cord*

1. The spinal cord ends at the level of
   _____ vertebra.

2. The segment of the meninges extending to the
   coccyx is the _____ _____ .

3. The cauda equina is composed of
   _____.

---

1. lumbar 2

2. filum terminale

3. nerves

PART II
BLOOD SUPPLY

Frame 9

There is not an extensive blood supply to the cord. The anterior and posterior spinal arteries branch from the vertebral and carotid arteries. Other blood supply comes from vessels which enter through each vertebral foramen with the spinal nerve. These are called radicular arteries. Unlike the brain, the collateral circulation of the cord is not well developed.

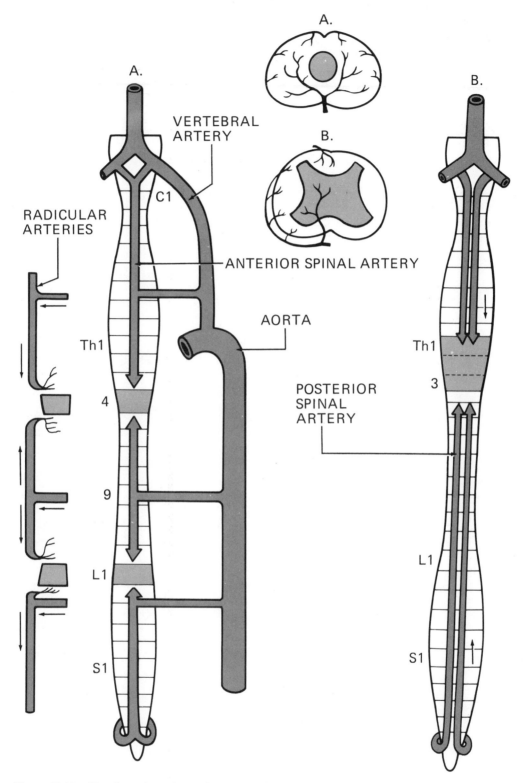

Figure 12.12. *Blood supply to the cord*

True or False:

1. _____ The vertebral artery is a main supplier of blood to the cord.

2. _____ When one artery in the cord is damaged, other arteries provide good collateral circulation.

3. _____ Each segment of the cord receives blood via the radicular arteries.

1. True

2. False

3. True

PART III
NERVE TRACTS

Sensory

Frame 10

The spinal cord serves as a pathway for transmission of impulses to and from the brain. Study the figure to find the important anatomic landmarks of the cord.

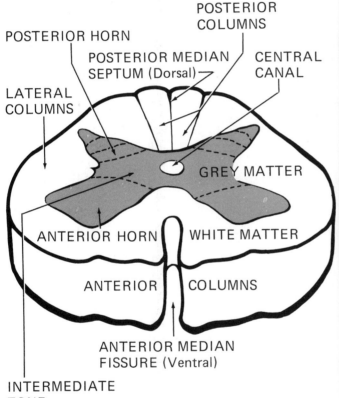

POSTERIOR COLUMNS

POSTERIOR HORN

POSTERIOR MEDIAN SEPTUM (Dorsal)

CENTRAL CANAL

LATERAL COLUMNS

GREY MATTER

ANTERIOR HORN

WHITE MATTER

ANTERIOR COLUMNS

ANTERIOR MEDIAN FISSURE (Ventral)

INTERMEDIATE ZONE

Figure 12.13. *Parts of the spinal cord*

1. The cord is divided in half by the _____ _____ fissure and the _____ _____ septum.

   1. anterior median, posterior median

2. The outer part of the cord is _____ matter.

   2. white

3. The inner grey matter is in the shape of the letter H. The "legs" of the H are called _____.

   3. horns

4. The horns and white matter positioned closer to the front of the body are called _____.

4. anterior

5. The _____ half of the cord is toward the back.

5. posterior

Frame 11

The spinal column is a relay system with temperature, pain, touch, vibration and proprioception impulses ascending from the periphery to the brain.

Recall that nerve fibers cross to the other side while traveling through the brain and cord. Sensory fibers cross

> immediately or soon after entering the cord
> or
> after entering the skull.

Therefore, sensation from the right side of the body is transmitted to the appropriate area in the left hemisphere.

True or False:

1. _____ All sensory fibers cross immediately after entering the cord.

1. False

2. _____ Sensory fibers terminate in the side of the brain opposite to the sensation.

2. True

Frame 12

The diagram depicts certain sensations being transmitted to the brain. Note the tracts that cross immediately upon entering the cord.

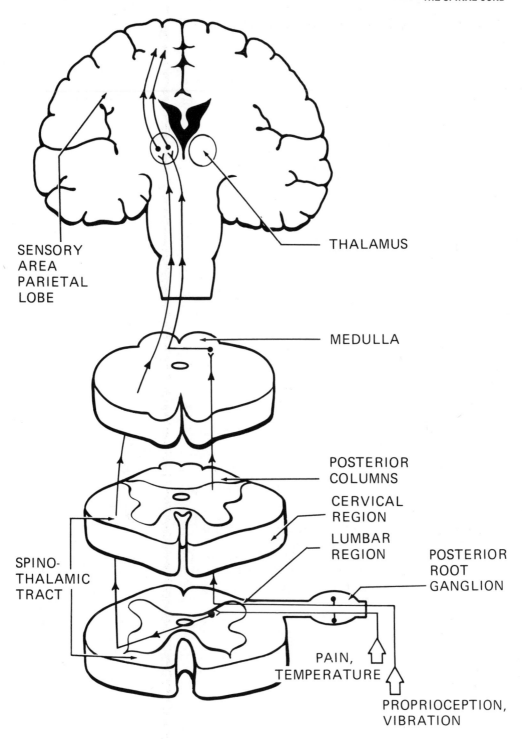

SENSORY
AREA
PARIETAL
LOBE

THALAMUS

MEDULLA

POSTERIOR
COLUMNS

CERVICAL
REGION

LUMBAR
REGION

POSTERIOR
ROOT
GANGLION

SPINO-
THALAMIC
TRACT

PAIN,
TEMPERATURE

PROPRIOCEPTION,
VIBRATION

Figure 12.14.   *Sensory tracts*

All sensory impulses enter the cord through the sensory portion of the spinal nerve.

Pain and temperature impulses synapse with other neurons. Shortly after entering the cord, they cross to the opposite side. The impulses then travel through the lateral spinothalamic tract (LST) to the thalamus.

True or False:

1. _____ The LST is a sensory tract.

2. _____ Sensations of pain and temperature enter the cord and are transmitted by the LST.

3. _____ Pain and temperature sensations do not cross in the cord.

4. _____ The LST ascends directly to the parietal lobe.

1. True

2. True

3. False

4. False, goes to the thalamus

Frame 13

Joe Carlson burns his right hand on his outdoor grill.

1. The sensations are carried in the _____ tract.

2. Sensations will _____ to the opposite side of the cord.

3. The _____ will recognize the stimulus and relay it to the sensory portion of the parietal lobe.

Don Hall has a transection of the left half of his spinal cord in the cervical area.

4. Pain and temperature sensations will not be transmitted from his _____ leg.

5. Sensation in the _____ leg will be normal.

1. LST

2. cross

3. thalamus

4. right

5. left

Frame 14

Refer again to Figure 12.14. Note that sensations of vibration and position (proprioception) travel on the same side in posterior columns to the medulla where they cross and proceed to the thalamus. The thalamus recognizes and sorts the impulses, relaying them to the appropriate localized area in the parietal lobe.

True or False:

1. _____ The posterior columns carry pain and temperature sensations.

2. _____ Vibration and proprioception are carried on uncrossed tracts.

3. _____ Posterior columns cross in the medulla.

1. False

2. True

3. True

Frame 15

Larry Link had trauma to the left posterior column of his cord. The effects would be:

1. loss of _____ and _____ sensations from his left leg

2. ability to sense vibrations in his _____ leg

3. unawareness of the _____ of his left leg

4. interpretation of sensations from the left side in the _____ parietal lobe.

1. vibration, proprioception

2. left

3. position

4. right

Frame 16

This diagram shows discrete sensory tracts in the cord. Note that the name of the tract indicates

location in the cord (lateral, anterior, posterior)
origination (spino)
termination (thalamic, cerebellar)

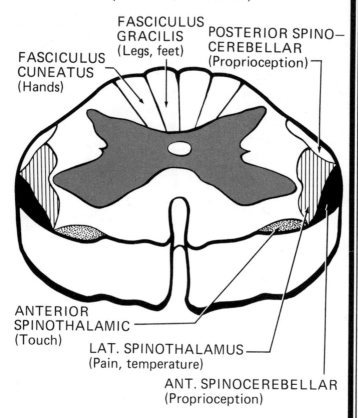

Figure 12.15. *Sensory tracts in the cord*

Frame 17

Figure 12.16 shows the areas of the body (dermatomes) specific to each peripheral nerve. The areas are not as discrete as pictured because damage to one nerve doesn't eliminate all sensory impulses from the area. Other nerves may contain a few fibers from the area.

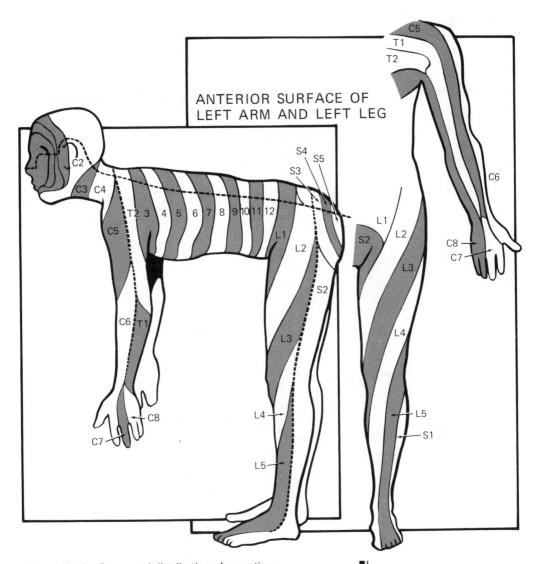

Figure 12.16. *Segmental distribution of sensation*

1. If S1 and S2 were cut, the (anterior/posterior) leg would be numb.

    1. posterior

2. Sensations from part of the hand travel via (C1-2-3/C6-7-8).

    2. C6-7-8

3. Sensory segments are (discrete/overlapping).

    3. overlapping

4. A patient who has damage to C4 and C5 would lack sensation in his (hands/shoulders).

    4. shoulders

Frame 18

Now put together what you know about sensory tracts and study the following figure.

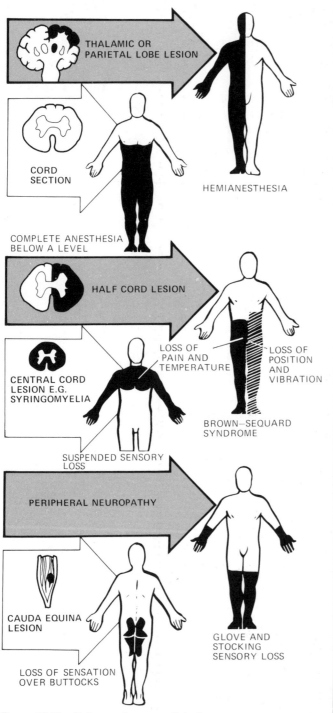

Figure 12.17. *Patterns of sensory disturbances*

True or False:

1. _____ If the thalamus is damaged, impulses are not relayed to the proper parietal area for sensation.

2. _____ A parietal tumor would disturb sensation on the same side as the lesion.

3. _____ If half of the cord is transected, position and vibration sense is lost on the same side.

4. _____ Because of early crossing of the pain and temperature impulses, loss of these sensations is contralateral.

5. _____ Central cord lesions interrupt pain and temperature impulse on both sides because fibers from both sides cross in the middle of the cord.

6. _____ A canda equina lesion interrupts impulses from S1 and S2.

1. True

2. False

3. True

4. True

5. True

6. False—S3, 4, 5

Motor

Frame 19

Motor tracts descend from the brain to the muscles of the body. Motor tracts cross in the medulla, therefore the left frontal lobe's motor strip controls movement on the right side of the body.

This drawing shows the descending motor tracts. Find the corticospinal tracts which transmit impulses for voluntary movement.

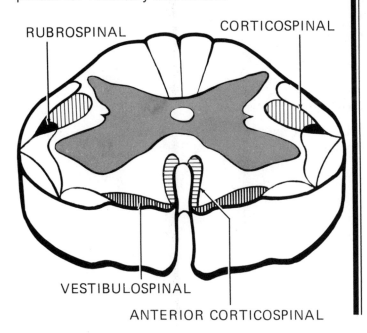

RUBROSPINAL   CORTICOSPINAL

VESTIBULOSPINAL

ANTERIOR CORTICOSPINAL

Figure 12.18. *Motor pathways in cord*

1. The corticospinal tracts originate in the _____ lobes of the brain.

   1. frontal

2. These carry impulses which control _____ _____.

   2. voluntary movement

3. They cross to the opposite side in the _____.

   3. medulla

4. Mr. Smith has a tumor in his right motor strip. He will be unable to move the corresponding part on his _____ side.

   4. left

5. Mr. Adams has damage to the corticospinal tract in the left side of his cord. He will be paralyzed on the _____ side.

   5. left (fibers cross in the medulla)

Extra-pyramidal Tracts

Frame 20

Look again at Figure 12.18 and find the rubrospinal, vestibulospinal and anterior corticospinal tracts. These tracts carry impulses which primarily control fine movements and muscle tone. These tracts originate in the basal ganglia of the brain.

True or False:

1. _____ Damage to the basal ganglia would cause problems with muscle tone and fine movement.

   1. True

2. _____ Extra-pyramidal tracts originate in the basal ganglia.

   2. True

3. _____ Damage to the rubrospinal tract would cause loss of sensation on the left.

   3. False

4. _____ Mrs. Wilson has Parkinson's disease which is due to dysfunction of the basal ganglia. She has rigidity due to increased muscle tone.

   4. True

5. _____ Fine tremors of Mrs. Wilson's hands are due to impulses from the basal ganglia transmitted by the extra-pyramidal tracts.

   5. True

Frame 21

Match the tracts with their functions.

1. _____ lateral spinothalamic	a. voluntary movement	1. c
2. _____ extra-pyramidal	b. simple touch	2. d
3. _____ posterior column	c. pain and temperature sense	3. e
4. _____ corticospinal	d. fine movements and muscle tone	4. a
	e. proprioception, vibration	

Match each brain area with its function.

5. _____ thalamus	f. facilitate or inhibit movement	5. h
6. _____ frontal lobe	g. voluntary motion	6. g
7. _____ parietal lobe	h. relay of sensory impulses to cortex	7. i
8. _____ basal ganglia	i. localize sensation	8. f

Frame 22

The spinal nerve as it exits from the vertebra is a mixed nerve containing both sensory and motor fibers. The posterior (sensory) root and the anterior (motor) root unite to form the spinal nerve. Both roots must be intact for a reflex to occur.

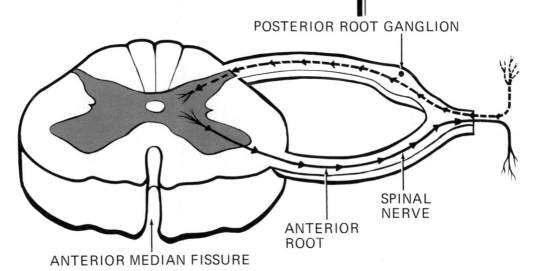

POSTERIOR ROOT GANGLION

SPINAL NERVE

ANTERIOR ROOT

ANTERIOR MEDIAN FISSURE

Figure 12.19. *Spinal nerve roots*

1. Cutting the _____root would relieve pain.

2. The anterior root contains _____fibers.

3. Cutting the anterior root would cause _____.

1. posterior

2. motor

3. paralysis

Frame 23

A reflex is a basic stimulus-response pattern that operates without voluntary or conscious control. Follow the pathways shown in the figure.

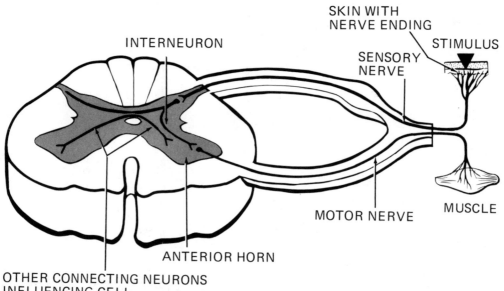

Sensations from the skin are sent via sensory fibers to the cord.

An interneuron connects the sensory and motor neurons.

The motor response travels through the motor fibers of the spinal nerve to the muscles, causing withdrawal from the stimulus.

This combination of the spinal nerve nucleus and fiber is called the lower motor neuron (LMN).

True or False:

1. _____ A reflex is voluntary.
2. _____ The cortex of the brain contributes to the lower motor neuron.
3. _____ If the motor fiber is destroyed the reflex will still be intact.
4. _____ Damage to the interneuron will disrupt the reflex arc.

1. False

2. False

3. False

4. True

Frame 24

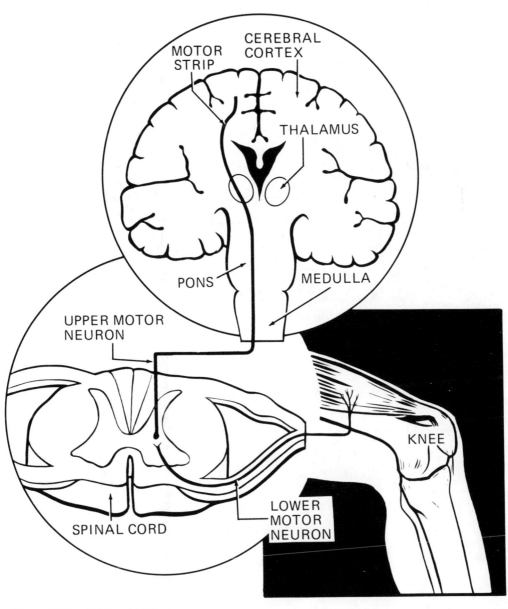

Figure 12.21. *UMN and LMN*

Motor neurons originate in the motor strip of the brain's frontal lobe. The fibers descend in the corticospinal tracts and synapse with an inter-neuron in the anterior horn cells of the spinal cord. The voluntary motor impulse is transmitted to the muscles by the motor fibers of the spinal nerve.

This combination of motor nerves in the cortex and the spinal cord fibers is called the upper motor neuron (UMN).

Indicate whether the following would cause UMN or LMN problems.

1. Damage to anterior root _____   1. LMN

2. Damage to motor strip _____   2. UMN

3. Damage to anterior horn cells _____   3. LMN

4. Damage to peripheral motor nerve _____   4. LMN

Frame 25

Remember that *upper* and *lower* refers to the neurons involved, not to how high in the cord the damage occurs.

True or False:

1. _____ A LMN injury can occur high in the cervical area of the cord.

1. True (damage to cervical spinal nerve)

2. _____ Any damage to the lower spinal cord (T12 to S5) is called LMN.

2. False (transection of descending tracts would be UMN)

PART IV
AUTONOMIC NERVOUS SYSTEM

Frame 26

The autonomic nervous system is a name given to a group of nerves that influence visceral activities in order to maintain a stable internal environment.

The neurons of the autonomic nervous system are made up of pre-ganglionic and post-ganglionic fibers. Pre-ganglionic fibers synapse with the post-ganglionic fibers to innervate the end organ. (Refer to Figures 12.22 and 12.23.)

True or False:

1. _____ The fibers of the autonomic nervous system within the spinal cord are pre-ganglionic fibers.

2. _____ Pre-ganglionic fibers synapse with post-ganglionic fibers.

3. _____ The autonomic nervous system regulates voluntary motor activity.

1. True

2. True

3. False

The autonomic system is most easily studied by dividing it into two systems, sympathetic and parasympathetic.

Sympathetic

Frame 27

The sympathetic system functions to prepare the body for fight or flight in stressful situations.

It stimulates the release of adrenalin which

—redirects blood flow to the most essential organs: brain, heart, lungs, skeletal muscles
—increases vascular volume and cardiac output
—mobilizes stored energy supplies to meet increased metabolic demands
—increases ventilation rate and volume.

Figure 12.22 shows the sympathetic system and the structures innervated. Note that the nerves are spinal in origin and exit between the vertebrae. The ganglia lie in a chain close to the cord.

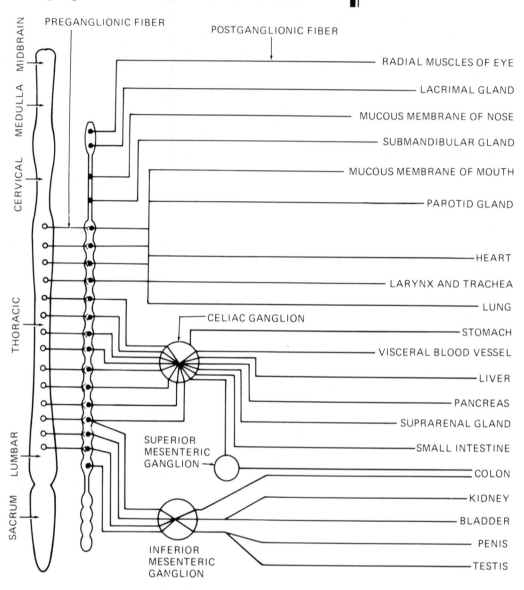

Figure 12.22. *Sympathetic system*

Parasympathetic

Frame 28

The parasympathetic nerves play a dominant role when the person is at rest. The regeneration of energy stores is its chief function, and its effects oppose those of the sympathetic system.

This drawing shows that the parasympathetic ganglia lie close to the end organ. Note also that all but one of the nerves is cranial in origin, and that the vagus (CN X) composes the largest segment of the system.

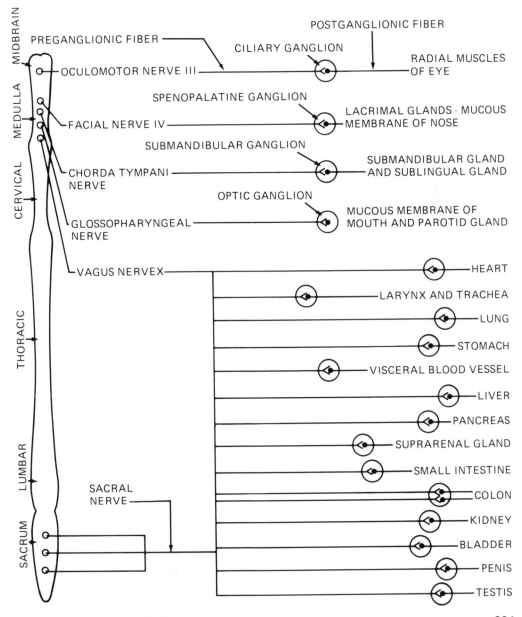

Figure 12.23. *Parasympathetic system*

Frame 29

The hypothalamus regulates and integrates the autonomic nervous system so that its effects precisely balance as the body's needs change.

Next review the effects of the autonomic system on major body structures.

Table 1. Functions of the Autonomic Nervous System

Structure	Sympathetic	Parasympathetic
Eye: Pupil	Dilatation	Contraction
Ciliary muscle	Relaxation and distance vision accommodation	Contraction and close-up vision accommodation
Glands: nasal, lacrimal, gastric, pancreatic, parotid, submaxillary	Vasoconstriction altering secretion	Increases thin, copious secretions
Sweat glands	Profuse sweating	No effect
Heart: Muscle	Increased rate and strength of contraction	Slows rate of contraction
Coronary arteries	Dilatation	Constriction
Lungs: Bronchi	Dilatation	Constriction
Blood vessels	Mild constriction	No effect
Intestine: Muscle	Decreased peristalsis	Increased peristalsis
Sphincter	Increased tone	Decreased tone
Liver	Glycogenolysis stimulated	No effect
Kidney	Output decreased	No effect
Penis	Ejaculation	Erection
Blood vessels: Abdominal	Constriction	No effect
External genitalia	Constriction	Dilatation
Skeletal muscle	Increased strength and glycogenolysis	No effect
Mental activity	Accelerated	No effect
Blood: Glucose	Increased	No effect
Coagulation	Increased	No effect

Source: Jones, D. et al, *Medical and Surgical Nursing,* NY: McGraw-Hill, 1978.

Frame 30

Write P for parasympathetic
    S for sympathetic

1._____	Raises cardiac output	1. S
2._____	Vagus nerve	2. P
3._____	Long pre-ganglionic fibers	3. P
4._____	Dilates pupil	4. S
5._____	Vasoconstriction	5. S
6._____	Dilates bronchi and increases ventilatory rate	6. S
7._____	Mobilizes stored glycogen	7. S
8._____	Increases peristalsis	8. P
9._____	Diaphoresis	9. S
10._____	Cranial and sacral nerves	10. P

CHAPTER 13

CAUSES OF SPINAL CORD DYSFUNCTION

Damage to the cord can result from many causes with either temporary or permanent loss of function. The symptoms depend on the area of the cord affected. Understanding the anatomy and pathology will enable you to provide knowledgeable nursing care.

At the conclusion of this chapter you will be able to:

1. List the major types of tumors found in the cord
2. Describe the differences found in flexion and extension injuries of the cervical spine
3. Differentiate section, compression, and contusion of the cord
4. Describe the basic mechanisms causing pathology in the spinal cord.

Chapter outline

Direct trauma to the cord
    Types of trauma
    Sequelae

Fractures of the cervical spine
    Flexion
    Extension

Tumors
    Kinds
    Sequelae

Herniated intervertebral disc

Interruption of blood supply

PART I
DIRECT TRAUMA
TO THE CORD

Types of Trauma

Spinal cord trauma is one of the main causes of disability in younger age groups. While trauma can occur at any level of the spinal column, injuries of the cervical vertebrae are most frequent.

Frame 1

Damage to the cord following trauma usually results from three mechanisms—contusion, laceration, or compression. Compression may be due to bone or tissue, blood clots, or edema pushing against the cord and interfering with the transmission of impulses. Relieving the compression may result in return of function if the period of compression has not been lengthy.

1. What are the three traumatic mechanisms which cause cord dysfunction?

   1. contusion, laceration, compression

2. What are three causes of cord compression?

   2. edema, hematoma, bone displacement

Frame 2

Contusion of the cord also occurs from trauma. The cord is more stable within the spinal column than the brain is within the skull so contusions from movement are less frequent. However, as portions of the vertebral column become dislodged, they often cause contusion of the cord. Because of poor collateral circulation in the cord, contusions often result in permanent damage.

The contused area is characterized by edema, petechial hemorrhages, and parenchymal tissue changes. Eventually demyelination and degeneration of the white matter takes place. The area becomes pale in appearance and tissues become soft and necrotic.

True or False:

1. _____ Contusions caused by movement of the cord are more common than contusions of the brain.

2. _____ The cord has good collateral circulation.

3. _____ Degeneration of white matter follows contusions.

4. _____ Edema following contusions interferes with blood supply to the area.

1. False

2. False

3. True

4. True

Frame 3

Less frequently than contusions, laceration or sectioning of the cord may result from trauma. Gunshot wounds and fracture-dislocations may cause laceration of the cord. The laceration results in permanent damage to the cord at the level of injury. Unfortunately cord tissue does not regenerate.

1. Transection of the spinal cord occurs (more/less) often than contusions.

2. Cord tissue (does/does not) regenerate.

1. less

2. does not

Frame 4

Trauma to the cord causes edema that interferes with the circulation to the cord and the transmission of impulses. It extends above and below the level of injury. Thus edema from an injury at C4 or C5 may result in respiratory difficulty because C2 and C3 segments are also affected. One method of treatment is to reduce edema by administration of corticosteroids.

1. What effect does edema have on the spinal cord?

1. interferes with circulation and transmission of impulses

2. What is one type of medication which will reduce edema?

2. corticosteroids

PART II
FRACTURES OF THE
CERVICAL SPINE

Flexion

Frame 5

Fractures of the cervical spinal column may be placed in two general categories: flexion injuries and extension injuries. Flexion fractures are the most frequent of the two. Figure 13.1 shows injury to the cord resulting from a flexion fracture-dislocation.

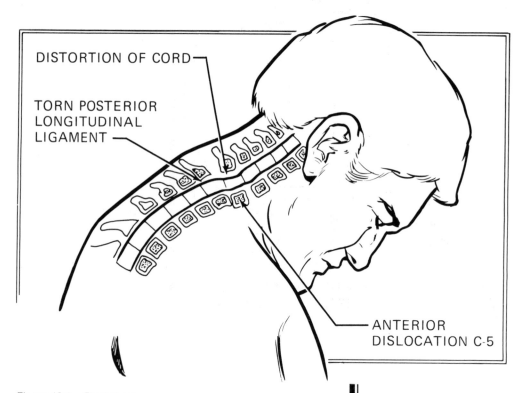

DISTORTION OF CORD

TORN POSTERIOR
LONGITUDINAL
LIGAMENT

ANTERIOR
DISLOCATION C-5

Figure 13.1. *Flexion injury*

Trauma which causes hyperflexion of the head may result in flexion fractures of the vertebrae and injuries to the cord. Processes involved include:

—The facets of the vertebrae may be dislocated forward and lock in place
—Fractures of spinous processes, pedicles, or lamina may occur and move to press against the cord

—The cord may be caught between two of the displaced vertebrae

—Disc fragments may be pushed out of place and against the cord.

Extension

Frame 6

Figure 13.2 depicts an injury to the spinal cord resulting from extension.

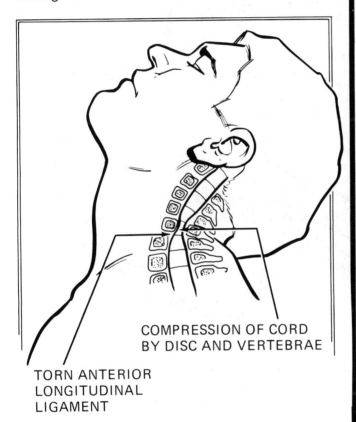

COMPRESSION OF CORD
BY DISC AND VERTEBRAE

TORN ANTERIOR
LONGITUDINAL
LIGAMENT

Figure 13.2. *Extension injury*

These result when the force is to the face and pushes the head backward. Damage to the anterior longitudinal ligament results in one vertebra being pushed backward while the vertebrae below remain more or less stable. Fractures of the vertebrae may or may not occur.

1. What ligament is injured in an extension injury?

1. anterior longitudinal

Would the following types of trauma result in a flexion (F) or extension (E) injury to the spine?

2. Diving accident in which back of head hits the diving board forcing the head forward.

2. F

3. Chin forced against the steering wheel in car accident.

3. E

4. Fall and striking back of head on stairs.

4. F

5. Blow under chin by attacker.

5. E

Frame 7

Not all injuries cause immediate damage to the cord. Sue Miles was in an automobile accident in which her head hit the windshield. She suffered an extension injury. Initially Sue had numbness over her entire body, but when admitted to the hospital no numbness or weakness was noted. While x-rays were being taken Sue's head was moved slightly, and she again experienced numbness and decreased strength in her hand grasp. Because the ligaments, especially the anterior ligaments, had been damaged, the spinal column was unstable and the cord was temporarily compressed. External stabilization of the vertebrae was needed to prevent cord damage.

1. Why is external stabilization needed in injuries to the spinal column when no cord damage has occurred?

1. To prevent it from occurring

Frame 8

Trauma to the lower spinal column is most frequent at T12, L1, L2. Direct violence to the area and forceful falls onto the feet or buttocks cause many of the injuries. The mechanisms for damage are similar to those in the cervical area.

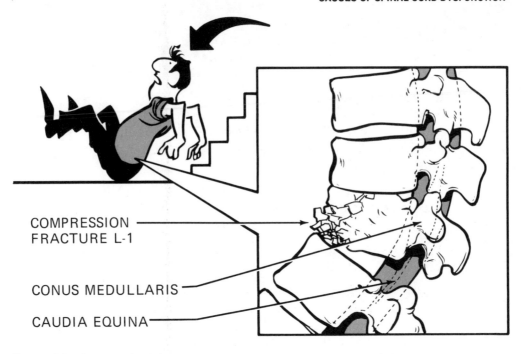

COMPRESSION FRACTURE L-1

CONUS MEDULLARIS

CAUDIA EQUINA

Figure 13.3. *Compression injury*

1. What thoracic vertebra is most frequently injured in a fall of several stories?

   1. T12

2. A fall onto buttocks would most likely cause damage of what lumbar vertebrae?

   2. L1, L2

Frame 9

Summary:

Mechanisms of damage due to trauma:

Compression → interference with impulse transmission, if relieved promptly function will return

Contusion → edema, hemorrhage, demyelination and degeneration of tissue, necrosis

Laceration → transection of nerve tracts with loss of function and no regeneration

Fractures of cervical spine:

Flexion: most frequent, due to blows to back of head. Damage due to locking of dislocated facets, dislocation of fractured parts, pinching of cord between dislocated segments, pressure of disc fragments

Extension: due to blows to the face. Damage to anterior longitudinal ligament causing instability of the vertebrae and pressure on the cord

Fractures of lower spine:

Most frequent at T12, L1 and L2 from falls onto feet or buttocks

Frame 10

Table 2 shows the motor dysfunction which occurs when specific levels of the spinal cord are damaged.

Table 2. Clinical Manifestations of Spinal Cord Damage

LEVEL OF CORD INJURY	MOTOR LOSS	SENSORY LOSS (PAIN, TOUCH, TEMPERATURE)	RESPIRATORY FUNCTIONING
Cervical			
C1 through C4	Complete quadriplegia	Complete sensory loss except for face	Complete loss of phrenic and intercostal nerve impulses to auxiliary muscles
C5	Complete quadriplegia with possible gross shoulder and wrist movement	Complete sensory loss below clavicles. Some sensation in lateral aspect of arms	Possible loss of phrenic and intercostal nerve stimulation to respiratory muscles
C6	Same as C5 with more control of wrist and shoulder movement	Same as C5 with additional sensation in arms and palmar surface of hands and thumb	Loss of intercostal nerve stimulation to auxiliary muscles of respiration
C7	Same as C6 with controlled flexion and minimally controlled extension of arms possible	Same as C6 with additional sensation in inner aspect of the arm and in the fingers	Same as C6
Thoracic			
T1 through T6	Paraplegia. Complete function of upper extremities; unable to assume standing position with braces	Loss of sensation on trunk and lower extremities at level of injury and below that level	Some interference with intercostal muscle functioning in high thoracic injuries
T7 through T12	Paraplegia. Increasingly able to control muscles of trunk; can assume standing position with brace support	Same as T1 through T6	No interference with respiratory function
Lumbar			
L1 through L2	Paraplegia. Increasingly controlled rotation of hip and flexion of leg as level of injury progresses from above down	Sensations to inner and anterior surfaces of thigh are supplied from above down by lumbar 1, 2, 3, and 4 sensory roots	No interference with respiratory function
Cauda Equina	Loss of ability to flex and extend foot. Loss of ability to rotate ankle and reduced ability to extend lower leg are possible alterations in motor functioning, depending on spinal nerve damaged	Alteration of sensation to outer and posterior surfaces of thighs and to the lower back and loss of perineal sensation can occur, depending on spinal nerve damaged	No alterations

Source: Moidel, H. et al, *Nursing Care of the Patient with Medical-Surgical Disorders*, NY: McGraw-Hill, 1976.

True or False:

1. _____ A complete section of the cord at C4 would necessitate assistance with respirations.

2. _____ A complete section of the cord at T3 would result in difficulty with hand movements.

3. _____ A complete lesion at the cauda equina would result in motor loss in the feet.

4. _____ Loss of sensation occurs at and below the level of injury.

1. True

2. False

3. True

4. True

PART III
TUMORS

Types

Frame 11

Tumors in the spinal column occur most frequently in the thoracic area of the spinal column. Several classification systems exist:

malignant or benign
intradural or extradural
intramedullary or extramedullary (inside or outside cord tissue)
primary or secondary malignant tumors.

Tumors may cause symptoms by pressure on the cord, pressure on the nerve roots, or interference with the blood supply.

This figure shows the location and frequency of various kinds of tumors.

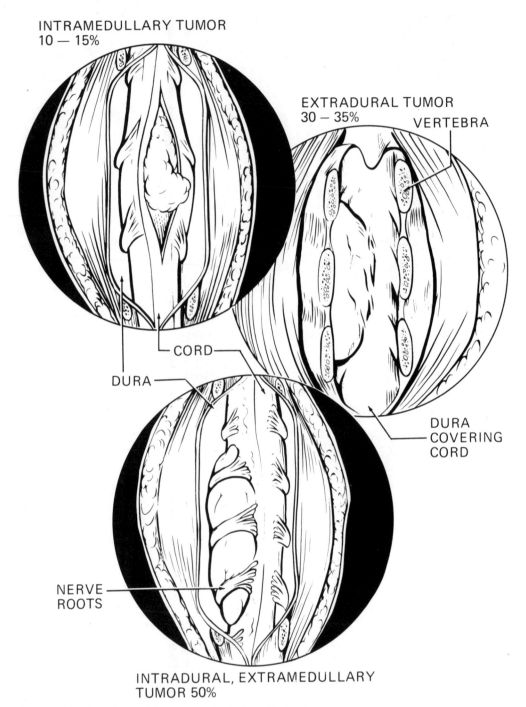

INTRAMEDULLARY TUMOR
10 — 15%

EXTRADURAL TUMOR
30 — 35%

VERTEBRA

CORD

DURA

DURA
COVERING
CORD

NERVE
ROOTS

INTRADURAL, EXTRAMEDULLARY
TUMOR 50%

Figure 13.4.   *Location and frequency of spinal cord tumors*

1. The most frequent level of cord tumors is in the (thoracic/lumbar) region.

1. thoracic

2. (Intramedullary/Extramedullary) location of tumors is most frequent.

2. Extramedullary

3. The following figure shows an (intradural/extradural) tumor.

3. intradural

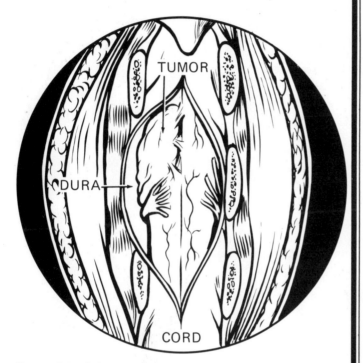

Figure 13.5. *Spinal cord tumor*

Frame 12

Characteristic findings for spinal cord tumors include:

  —Pain which is increased when the person reclines
  —Tingling, numbness, and coldness begin in one extremity progressing gradually up to the level of the tumor
  —Increasing clumsiness, weakness, and spasticity which correspond to the sensory spread
  —Urinary problem: initially urgency, followed by retention and overflow.

True or False:

1. _____ Pain in cord tumors is most intense in a sitting position.

1. False

2. _____ Initial bladder problems in a cord tumor include dribbling from overflow.

    2. False

3. _____ Numbness is found below the level of the tumor.

    3. True

Frame 13

Metastatic malignant tumors are common. The bony structures of the spinal column are frequent sites for metastasis because of the rich blood flow to the vertebral bodies. Primary sites include the breast, prostate, kidney and lung. Lymphomas are also common.

Tumors cause cord damage in two ways:

    a. Increased bone cell production with pressure on the cord (osteoblastic tumors)
    b. Bone destruction with collapse of vertebrae and spinal instability (osteoclastic tumors).

Metastatic tumors grow rapidly and the time period from initial pain from nerve root irritation to paralysis from cord compression may be only days.

1. List four common sites from which malignant tumors metastasize to the spinal column.

    1. breast, lung, prostate, kidney

2. Why is the spinal column prone to metastatic invasions?

    2. rich blood supply in bone

3. What are the two ways bone in the spinal column is affected by metastatic tumors?

    3. increased bone cell production, destruction of vertebrae

Frame 14

An example of a primary malignant extradural tumor is multiple myeloma. Tumor cells replace the cancellous bone of the vertebrae, weakening the structures. Compression of the vertebral bodies causes pinched nerve roots and eventual pressure on the cord.

True or False:

1. _____ Multiple myeloma replaces bone cells with tumor in the vertebral column.

   1. True

2. _____ Collapse of vertebral structures would compress the cord.

   2. True

Frame 15

Agnes Black entered the hospital because of severe back pain and some numbness and weakness in lower extremities. The neuro exam and diagnostic tests revealed a lesion at T8, 10. An intradural, extramedullary meningioma was found. Figure 13.4 in Frame 11 shows the tumor. Mrs. Black should get return of function unless the pressure on the cord caused permanent damage. Several nerve roots may have to be cut to remove the tumor but because they are in the thoracic region no difficulty should result from the surgery.

1. The nerve roots for T8,10 innervate the (diaphragm/intercostals).

   1. intercostals

2. Meningiomas (compress/invade) the cord.

   2. compress

3. Weakness in the lower extremities would be caused by pressure on the (lateral spinothalamic/corticospinal) tract.

   3. corticospinal (motor, refer to Chapter 12, Frame 19)

Frame 16

Intramedullary tumors arise from cells within the cord. They include angiomas, lipomas, dermoids, gliomas, and ependymomas. Ependymomas are the most common type.

Initial symptoms include bilateral impairment of pain and temperature sense below the level of the tumor. The tumors are very slow growing. Eventually muscle spasticity and fibrillations occur. Intramedullary tumors are extremely difficult to remove surgically without further damaging the cord. Even very small intramedullary tumors cause symptoms.

1. The most common type of an intramedullary tumor is the _____.

1. ependymoma

2. A person with an intramedullary glioma would initially experience a decrease in _____ and _____ sense below the level of the lesion.

2. pain, temperature

PART IV
HERNIATED
INTERVERTEBRAL DISCS

Frame 17

Herniated intervertebral discs are most common in the lumbar area as this part of the spinal column bears the strain of lifting, bending and other weight-bearing. Trauma may also cause an acute disc protrusion. L4 and L5 are the spaces where protruded discs are most likely to occur. Symptoms result from pressure on the nerve root. A disc at the L4,5 space causes radiating pain down the buttocks and posterolateral leg and paresthesia in the outer aspect of the calf, foot, and toes. A large protruded disc may cause paralysis. If a medical regimen of bedrest and traction does not relieve the symptoms, the disc is removed surgically. Since the nerve root was compressed, immediate elimination of symptoms may not occur.

True or False:

1. _____ L2 is the most common site for protruded discs.

1. False

2. _____ An accident may cause an acute disc protrusion.

2. True

3. _____ Buttock pain is found with an L4,5 disc protrusion.

3. True

4. _____ Surgical removal of the disc results in immediate resolution of symptoms.

4. False

PART V
INTERRUPTION OF BLOOD SUPPLY

Frame 18

Dissecting abdominal aortic aneurysms or clamping of vessels for vascular surgery may cause paralysis. If blood supply to the cord can be quickly restored, permanent paralysis will not occur. Because the cord does not have good collateral circulation, interruption of the blood supply poses extreme danger to cord function.

Trauma, tumors and vascular conditions also interrupt adequate blood flow to the cord.

1. What type of surgery may endanger blood supply to the cord?

1. repair of abdominal aortic aneurysm

2. Why is the cord more affected by interruption of blood supply than is the brain?

2. poor collateral circulation

Frame 19

Summary:

Tumors
Occur most often in thoracic area. May be:
—extradural, intradural or intramedullary.
—malignant or benign
—primary or secondary.
Damage due to pressure on cord and nerve roots or interference with blood supply
Symptoms: pain, paresthesias, motor difficulty, urinary problems

Herniated intervertebral discs
Most common in lumbar area due to trauma, lifting
Damage due to pressure on nerve root
Symptoms: pain and paresthesia along nerve root distribution, possible paralysis

Interruption of blood flow
   Due to dissecting abdominal aortic aneurysm or clamping of aorta for vascular surgery
   Results depend on length of interruption
   Cord has poor collateral circulation

CHAPTER 14

SPINAL CORD INJURY: NURSING ASSESSMENT AND INTERVENTION

Nursing assessment and care contribute much to the overall welfare of the cord-injured patient. Both physiologic and psychologic reactions require expert assessment and skilled interventions.

At the conclusion of this chapter you will be able to:

1. Associate physiologic findings with levels of dysfunction
2. Recognize changes indicative of deteriorating cord function
3. State the components of a nursing assessment for a patient with suspected active cord trauma
4. Define a reflex
5. Describe findings in spinal shock
6. Differentiate signs of upper motor neuron (UMN) and lower motor neuron (LMN) dysfunction
7. Identify the causes of autonomic hyperreflexia
8. Recognize the signs and symptoms of autonomic hyperreflexia
9. Describe typical psychologic reactions found in persons with paraplegia or quadriplegia

Chapter outline

Disruption of motor and sensory tracts
    Voluntary movement
    Sensation
    Reflex activity
        Spinal shock
        Spastic and flaccid paralysis
        Bladder and bowel function
        Sexual function

Respiratory status
    Respiratory muscle paralysis
    Nursing assessment
    Implications

Control of internal environment
    Cardiovascular regulation
    Temperature control
    GI motility
    Autonomic hyperreflexia

Psychologic reactions
    Shock
    Denial
    Regression
    Depression

PART I
DISRUPTION OF MOTOR
AND SENSORY TRACTS

Panel 1

Terry Brown, age 17, was admitted with an unstable fracture of C6, 7 sustained during a tumbling exercise at school. Immediately after the accident Terry said he felt numb all over and couldn't move anything. This lasted for only a few minutes. He had no motor or sensory deficits on admission to the hospital.

Emergency care included keeping Terry's neck in alignment and immobilizing him on a back-board. Initial movement of the patient is critical to preventing permanent cord damage. Terry was not moved until the paramedics arrived. One paramedic maintained Terry's head in alignment and prevented flexion and extension. The others lifted Terry onto a back-board and secured his head to the board to prevent movement.

If professional assistance in moving a back-injured person is not available, a door or a solid frame can be used for a back-board. The person's head is secured to the board with towels or strips of cloth. Sandbags, shoes filled with sand, or other solid objects can be used to maintain alignment.

X-rays showed an anterior inferior fracture of C6. Trauma to the cord could be caused by shifting of bone fragments which would press against the cord. Early detection of the signs of cord compression will allow the physician to readjust the traction and immobilization of the area.

Frame 1

1. Choose the most important consideration in giving emergency care to a person with possible back injury:

   a. Monitor vital signs
   b. Immobilize the head and spine before transporting
   c. Keep the neck flexed
   d. Test to see how well the patient can move his legs

1. b

2. Why were the paramedics careful to maintain alignment of Terry's head?

   a. Movement could cause loss of consciousness
   b. To prevent unnecessary pain
   c. To prevent movement of vertebral bone fragments

2. c

Voluntary Movement

Frame 2

Terry was admitted to the neuro ICU and Jill Collins, R.N., was responsible for his care. She monitored him closely for changes in voluntary movement, sensation, reflex activity and sphincter control.

To test voluntary movement of arms and legs, Jill used the techniques you learned in Chapter 5, Frame 38. She asked Terry to squeeze her hands and move each arm and leg. In addition she checked the spinal nerves which emerge from C6–7 by having Terry rotate his arms externally and extend his elbow and wrist.

Table 1. Assessment Guide to Determine Approximate Level of Spinal Cord Lesion

Cord Level Associated With Motion	Movement To Be Requested of the Patient	Body Part To Be Observed	Cord Level Associated With Sensation in Each Listed Body Part*
S2-S4	Tighten the muscle around my finger (finger in anal sphincter)	Perineum	S5
L5, S1, and S2	Bend and straighten your toes	Toes	L5
L2-L4	Straighten your leg	Knees	L3
L1-L3	Bend (flex) your hip	Hips	L2
T5-T12	Tighten your abdomen	Abdomen Pubis Navel Nipple line	L1 T10 T4
C8-T1	Oppose your thumb to each finger tip; make a fist	Thumb, first two digits, little finger	C6 C7 T1
C6	Bend your wrist up (only the radial wrist extensor will contract)	Wrist	C6 (thumb side of wrist)
C5	Bend your elbow	Elbow	Radial side C6 Ulnar side T1
C3, C4, and C5	Shrug your shoulders; take a deep breath (diaphragm descends causing abdomen to bulge; upper chest does not move)	Shoulder, chest, and abdomen	C4

*Light touch, pinprick, position.

Source: Jones, D. et al, Medical and Surgical Nursing, NY: McGraw-Hill, 1978.

1. If a motor nerve root is damaged, motion is decreased:

    a. on the same side
    b. on the opposite side

    1. a

2. If Terry had weakness in making a fist with his right hand, Jill should:

    a. not be surprised as this is expected with his level of damage
    b. notify the physician
    c. institute a regimen of active exercise

    2. b (he had no motor deficit on admission)

3. Which of the following processes could cause pressure on the cord and motor deficits?

    a. edema
    b. hematoma formation
    c. displacement of bone fragments
    d. disc protrusion

    3. all

4. Weakness of one side, or of the entire body below the arms, would indicate pressure on the:

    a. ventral or anterior cord
    b. dorsal roots

    4. a

5. Which of the following tests would detect dysfunction at the T-1 level?

    a. tighten abdominal muscles
    b. shrug shoulders
    c. make a fist
    d. bend elbow

    5. c

Sensation

Frame 3

Jill checked Terry's response to pain, light touch, and proprioception at various levels of his body. She asked Terry to look away and to tell her when he felt her touch. She used both firm pressure and light touch to all extremities and his trunk.

Jill then asked Terry to close his eyes. She flexed and extended one finger of each hand and a toe on each foot asking Terry to tell her if it was straight or flexed. This tests proprioception (position sense).

1. If Terry were unable to sense pain in his legs, there would be damage to the (spinothalamic/ corticospinal) tract.

1. spinothalamic

2. Loss of proprioception on the right would indicate pressure on the (posterior/anterior) columns on the same side.

2. posterior

3. Bill Stein has a spinal cord transection at T-1. He would have complete loss of sensation on (one side/both sides) of the body below the lesion.

3. both sides

4. Mr. Stein has to look at his foot to tell if it is caught under the foot rest of his wheelchair. This is due to loss of (proprioception/ cerebellar inhibition).

4. proprioception

Frame 4

Bill Stein's loss of motion and sensation has important implications for nursing care.

1. Choose the nursing problems you would expect.

1. all

   a. alteration in body image
   b. disuse phenomena
   c. injury to extremities—excessive heat, cold, trauma

2. Which of the following actions should be included in the care plan?

2. a, b, d

   a. teach patient to visually check position of extremities
   b. turning schedule and inspection of skin over bony prominences
   c. use of hot water bottles for warmth
   d. passive range of motion
   e. check for sensation of pain by pricking the skin with a pin

Reflex Activity

Frame 5

Immediately after a spinal injury at any level there is usually flaccid paralysis and retention of urine. This is called spinal shock. It is thought that sudden interruption of impulses from the brain causes cessation of all cord functions below the injury. Spinal shock may last from a few days to several weeks or persist for several months. The return of reflex activity indicates the end of spinal shock.

True or False:

1. _____ Spinal shock causes increased reflex activity.

2. _____ Spinal shock is an immediate result of cord injury.

1. False

2. True

Frame 6

Reflex activity returns and becomes hyperactive, causing spastic contraction of muscles. This is often mistaken for return of voluntary movement by the patient and needs to be explained. Patients with cervical injury usually have a return of reflex activity in 4-6 weeks.

True or False:

1. _____ Spasticity is not indicative of return of voluntary movement.

2. _____ Mr. Stein (transection at T1) begins to have involuntary, uncoordinated movements of his legs. This indicates that spinal shock is over.

1. True

2. True

Frame 7

Transection of the cord results ultimately in spasticity below the level of injury. Sensory impulses come into the cord and connect with the motor segment. Contact with the inhibitory fibers from the brain is lost so the resulting muscle contraction is intense and uncoordinated.

True or False:

1. _____ A patient with spinal cord damage has hypertonic reflexes because they are not suppressed by impulses from the brain.

2. _____ The corticospinal and extra-pyramidal tracts carry impulses to inhibit and coordinate reflect movements.

3. _____ A patient with cord transection at L2 would have permanent flaccid paralysis of his legs.

1. True

2. True

3. False

359

Frame 8

Bowel and bladder function are also reflex activities which are abnormal in cord injury.

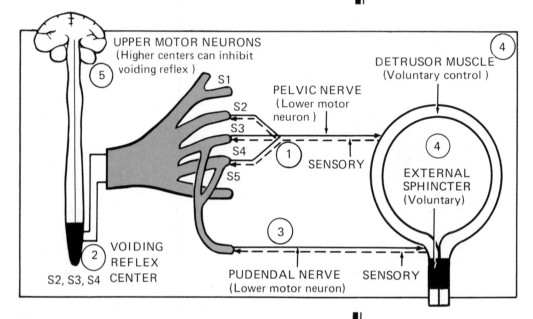

Figure 14.1. *Normal voiding reflex*

Normally, bladder distention (250–400 ml) causes stretch receptors in the detrusor muscle to send impulses through the pelvic nerves to the S2,3,4 segments of the cord (1,2). The external and internal sphincters are connected via the pudendal nerves to S3 and 4. Voiding occurs when the detrusor muscles contract and the sphincter relaxes (4). The frontal lobe of the brain provides voluntary control over voiding (5).

1. Which two spinal nerves are needed for voiding?

2. What is the role of the frontal lobe in micturition?

3. Where in the spinal column is the voiding reflex center.

1. pudendal, pelvic

2. voluntary control

3. S2,3,5

Frame 9

During spinal shock there is no reflex activity in the cord. The flaccid bladder distends to retain large amounts of urine. The normal sensations of fullness are lost. Small amounts of urine are voided, but the bladder remains distended. This is called retention with overflow. Drainage by catheter is necessary to prevent damage to the bladder wall and infection.

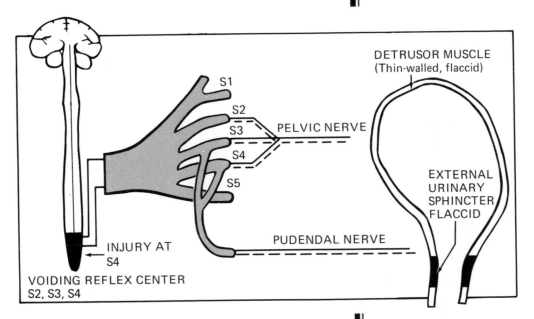

Figure 14.2. *Flaccid bladder during spinal shock*

True or False:

1. _____ During this period the nurse should keep careful intake and output records.

2. _____ During spinal shock a patient might void 50 ml and retain 500 ml in his bladder.

3. _____ Catheterization would not be necessary during this period.

4. _____ Palpation of the abdomen for bladder distention should be done at intervals.

1. True

2. True

3. False

4. True

If the spinal nerves (pudendal and pelvic) were severed the patient would have a flaccid bladder permanently.

Frame 10

After spinal shock ends, reflex activity returns but the pathways to the brain are not intact. The patient has no control over voiding.

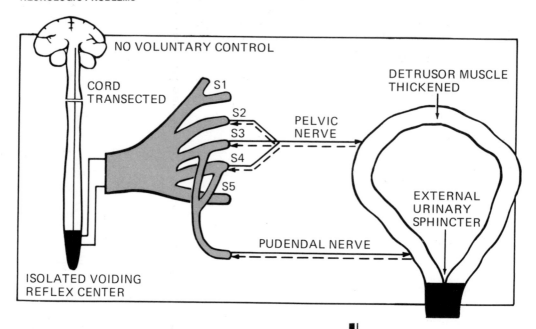

Figure 14.3. *Spastic bladder*

Bladder function is characterized by:

small capacity
hyperirritable detrusor muscle and sphincter
loss of inhibition of reflex from the brain.

The patient will have frequent, incomplete void-ings of urine because sphincter relaxation is not coordinated with bladder contraction.

1. What would be expected in a patient with spi-nal cord transection at C6?

    a. voids 100 ml q2h
    b. voids 200 ml q24h
    c. voids 600 ml q12h

1. a

Frame 11

Several simple tests may be done to evaluate bladder function. Check the integrity of the pelvic nerve by instilling cold sterile saline via a straight catheter. If the pelvic nerve reflex is not damaged, the catheter and saline will be forcefully expelled. The integrity of the pudendal nerve reflex is eval-uated by inserting a finger into the rectum to see if the rectal sphincter contracts.

True or False:

1. _____ Expulsion of the catheter in the ice test
indicates that the pelvic nerve is intact.

1. True

2. _____ Contraction of the rectal sphincter when a finger is inserted indicates damage to the pudendal nerve.

3. _____ A patient with a C6 lesion will be able to voluntarily control urination.

2. False

3. False

Frame 12

Urinary retention increases the risk of bladder infection in both flaccid and spastic bladder conditions.

1. List all the nursing measures you can think of to prevent infection.

1. Sterile technique with catheter and drainage, perineal care, encourage fluids, careful intake and output records, keep urine pH acidic

Frame 13

Because voluntary control of bowel evacuation may be lost, regulation of bowel movements is accomplished by adequate fecal bulk, timing and artificial stimulation of the reflex. A diet adequate in fiber results in formed feces which stimulates the sphincter to relax. Suppositories or digital stimulation may also be used to promote defecation. Records of bowel movements are kept so that impaction and distention are recognized and prevented.

1. Why does the patient have bowel movements even if the corticospinal tract is interrupted?

1. fecal bulk stimulates the sphincter to relax

Frame 14

Mike Murphy, a construction worker, fell several stories from a building ledge and landed on his feet on a concrete surface. Mike suffered a comminuted or "bursting fracture" of the bodies of L2 and L3 vertebrae. He had a complete cord lesion at this level.

1. What deficits would you find in Mr. Murphy? (Hint: Review Chapter 13, Frame 10.)

   1. Loss of bowel and bladder control, paralysis of legs

2. For several days after admission you would expect him to have what kind of bladder problems?

   2. flaccid bladder with retention and overflow

3. After spinal shock is over, what kind of bladder problems would occur?

   3. spastic bladder with frequent incomplete voiding

Frame 15

The ability for sexual functioning cannot be predicted immediately. Since Mr. Murphy's trauma was in the lumbar area, damage to the nerves for erection may have occurred. S2,3,4 nerves control erection. T11 to L2 contains the sympathetic fibers for seminal emission. Ejaculation is controlled by sacral nerves S2,3,4.

If the sacral reflex arc is not damaged, Mr. Murphy can have reflex erections. Most quadriplegics and paraplegics are able to have reflex erections. They do not, however, have any sensation. Only a small percentage, about 10%, have ejaculation.

The female will have menstrual periods, be able to become pregnant and have a vaginal delivery.

1. Why may Mike be unable to have an erection?

   1. Sacral nerves may have been damaged in lumbar area

2. Why is there question about his ability to have children?

   2. Seminal emission is controlled by T11-L2

Frame 16

Summary:

Emergency care: keep spine in alignment, prevent neck flexion/extension, immobilize patient to prevent cord injury from shifting of bone fragments.

Disruption of motor and sensory tracts
Assess: voluntary movement, strength, specific movements controlled by involved spinal segment
sensation of pain and light touch and proprioception

Plan: to prevent traumatic injury and disuse phenomena.

Reflexes

Spinal shock: period of flaccid paralysis and complete retention of urine lasting days to months after injury
Return of reflexes: spastic paralysis, hypertonic reflexes, due to loss of brain inhibition and coordination

Bladder and bowel function

Flaccid bladder: retention and overflow
Spastic bladder: small capacity, frequent voiding with retention due to uncoordinated reflex

Plan: to prevent bladder infection

Bowel evacuation: involuntary, due to stimulation of defecation reflex

Sexual function

Male: S2,3,4 controls erection and ejaculation. T11 to L2 control seminal emission. May have reflex erection, 10% have ejaculation. No sensation.
Female: Normal menstruation and child-bearing capacity, no sensation.

PART II
RESPIRATORY STATUS

Panel 2

Another patient on the acute neuro unit is Mary Anderson, age 20. Mary was injured in a diving accident, and has a fracture dislocation at C5 with paralysis and anesthesia below that segment. She is still in the period of spinal shock with flaccid paralysis, absent reflexes, and a flaccid bladder.

Respiratory function is a prime concern for Mary. There are several factors which affect respiratory status in patients with cervical spine injuries.

The phrenic nerve to the diaphragm exits at C3–4. Ascending edema may temporarily affect these segments of Mary's cord, paralyzing the diaphragm and significantly decreasing ventilation.

A complete cervical spine lesion results in paralysis of the intercostal and abdominal muscles. The role of the intercostal muscles in respiration is to assist in expansion of the rib cage for inspiration. Paralysis of the intercostals causes a 60% decrease in effective ventilation. The abdominal muscles assist primarily with expiration, which blows off CO_2.

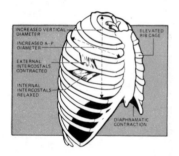

Figure 14.4. *Muscles of inspiration*

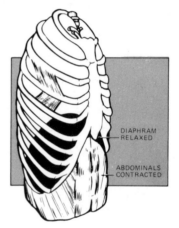

Figure 14.5. *Muscles of expiration*

Diaphragm (C3–4)
External intercostals (T2–L1)
Sternocleidomastoids (CN XI)
Scapular elevators plus anterior
  Serrati (C5–6)
Scalene (C6–8)
Erectus muscles of spine

Abdominals (T7–12)
Internal intercostals (T2–L1)
Posterior inferior serrati (C5–6)

Patients with cervical cord injuries also have difficulty coughing which increases chances of respiratory problems. Coughing relies on action of the abdominal and intercostal muscles to build up pressure in the chest and abdominal cavities in order to force air through the larynx. Inability to cough up secretions makes the patient susceptible to pulmonary complications.

There are two respiratory control centers in the CNS:

> *Voluntary center—cortex of the brain*
> *Involuntary center—brainstem (pons and medulla)*

Because the corticospinal tracts carry both voluntary and involuntary fibers, results of damage may vary. Some patients may lose involuntary respiratory control and still be able to maintain voluntary control.

Effects of cord transection:

> *Above C3—apnea and respiratory arrest*
> *C3 to C4—damage to the phrenic nerve which exits at this segment of the cord*
> *T12 and above—paralysis of abdominal and intercostal muscles*

Respiratory Muscle Paralysis

Frame 17

Panel 2 will help you answer these questions.

1. If a patient's transection is at C4, this results in:

   a. apnea
   b. paralysis of the diaphragm
   c. paralysis of abdominal muscles
   d. paralysis of intercostal muscles

1. b, c, d

2. Mary's loss of the abdominal and intercostal muscles will decrease respiration by:

   a. 100%
   b. 60%
   c. 40%
   d. 10%

2. b

3. Which muscles of respiration have not been affected by her C5 lesion?

   a. diaphragm
   b. abdominal and intercostal
   c. sternocleidomastoid
   d. scaleni

3. a, c, d

4. Will Mary be able to cough effectively?

   a. yes, because her diaphragm is not involved
   b. yes, because all muscles needed for cough are innervated
   c. no, because she lacks abdominal and intercostal innervation

4. c

Nursing Assessment

Frame 18

When Jill Collins assessed Mary Anderson's respiratory status she noted:

Muscles used in ventilation:

Mary was using her neck and shoulder muscles to elevate her ribs. These are called the accessory muscles for ventilation. More energy (and therefore oxygen) is used when the work of breathing is increased.

Mental status:

One of the first signs of hypoxia is restlessness progressing to confusion. CO_2 retention causes lethargy and headache.

Color and respiratory pattern:

More rapid rate, ashen or cyanotic skin and fatigue indicate hypoxia and/or CO_2 retention.

Vital capacity (V.C.):

A spirometer can be used for measurement or V.C. can be estimated. Jill asked Mary to take a deep breath and count out loud, fast and distinctly without taking a second breath. Each number represents about 100 ml of V.C. Vital capacity below 100 ml should be reported to the physician.

Arterial blood gases:

Blood is drawn for this purpose if there are any signs of hypoxia.

Normal values:
PO_2 = 80–100 mm Hg
PCO_2 = 35–45 mm Hg
O_2 saturation = 95% or greater

Breath sounds

Jill listened for abnormal or absent breath sounds over Mary's lung fields twice each shift.

1. An early sign of hypoxia is _____.

1. restlessness

2. The neck and shoulder muscles are called _____ muscles of respiration.

    2. accessory

3. Mary can count to 3 on one breath. Her V.C. is about _____ ml.

    3. 300

Implications

Frame 19

Spinal cord patients who have respiratory in-adequacy are treated with

artificial ventilation
phrenic nerve pacing for high cervical lesions in which the phrenic nerve is intact.

1. Jill's nursing care plan for Mary should include what nursing actions to maintain respiratory adequacy?

    1. frequent turning, suctioning if necessary, humidifier in room and good fluid intake to keep secretions moist, chest percussion to loosen secretions, intermittent positive pressure breathing, teach breathing exercises

Frame 20

Summary:

Spinal cord injury disrupts respiratory function
above C3—apnea and respiratory arrest
C3 to C4—damage to phrenic nerve with paralysis of diaphragm
T12 and above—paralysis of abdominal and intercostal muscles needed for chest movements and coughing

Assessment: use of accessory muscles, mental status, color, respiratory pattern, vital capacity, arterial blood gases, breath sounds

Plan: to prevent airway obstruction, prevent pooling of secretions, assist chest expansion

PART III
CONTROL OF INTERNAL ENVIRONMENT

Cardiovascular Regulation

Frame 21

Hypotension is common in patients with spinal cord injuries. Mary's BP was 80/50. Because of paralysis of the sympathetic chain of ganglia, vasodilation and loss of the vasomotor reflex occur. Decreased or absent muscle tone eliminates the muscles' contribution to venous return from the legs. Elastic stockings or ace bandages help to reduce peripheral venous pooling.

1. What are two causes of hypotension in Mary's case?

   1. vasodilation, lack of muscle tone

2. What nursing intervention would help elevate the BP?

   2. application of elastic hose or ace bandages

Frame 22

Orthostatic hypotension is a serious problem. Methods used to accustom the patient to upright posture include:

   —very gradual tilting of the CircOlectric bed or tilt table, slowly increasing the angle of incline and time spent upright

   —use of an anti-gravity suit (space suit) when upright, or

   —elastic hose and abdominal binder to prevent venous pooling.

1. Mary Anderson is on a CircOlectric bed and is upright briefly as the bed is turned. This (will/will not) be a hazard.

   1. will

2. Orthostatic hypotension causes (fainting/papilledema).

3. What nursing actions should be planned when turning Mary?

2. fainting

3. Use elastic hose and abdominal binder, turn bed very gradually and monitor BP, pulse, and subjective signs carefully

Frame 23

Venous thrombosis is another hazard for Mary because of:

immobilization
muscle paralysis
vasomotor paralysis
venous stasis of blood.

Because Mary is unable to detect pain in her calf or thigh, Jill will inspect these areas for redness and warmth. She measures Mary's legs in the calf area. In thrombophlebitis, edema causes increased circumference. In addition, she will be careful to prevent trauma to Mary's legs during position changes and hygienic care.

Pulmonary embolism is a serious sequela of venous thrombosis that further diminishes respiratory capacity.

1. Two indications of thrombosis in a leg are _____ and _____ of skin.

1. redness, warmth

2. Respiratory difficulties could result from a _____ _____.

2. pulmonary embolus

3. What nursing actions can prevent venous thrombosis?

3. Use of elastic hose, range of motion and position changes, prevent trauma by careful handling of extremities

Temperature Control

Frame 24

During spinal shock, the skin of Mary's arms, trunk and legs is dry and cool. Trauma to her spinal cord at C5 disrupted the sympathetic connections between the midbrain and peripheral nerve ganglia. As a result, Mary's body has lost the ability to automatically adjust to changes in internal and external temperature.

Factors reducing heat loss	Factors increasing heat loss
Inability to sweat below the level of the lesion Reduced ventilatory volume	Vasodilation (due to loss of sympathetic influence)

Jill Collins needs to assess Mary's temperature as well as the environmental temperature, and to take actions to reduce wide fluctuations.

True or False:

1. _____ The only body area where Mary perspires is on her head and neck.

2. _____ Mary has a bladder infection with temperature spikes to 103°F. A hypothermia blanket would not be useful to lower her temperature.

3. _____ Since the ICU is kept very cool, Jill should cover Mary with extra blankets to prevent heat loss if her body temperature is normal.

4. _____ Mary's temperature should be taken twice a day.

1. True

2. False

3. True

4. False—q2–4h

GI Motility

Frame 25

Paralytic ileus frequently occurs in patients with spinal cord trauma because of disruption of the autonomic nervous system.

Abdominal distention may contribute to decreased lung expansion and respiratory problems.

Constipation and impaction are frequent problems.

Distention decreases the blood supply to the intestinal wall and leads to venous thrombosis and necrosis of the bowel wall.

Distention also interferes with absorption of vital nutrients from the small intestine.

Assessment includes observation for distention and listening for bowel sounds.

1. Paralytic ileus is a result of interruption of the (autonomic/motor) system.

2. In paralytic ileus there are (increased/decreased) bowel sounds.

3. Blood supply to the bowel wall (is/is not) affected.

4. Malabsorption of nutrients increases development of (disuse phenomena/spasticity).

1. autonomic

2. decreased

3. is

4. disuse phenomena

Frame 26

Bowel motility is encouraged by:

diet adequate in bulk
reduced amount of gas-forming food in diet
daily bowel program with artificial stimulation of defecation reflex
adequate fluid intake.

1. Establishing a bowel routine for Mary will include

    a. Use of suppositories or digital stimulation of the rectal sphincter
    b. Varying the time of day for the program
    c. Recording fluid intake, number and character of bowel movements
    d. Waiting until the spinal shock period is over to plan a bowel program

1. a, c

Frame 27

Summary:

Cardiovascular

Hypotension—paralysis of sympathetic chain with vasodilation and loss of vasomotor reflex and ↓ muscle tone → poor venous return, orthostatic hypotension, venous thrombosis

Assess: BP, P, toleration of upright position, signs of thrombosis in legs

Plan: to prevent venous stasis and trauma to legs, to gradually accustom the patient to upright position.

Temperature Control

Loss of sympathetic influences causes inability to sweat below the lesion and vasodilation. Body cannot automatically adjust to temperature changes.

Assess: body and room temperatures
Plan: to artificially reduce high temperature; to prevent heat loss

GI Motility

Loss of autonomic innervation to the small and large intestine causes paralytic ileus, venous thrombosis, ischemia of bowel wall, malabsorption, constipation and impaction.

Assess: Bowel sounds, abdominal distention, adequacy of elimination

Plan: Bowel program to promote elimination.

Autonomic Hyperreflexia

Panel 3

Cedric Burns suffered high thoracic cord trauma one year ago. He returned to the hospital two weeks ago to have surgery to stabilize his spine. Cedric was sitting in his wheel chair when Jill Collins entered his room to answer the light. She noted that he was diaphoretic and his face was flushed. Cedric said, "My head feels like a million hammers are in it." His blood pressure was 260/148 and his pulse was 46. In addition, Cedric had piloerection (hair on the body erect). Jill recognized these symptoms as autonomic hyperreflexia, notified the physician immediately, and began to assess the cause.

The symptoms of autonomic hyperreflexia, a dire threat to some patients with spinal cord injury, are triggered by distention or contraction of the bladder or rectum, stimulation of pain receptors, or stimulation of the skin. Immediate removal of the triggering factor is the essential treatment.

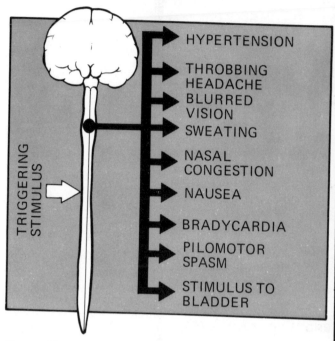

Figure 14.6. *Autonomic hyperreflexia*

Frame 28

The mechanism for autonomic hyperreflexia occurs as follows:

A. Sensory receptors below the level of the cord lesion are stimulated.
B. The intact autonomic reflex arc causes reflex arteriolar spasm and elevation of blood pressure. There is profuse sweating above the level of the lesion.
C. The baroreceptors in the carotid sinus, aorta, and cerebral vessels detect the elevated BP and stimulate CN IX and CN X for the parasympathetic action to decrease BP. The heart rate is slowed but because of the cord lesion efferent impulses cannot reach the visceral and peripheral vessels to initiate vasodilation.

Notice that stimuli such as:

distention or contraction of the bladder or rectum

stimulation of pain receptors
stimulation of the skin

cause autonomic hyperreflexia. The stimulus must be intense and constant to trigger autonomic hyperreflexia.

1. Number these statements from 1 to 4 in order of occurrence in autonomic hyperreflexia.

_____ Baroreceptors detect elevated BP and seek to lower it

3

_____ Strong, constant stimulus below level of lesion

1

_____ Impulses to peripheral and visceral vessels for vasodilation are blocked

4

_____ The autonomic system responds to the stimulus with profuse sweating and elevation of blood pressure

2

Frame 29

Because the autonomic system is disrupted, the usual response mechanisms to triggering stimuli are prevented.

This is one of the most serious emergencies that can develop in the cord-injured patient.

1. Which of these problems could cause Cedric's symptoms?

1. all

a. fecal impaction
b. sitting in a draft
c. kinking of the catheter tubing with urinary retention
d. genito-urinary infection
e. pressure on the testicle
f. sharp objects pressing on the skin

2. What action should be taken when the symptoms are noted?

2. b, d

a. Wait and observe to see if the hyperreflexia symptoms are repeated
b. Immediately notify the physician
c. Talk with the patient so that these anxiety-induced symptoms are relieved
d. Look for the triggering stimulus

Frame 30

Nursing assessment focuses on determining the triggering stimulus. A distended bladder from a plugged catheter is the most common cause. Jill was gentle in palpating the abdomen to check for distention as this may increase stimulation. She checked to see if the catheter tubing was kinked. Then she slowly irrigated the catheter with 30 ml sterile saline. She found that Mr. Burn's catheter was plugged and the saline irrigation opened it. Four hundred ml of urine drained into the collector.

1. Name two causes of bladder distention.

2. Why is it essential to gently irrigate the catheter?

1. tubing kinked, tubing or catheter plugged with sediment

2. Vigorous stimulation will increase BP and other symptoms

Frame 31

Impaction may be the cause of autonomic hyperreflexia. Before doing a digital exam, Nupercainol ointment should be inserted because rectal stimulation may increase symptoms. Evacuation of the impaction should be done only after the BP has been lowered by medication.

To prevent impaction the nurse or the patient should keep track of bowel movements and an effective bowel routine should be planned. Patients need to know that small watery stools may be a sign of impaction and not of diarrhea.

True or False:

1. _____ When impaction is the cause of hyperreflexia, the most important action is to immediately remove the feces.

2. _____ Nupercainol ointment should be applied to the gloved finger before examining the patient.

3. _____ Loose, watery stools may be indicative of impaction.

1. False

2. True

3. True

Frame 32

When Mr. Burns' physician was notified, she ordered a ganglionic blocking agent, hydralazine (Apresoline), to lower the blood pressure. She explained that the high blood pressure makes Mr. Burns prone to a cerebral vascular accident. Occasionally it is necessary to maintain the patient on hydralazine for a period of time because hypersensitivity to triggering stimuli may persist.

1. What classification of drug is used to lower the BP in autonomic hyperreflexia?

2. Hypertension puts the patient at risk for what complication?

1. Ganglionic blocker

2. CVA

Frame 33

The nurse must be alert to early symptoms and signs of autonomic hyperreflexia. Most of all, prevention by means of assessing and maintaining a record of bowel and bladder function is essential. Because patients with cord trauma above T6-8 are susceptible to autonomic hyperreflexia, the patient and the family need to be taught the symptoms of autonomic hyperreflexia and the means of relieving them. One method for helping to decrease the BP is to place the patient in a sitting position so that blood will flow to the extremities.

1. Who would be most prone to autonomic hyperreflexia?

   a. Sue with a lesion at T10
   b. Tom with a lesion at C7,8
   c. Mark with a S2,3 sacral lesion

2. Which of the following would help decrease the BP?

   a. decreasing sensory stimulation
   b. putting warm blankets on the patient
   c. sitting the patient up in bed
   d. removing constrictive clothing

1. b

2. a, c, d

Frame 34

Summary:

Autonomic hyperreflexia is an excessive autonomic response to stimuli such as bladder or bowel distention, skin stimulation, pain stimuli

Symptoms: hypertension, throbbing headache, blurred vision, sweating above the level of lesion, bradycardia, nausea, nasal congestion, pilomotor spasm

Care: Notify physician, observe bladder for distention, catheter for proper drainage, assess bowel elimination pattern for impaction (use Nupercainol for rectal exam), place patient in sitting position, administer ganglionic blocking agent as ordered.

Teach patient and family how to prevent and treat the condition.

Frame 35

Meticulous, frequent assessment of the skin is essential to prevention of skin breakdown. Immobilization, loss of sensation, decreased peripheral circulation, and venous stasis all threaten skin integrity. Turning at least q2h and skin massage with special attention to bony prominences are necessary. The nurse assumes major responsibility for assessing and maintaining skin integrity.

1. List three reasons why skin should be assessed q2h.

2. List at least three body areas to which the nurse should give special attention for skin care.

1. immobilization, loss of sensation, peripheral pooling of blood

2. sacrum, hips, knees, ankles, heels, scapula, elbows, ears

PART IV PSYCHOLOGIC REACTIONS

Frame 36

Nursing assessment of the patient with spinal cord trauma would not be complete without attention to the psychologic state. Reactions to the paralysis include: shock, partial recognition, initial stabilization, regression, denial, depression, and social recovery. The patient may not necessarily follow this sequence.

Shock

Shock follows the trauma. Assessment reveals a flat affect, slow mental processing, unresponsiveness, and possible confusion. The patient is quiet and withdrawn. This gradually gives way to the patient asking some questions, focusing on the present. The person is more aware of outside stimuli and adjustment seems to be taking place. Unless demands are made on the patient, he appears able to deal with day-to-day activities.

1. Which of the following are indicative of shock following cervical trauma?

   a. loud laughter
   b. slow response to questions
   c. undue demands
   d. eyes closed much of the time
   e. rarely smiles

1. b, d, e
   (a and c are not withdrawn behaviors)

Denial

Frame 37

Denial is a common reaction, and it's purpose is to protect a person from the overwhelming impact of reality. By the use of denial, the patient can take reality in bits and pieces, as much as he can accept.

Ken Shilling has been in ICU following a C6 transection. One day he told Jill, "You know, all of this care isn't necessary. In a few weeks I'll be able to sit up and then walk. I've seen it in movies, and because I'm young and strong it will surely happen that way to me, too."

1. Which response would reflect reality without making Ken defensive?

   a. Surely you don't believe everything you see in movies!
   b. You have to be realistic about this. Remember what the doctors told you about the injury and the effects that it has.
   c. Well, we'll get busy now with the care you need, and see what happens.

1. c—focuses on the present
   (a—ridicules
   b—confronts)

2. Ken replied, "You don't believe in miracles. You probably think I'm wrong, just like the others." Which would be the best response?

   a. You are right. I'm glad you are coming around to our point of view.
   b. I don't know for sure what will be possible for you, but I'm willing to work with you on your goals.
   c. Nobody thinks you're wrong, just unrealistic.

2. b
   (a—"We're right and you're wrong"
   c—negative judgment of his opinion)

The key point in dealing with denial is to reflect reality gently, but not to force the patient into defending his unrealistic ideas.

Most patients observe other patients closely and will accept reality at an individual pace.

Frame 38

Ken continued to talk about his belief in a complete recovery. One day he told Jill that he would "not waste my energy on another bedside physical therapy session. It's silly to do all this fooling around. In a few days I'll be better."

1. Ken's pattern of denial

   a. is a normal reaction to severe stress
   b. is interfering with his care
   c. is a sign of psychosis
   d. should be dealt with forcefully

1. a, b

Dealing with denial that interferes with care is difficult. Sometimes it is helpful to:

> offer alternatives acceptable to the patient's belief system
> encourage future orientation.

2. Which response(s) might help Ken to accept care?

   a. If you don't do your P.T., we will have to eliminate evening visiting hours.
   b. It's up to you. The therapist has other patients who want to get well.
   c. The P.T. exercises build up strength in your arms. This will allow you to do many things whether you walk or not.
   d. Think of what you want to do in the future. You can't do it if you let your muscles get weak now.

2. c, d
(a—punitive
b—uncaring)

Regression

Frame 39

Regression is another reaction that can occur with denial, or separately. Behavior indicative of regression includes: helplessness, self-pity, self-concern and egocentric demands.

Later Ken stated, "My old self has died. What's the use of hoping or trying? People will just have to take care of me. I can't do anything." Ken began making many small demands for care and attention, and talked only of himself and his needs.

1. What are some strategies that might help?

   a. Tell Ken he's acting like a baby and nobody wants to take care of him anymore.
   b. Set limits by telling Ken when you will return and how long you will have with him. Stick to the schedule.
   c. Decrease the time and attention he gets until he behaves better.
   d. Ask the physician to speak to him about it.
   e. Give feedback about small improvements in his condition from day to day.
   f. Provide opportunities for obvious success.

1. b, e, f (d may also help)
   (a—punitive, sarcastic
   c—withdrawing)

Depression

Frame 40

Depression is also frequent in the acute period. Moodiness, pessimism, quietness and statements of worthlessness are behaviors indicative of depression. One would expect the patient to mourn the loss of body function, but when this reaction extends over long periods of time it is not healthy.

1. Which of the following statements would be characteristic of a patient who is depressed?

   a. "I'll walk again."
   b. "What's left in life for me?"
   c. "The best thing that could happen to me is to fall out of a window."
   d. "A wheelchair—I'll never be able to live in a wheelchair."

1 b, c, d
(a—hopeful)

Therapeutic interventions for depression include:

allow the person to express his discomfort
accept feelings without endorsing them
convey your belief that life is worthwhile and there is something the patient can do to cope with the situation
gradually give the patient some sense of power; give him a chance to say no, to choose and direct.

The assessment and skillful handling of Ken's psychologic state will help Jill Collins to:

> keep track of his level of motivation and try to influence it

> recognize when he is ready to learn about his disability and self-care

> give feedback so he can adjust.

Frame 41

Summary:
Psychologic reactions frequently seen in acute care are:
Shock—↓ intake of information, ↓ attention and responsiveness
Denial—protective, belief in miraculous cure
Care: reflect reality without putting patient on the defensive

Regression—self-centered, self-pitying, demanding, helpless
Care: Set limits, give feedback on progress, plan activities likely to be successful
Depression—pessimistic, feels worthless, sad, tired
Care: Accept feelings without endorsement, convey what he can do to control the situation

CHAPTER 15

STABILIZATION OF THE SPINE

Much of the immediate treatment and care of the patient with cord trauma is related to attaining and maintaining stabilization of the spine. This necessitates immobilization. You will learn about application of skeletal traction, use of turning frames, and related nursing responsibilities. Don't forget that prevention of the disuse phenomena is also an important nursing goal.

At the conclusion of this chapter you will be able to:

1. Describe the procedure for insertion of tongs
2. Identify factors to assess in a patient with tongs
3. Choose nursing interventions for a patient with tongs
4. List the safety considerations for turning a CircOlectric bed
5. State methods other than tongs used for stabilization of injured vertebrae.

Chapter outline

Skeletal traction
   Insertion of tongs
   Nursing assessment
   Nursing care of traction site

Turning Frames
   CircOlectric bed
   Stryker frame
   Nursing considerations

Hyperextension

Surgical fusion

PART I
SKELETAL TRACTION

Frame 1

Patients who have sustained trauma to the cord, regardless of level, are frequently immobilized. If the patient has motor and sensory function, immobilization is still needed to prevent further damage to the cord. This may take the form of bed rest, use of a CircOlectric bed, Stryker or Foster frame, traction, or braces. Immobilization serves several purposes. It reduces tissue damage from unstable bone fragments. Alignment of the vertebrae allows for healing and repair of the vertebral structures and ligaments.

True or False:

1. _____ Immobilization reduces damage to tissues surrounding the fracture.

2. _____ Braces are a form of immobilization.

3. _____ Repair of ligaments is a major purpose of immobilization.

4. _____ Traction is used to attain alignment.

1. True

2. True

3. True

4. True

Insertion of Tongs

Frame 2

When the injury is in the cervical spine, skeletal traction with tongs inserted into the skull is used to maintain alignment and achieve stabilization. There are many types of tongs: Crutchfield, Vinke, Barton, and Gardner-Wells. Physician preference dictates the type of tongs used. Assessment and care is essentially the same for all tongs.

True or False:

1. _____ Tongs are a form of skin traction.

2. _____ The type of injury dictates the type of tongs used.

3. _____ Tongs help achieve alignment.

4. _____ Patients with cervical fractures often have tongs to maintain traction.

1. False

2. False

3. True

4. True

Frame 3

Now review the procedure for inserting Crutchfield tongs.

—The patient is placed on CircOlectric bed or Stryker frame.
—Hair is shaved in the temporal area.
—The area is cleansed with soap and antiseptic solution.
—A local anesthetic such as xylocaine is injected.
—A small incision is made and bleeding is controlled.
—The scalp muscles and periosteum are retracted to expose the bone.
—A drill is used to make an opening into the outer table of the skull bone.
—Tongs are inserted and tightened.
—A small gauze dressing is applied around the tongs.

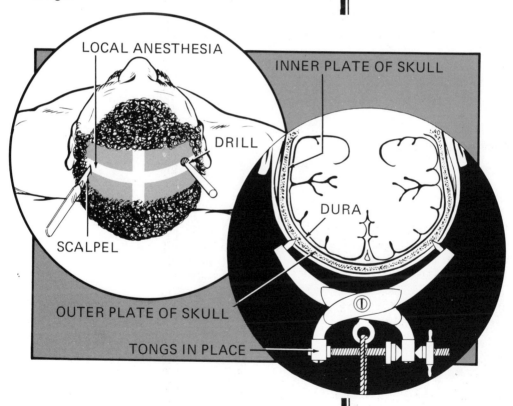

Figure 15.1. *Insertion of Crutchfield tongs*

True or False:

1. _____ General anesthesia is used for inserting the tongs.

1. False

2. _____ A hole is made all the way through the skull.

3. _____ The entire head is shaved.

4. _____ Tongs are tightened after insertion.

2. False

3. False

4. True

Frame 4

Gardner-Wells tongs differ in the following ways:
  —They are inserted lower on the temporal bone

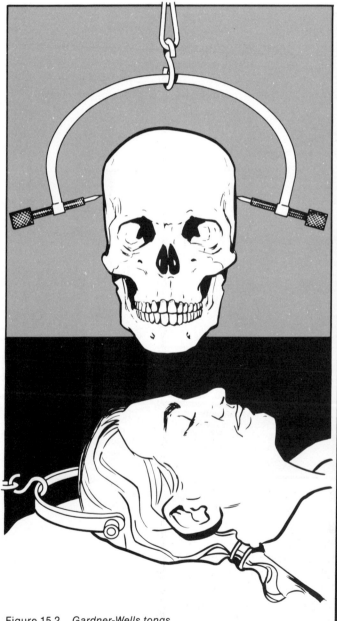

Figure 15.2. *Gardner-Wells tongs*

—The scalp is not shaved. Hair is clipped around the site, which is then prepared with antiseptic

—After local infiltration of anesthetic, the tongs are applied to the skull just above and in front of the ear. The points are advanced until the spring-loaded point shows that the proper pressure is being exerted. The tongs are then tilted back and forth to seat the points

—The pressure causes the outer table of the bone to atrophy, so that the points advance slightly and seat themselves in about 24 hours.

1. Choose facts about Gardner-Wells tongs which are advantages over Crutchfield tongs:

   a. Short scalp incision
   b. No burr holes are drilled in the skull
   c. Because the points are angled in the direction of the pull, the traction would tend to hold them in place
   d. Anesthetic is not required

1. b, c
   (a—there is no scalp incision)

Nursing Assessment

Frame 5

Weights are applied to the tongs, and x-rays are taken to determine if alignment is attained. The amount of weight is determined by the number of pounds needed to overcome muscle spasm and keep the bone in good alignment, usually 25 to 40 pounds.

Important Observations:

—Neuro checks—Over-reduction may occur, which could cause or increase neuro deficits

—Weights should hang freely

—The knot in the traction rope should not rest against the pulley. This negates the weights.

—The patient may be pulled toward the head of the bed by the weights. Repositioning is required. Sometimes the head of the bed is put on shock blocks to provide countertraction.

Figure 15.3 demonstrates correct positioning. Sandbags may be placed on each side of the head to prevent rotation.

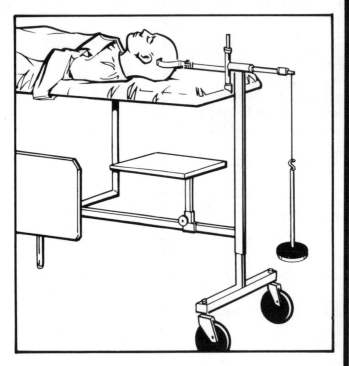

Figure 15.3. *Position for traction*

True or False:

1. _____ In order for traction to be effective the tongs, rope, and weights must be freely suspended.

2. _____ Counter-traction is never used with skeletal traction.

3. _____ Neuro deficits would indicate that the traction should be re-evaluated.

1. True

2. False

3. True

Frame 6

In addition to checking the weights, the nurse should frequently assess the tongs for tightness and placement.

The tongs should be secure in the skull with no movement to prevent dislodgement. If tongs do pull out, sandbags should be placed next to the patient's head to maintain alignment while the physician is notified.

Tongs may erode the bone and slip into the muscle. The patient feels a jolt and pain because scalp muscle has sensory receptors for pain. Erosion of bone is more common in older persons who have tongs in place for a long period of time.

1. What two things should you do if tongs accidentally come out of the patient's skull?

2. What would be an indication that the tongs had slipped out of the bone into the muscle?

3. In what patient population is erosion more common?

1. place sandbags by head; call physician

2. pain

3. older persons

Nursing Care of Traction Site

Frame 7

The scalp around the tongs is cleansed each shift with hydrogen peroxide and an antiseptic solution. Small gauze dressings may be applied. While doing the cleansing the nurse notes any redness or drainage. Occasionally tongs perforate through the inner layer of the skull and tear the dura. CSF escapes and a channel for organisms to enter the subarachnoid space is created. Checking drainage for sugar content will establish if it is CSF.

1. How could you differentiate CSF from other drainage at tong sites?

2. How often is tong care done?

1. use testape and check for sugar

2. each shift

Frame 8

The time tongs are left in place varies for each patient depending on the type of injury, the stability of the spine, and the medical treatment plan.

Followup x-rays are done, and the weights are gradually reduced to 5–10 pounds. Stability is usually reached in 2–6 weeks.

Types of immobilization used following the removal of tongs include:

Minerva jacket—a plaster cast which extends from the waist to the top of the head

Halo brace—the frame is attached to the skull and extends to the waist

Peterson brace—extends around chest with chin and occiput firmly held by bars.

The nature of the injury and the physician's preference determine the type of immobilization employed. Continued immobilization may be required for 3 to 6 months.

A surgical fusion may be done to increase stability.

True or False:

1. _____ A minerva jacket is a cast applied for maintaining stability of the cervical spine.

2. _____ Tongs are always left in until the vertebrae completely heal.

3. _____ The halo brace allows for free movement of the head.

1. True

2. False

3. False

Frame 9

Summary:

Skeletal traction, by means of tongs is used to maintain alignment of fractured cervical vertebrae.

Tongs are inserted into the outer plate of the skull bone and the sites may be covered by small dressings. Weights are applied to maintain alignment.

Assessment: neuro checks, freely hanging weights, correct patient position, tongs: tightness, correct placement

Complications: over-reduction with ↑ neuro deficits, dislodgment of tongs, bone erosion with perforation of dura

Nursing Care: Clean tong sites each shift with hydrogen peroxide and antiseptic. Observe sites for infection, tong placement and CSF drainage.

Casts, braces, and surgical fusion are methods used to maintain stabilization when tongs are removed.

PART II
TURNING FRAMES

Turning frames, such as the CircOlectric bed, Stryker frame and Roto rest bed, are used for patients in cervical traction and for patients with trauma in other areas of the spinal column. Patient comfort is promoted and anxiety is reduced when the nursing staff exhibits expertise in turning the frame and managing care.

Review use of the most common frames and the safety considerations. Before you carry out these procedures independently you will need to:

> read your hospital's procedure and
> ask a nurse who is familiar with the procedure to demonstrate and assist you.

CircOlectric Bed

Panel 1
Turning the CircOlectric bed

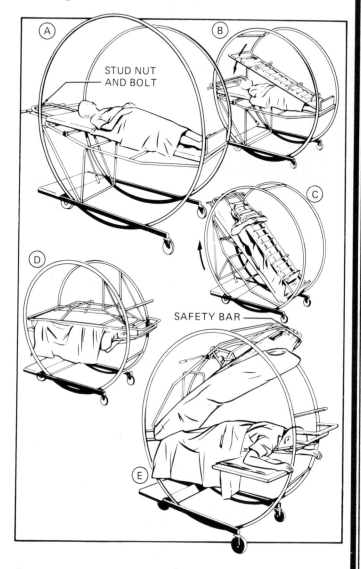

A, The patient is in back-lying position, with the hips centered at the gatch. The footboard is adjusted to prevent the patient from sliding downward during transfer. The pillow is used to pad the patient's legs and knees. A sponge rubber face mask is applied to protect the face. **B,** The anterior frame is installed and locked in place with a stud nut and bolt. **C,** After telling the patient the direction that he will be turned, the nurse rotates the bed electrically. Safety straps are necessary if the patient is unable to control his arms. **D,** The posterior stud nut is removed from the head of the frame, and the safety bar is pulled forward to disengage the posterior section. **E,** The posterior section is raised high overhead and locked into the circle frame with the safety bar. (Courtesy Stryker Corp., Kalamazoo, Mich.)

Figure 15.4. *Turning the CircOlectric bed*

Stryker Frame

Panel 2
Turning the Stryker Wedge Frame

STABILIZATION OF THE SPINE

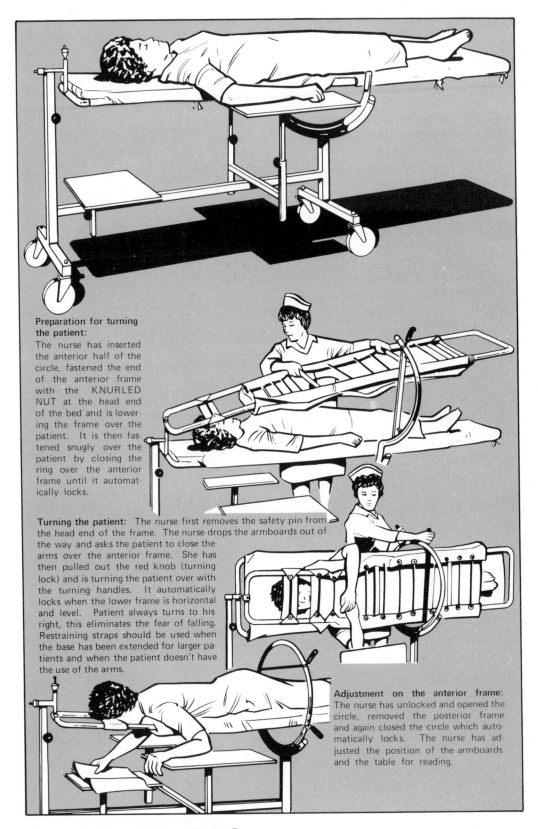

Preparation for turning the patient:
The nurse has inserted the anterior half of the circle, fastened the end of the anterior frame with the KNURLED NUT at the head end of the bed and is lowering the frame over the patient. It is then fastened snugly over the patient by closing the ring over the anterior frame until it automatically locks.

Turning the patient: The nurse first removes the safety pin from the head end of the frame. The nurse drops the armboards out of the way and asks the patient to close the arms over the anterior frame. She has then pulled out the red knob (turning lock) and is turning the patient over with the turning handles. It automatically locks when the lower frame is horizontal and level. Patient always turns to his right, this eliminates the fear of falling. Restraining straps should be used when the base has been extended for larger patients and when the patient doesn't have the use of the arms.

Adjustment on the anterior frame:
The nurse has unlocked and opened the circle, removed the posterior frame and again closed the circle which automatically locks. The nurse has adjusted the position of the armboards and the table for reading.

Figure 15.5. *Turning the Stryker Wedge Frame*

Frame 10

General safety considerations for all turning frames:

- —Adjust padding over body prominences and for patient comfort.
- —Make sure feet are in proper alignment and away from turning mechanisms.
- —Lock top frame securely.
- —Use straps to secure the patient between the frames. Be sure arms are secured safely.
- —Tell the patient which direction he will be turned and prepare him for changes in sensation which may occur.
- —Plug the CircOLectric bed into the outlet only when turning.
- —Be sure traction weights are hanging freely at all times.
- —Plan the turn to prevent dislodgment of IV and monitoring lines.
- —Have enough help.

1. It was a busy day on the acute neuro unit. A new nurse was caring for Mary Anderson. She had never turned a CircOlectric bed before. She read the procedure and decided to attempt it without help, rather than bother the other nurses. Do you agree with this decision?

   1. No, not safe for the patient

2. Jill Collins asked another nurse to turn her on a Stryker frame so that she could know what it felt like. Is this a good idea?

   2. Yes, it increases her understanding and ability to teach patients about the frame

3. On another very busy day, the safety straps were missing from a patient's room. The nurses decided that straps weren't necessary, and turned the patient without them. Do you agree?

   3. No, this is taking unnecessary chances

Frame 11

Establishment of a turning schedule is important in coordinating care. This should be posted by the bed. Points to consider in determining the schedule include:

—Length of time tolerated on abdomen. While it is best to be two hours on the back and two hours on the abdomen, many persons initially cannot tolerate long periods on the abdomen.
—In what position does the patient prefer to eat his meals?
—Are there favorite television programs the patient likes to watch?

Allowing the patient to have input into the schedule gives him a feeling of control over some aspects of care.

1. List three factors to consider in establishing a turning schedule for a patient.

   1. time tolerated on abdomen, where he likes to eat meals, TV programs he likes to watch

397

Nursing Considerations

Frame 12

Patients immobilized with tongs on a CircOlectric bed feel restrained and isolated. Nursing interventions can help to reduce these feelings.

The visual field is greatly reduced because the patient cannot turn his head. When entering the room walk over to the bed so that the patient can see you. Patients may have feelings of distrust and apprehension when they hear someone in the room and don't know who it is. Always make sure the call light is within the patient's reach. Place needed articles close by and have the patient feel where they are.

Sensory input may also be increased with prism glasses which allow for TV viewing. Some of the newer beds have an attachment for a small TV on the bed. A tape recorder or a radio placed so the patient can activate it are helpful. Books on film which project on the ceiling may be used.

1. Which of the following would help decrease sensory deprivation in the patient on a CircOlectric bed?

   a. keep the radio going constantly
   b. place interesting posters on the ceiling and change them periodically
   c. have a roommate who is alert and talkative
   d. obtain prism glasses

2. Before leaving the patient's bedside, the nurse should:

   a. place the call light so the patient can use it
   b. move the tray table within reach
   c. put kleenex on tray table
   d. tell the patient when he will be turned the next time

1. b, c, d

2. all

Panel 3
The Roto Rest Bed

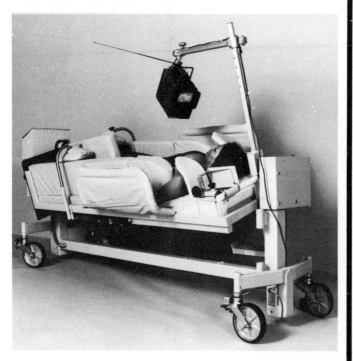

Figure 15.6. *Roto Rest bed*

This bed rotates automatically 14 times per hour. The patient is slowly turned from side to side. Traction apparatus can be attached, and arm and leg hatches can be opened for range of motion exercises.

Nursing Care: *Use padded accessories to hold the patient securely in place to prevent shearing.*

Benefits: *Reduces uneven movements and jolts often present with normal turning frames.*
Sleep is not interrupted.
More frequent position changes occur than is practical with manual methods.

PART III
HYPEREXTENSION

Frame 13

In some types of injury, hyperextension of the spine is needed to attain vertebral alignment.

This may be accomplished by placing folded sheets under the patient's back or a blanket roll under the mattress at the level which will hyperextend the fracture site.

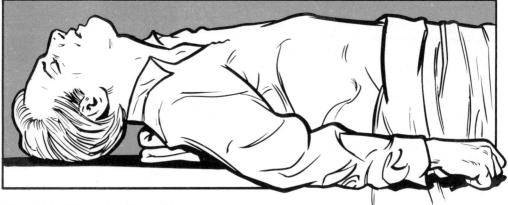

Figure 15.7. *Hyperextension position*

Remember to indicate on the nursing care plan exactly how the patient is to be positioned: the number of rolls or sheets and their placement.

1. To achieve hyperextension of the neck, sheets or rolls would be placed under the patient's (head/shoulders).

2. Hyperextension is used to achieve (alignment/traction) of the fracture.

1. shoulders

2. alignment

PART IV
SURGICAL FUSION

Frame 14

In some injuries, surgical removal of part of a vertebra may be done. Some indications for surgery include:

> progression of neurologic deficit
> partial or complete blockage of CSF flow
> penetrating wounds
> presence of bone fragments or foreign bodies in the cord
> persistent dislocation

If the surgeon anticipates movement of the vertebrae during weight bearing, a posterior fusion and/or anterior fusion is done using bone grafts or steel rods to stabilize the area. Bone grafts are usually taken from the iliac crest and shaped to fit across the unstable area. The graft may be wired to normal vertebrae above and below. Tongs are left in place until the bone begins to fuse. Eventually the whole area forms a solid bony bridge. A brace or cervical collar is worn until the fusion is solid.

Frame 15

Summary:

Turning frames are used to reposition patients without interfering with traction and cervical immobilization.

Safety considerations: Pad and protect bony prominences and extremities, securely lock the frames, use safety straps, tell the patient which direction he will turn, plug in the CircOlectric bed only when turning, be sure weights hang freely.

Nursing Care: establish effective turning schedule
recognize limitation of visual field
provide diversionary activities

Hyperextension of the spine is indicated in some injuries.

Surgical stabilization is used to relieve pressure on the cord, remove bone fragments and fuse unstable vertebrae.

CHAPTER 16

CASE STUDY: SPINAL CORD INJURY

Cervical trauma results in both physiologic and psychologic shock. The patient finds himself totally dependent upon health professionals for all aspects of care. Nursing care plays an important role in maintenance of life and in rehabilitation. While studying the care of David Norris, who is paraplegic following an accident, you'll have an opportunity to apply the material from previous chapters. Your focus will be planning care for David during the period immediately following his trauma and later in his hospitalization.

At the conclusion of this chapter you will be able to:

1. Identify the priorities of immediate care following cervical trauma
2. Develop a nursing care plan for a patient with cervical trauma
3. Choose nursing interventions which will help a patient adapt to his paraplegic state
4. Relate nursing care required to physiologic findings
5. Select interventions to assist the family in dealing with the crisis.

Chapter outline

Initial Care

Nursing care plan

Intermediate Care
    Goals of the therapeutic plan
    Signs and symptoms of complications
    Recovery from spinal shock
    Patient and family teaching

PART I
INITIAL CARE

Case Presentation

David Norris, age 23, fell from a scaffolding while he was working as a brick-layer constructing a university dormitory. The foreman immediately called an ambulance and did not allow anyone to move David. The paramedics transported him to the emergency room of the nearby university hospital.

From the time of the accident David could not feel or move his lower body. X-rays taken on admission showed a fracture of C7 with C6–7 subluxation. X-rays of the skull and shoulders revealed no fractures of these areas.

David was placed on a Stryker frame and Gardner-Wells tongs were inserted. Fifteen pounds of weight were applied. Two folded sheets were placed under David's shoulders to keep his neck in hyperextension.

An IV was started and 5% dextrose in Ringers lactate (D₅RL) begun. A Foley catheter was inserted. David was transported to the neurosurgical intensive care unit. Orders included:

D₅RL 2500 ml q24h
NPO
Intake and output—call if output less than 30 ml an hour
I PPB treatment q4h
Cough and deep breathe q2h
Vital signs and neuro check q1h
Elastic stockings
Tong care tid
Catheter care tid
Range of motion exercise tid
Turn q2h—stomach 1 hour, back 2 hours
Diazepam (Valium) 10 mg IM q6h
Codeine ¼ gr. IM q4h PRN
Dexamethasone (Decadron) 10 mg IV stat and 4 mg IV q6h

On admission to the ICU, David had no sensation or movement below C6. His legs were flaccid. Bowel sounds were absent. His hand grasp was very weak. David complained of chilling despite being covered with two blankets. His skin was cool and dry. Vital signs were:

T   98°F
BP   90/60
P   56
R   24

David kept his eyes closed most of the time but would respond to questions. He didn't like being turned to his abdomen.

David lived at home with his parents, 2 brothers, and 4 sisters. He was the second eldest. The family has lived in a nearby small town all of their lives and have many friends and relatives in the area. David had a girl friend; they had been going together for about a year. She was married previously and had a 4-year-old daughter.

His mother described David as "quiet and keeps everything inside." David liked sports; mostly he liked to watch and not participate. He smoked one package of cigarettes a day and drinks alcohol occasionally. After graduating from high school, David began to work as a brick-layer for the Delaney Company.

Discussion

Frame 1

1. Which of the following symptoms would indicate that David is in spinal shock?

   a. Flaccid extremities
   b. Weak grasp with hands
   c. BP 90/60
   d. Complaints of chilling
   e. Absent bowel sounds
   f. No sensation below C6
   g. Respirations = 24
   h. Skin cool and dry

1. a, d, e, h
   (maybe c depending on his normal range; a, f and g may be present but are not indicative of spinal shock)

Nursing Care Plan

At this point in David's hospitalization, he had many needs. Jill Collins chose four goals which were priorities for his immediate care. The goals were:

Prevent neuro deterioration
Maintain skin integrity
Prevent respiratory complications
Promote comfort

PREVENT NEURO DETERIORATION

Frame 2

1. Which of the following nursing actions would help achieve this goal?

   a. Keeping two sheets under David's shoulders
   b. Not turning the bed

1. a, c, d

   c. Checking the rope on the tongs so the knot
     doesn't touch the bed
   d. Administering Decadron on time
   e. Restricting movement of upper extremities

Frame 3

Outcome criteria are used to determine if a goal is
achieved.

1. Which of the following would be criteria for
determining if spinal cord deterioration has
been prevented?   1. a, b

   a. 24 hours after accident, the hand grasp is
     the same
   b. respiratory status remains normal
   c. no decubitus ulcer
   d. able to answer all questions

SKIN INTEGRITY

Frame 4

Recall the many pathologic findings in the patient
with cord trauma which make maintaining skin
integrity a major problem.

1. Which of the following mechanisms contribute
to this difficulty?   1. a, b, c, d

   a. dilation of peripheral vessels
   b. absence of muscle tone in lower extremities
   c. absence of voluntary movement in legs
   d. absence of sensation
   e. absence of perspiration below C8

Frame 5

Another contributing factor is nutrition. During
the days immediately following the accident,
David was not given food to eat because of paralytic ileus. IV's provide water, carbohydrates, vitamins and minerals, but no protein for cell repair.

1. David will probably have (more/less) cell
breakdown than cell repair.   1. more

2. If pressure on his skin causes microscopic tissue damage, repair will be (fast/slow).   2. slow

3. Decubitus ulcers (could/could not) begin during the first hospital day.   3. could

Frame 6

David smokes a pack of cigarettes a day. He kept asking to be allowed to smoke to "calm my nerves." Jill told David about the restrictions on smoking because oxygen is used in the intensive care unit. He said "Okay," but the next time she went to his bed he asked again for a cigarette. She repeated the explanation and told him that his respiratory capacity is also decreased. She then heard David asking his family for cigarettes.

1. What response would be best?

    a. I can't believe you still want to smoke when I've told you why you can't.
    b. It's difficult when everything is changed or taken away. Would a mint or gum help?
    c. Maybe tomorrow you'll be transferred and can smoke all you want to.

1. b
(a—treats patient as a child
c—avoids issue)

Frame 7

The next day David's respirations were very rapid and sounded moist. Pulmonary edema may occur in patients with cord trauma because the vasodilation of vessels allows fluid to seep out of vessels and into the lung tissue. Fluid intake must be closely monitored, as fluid overload increases the possibility of pulmonary edema. The period of rapid respirations lasted for only an hour.

1. Which nursing actions would promote adequate ventilatory and respiratory function?

    a. check his abdomen to see if it is distended
    b. maintain adequate fluid intake
    c. reduce anxiety
    d. use the incentive spirometer only when he is on his back
    e. change position often

1. a, b, c, e

Frame 8

David's father asked, "The doctor said David's breathing has to be watched closely. How can we tell he's breathing okay?"

1. Which signs determine adequacy of respiration?

   a. color of mucous membranes
   b. degree of tiredness
   c. rate of respirations
   d. depth of respirations
   e. level of alertness
   f. appetite

1. a, b, c, d, e

Frame 9

Despite efforts of the staff, David developed a pulmonary infiltrate. His temperature was elevated to 101.4°F. An antibiotic (Keflin 500 mg q6h IV) was begun. David didn't like to cough and his attempts required much effort.

1. What approach would be best to gain David's cooperation in carrying out respiratory hygiene?

   a. You'll just have to cough. You can if you want to.
   b. I'll help you cough by putting some pressure on your diaphragm.
   c. Let's try the coughing and therapy after you've had your nap.
   d. If you don't cough it up, we'll have to suction the material out.

1. b, c,
  (a—authoritarian
  d—threatening)

Frame 10

The suddeness of the accident and the immediate switch from independence to complete dependence places great stress on the individual. David reacted to the stress in a typical manner: withdrawal, keeping his eyes closed and being quiet. While there are no ways Jill can change David's present state to one of independence, there are many actions that will promote comfort and convey concern and care.

David didn't like to be on his abdomen. "I can't sleep. I can't do anything except look at the floor while I'm over. Why can't you let me be on my back longer?"

1. Which activities could be done while David is on his abdomen to allow more time for sleep when he's on his back?

   a. oral hygiene
   b. range of motion exercises
   c. incentive spirometer
   d. tong care
   e. catheter care

1. a, c, d
   (b—partially)

Frame 11

Immobilization can predispose to confusion and restlessness.

1. Why should the nurse seek ways to prevent confusion and restlessness?

1. A patient may disrupt traction

2. Indicate which of the following would be therapeutic for reducing chances of confusion.

   a. placing articles in the same place in the bedside area.
   b. informing David of who you are and walking to the bed so he can see you
   c. placing a watch or clock close at hand
   d. reducing family visits to twice a day
   e. plan for uninterrupted periods of sleep

2. a, b, c, e

Frame 12

Personal hygiene aids in preventing infection and also promotes comfort.

1. In establishing a plan of care for David, which information should Jill secure?

   a. type of razor he uses
   b. type of deodorant
   c. how often he bathes
   d. when he prefers to have his bath
   e. allergies

1. a, b, d, e

Frame 13

David's constant complaint was of "being cold". His mother asked why hot water bottles can't be used on his feet to warm him up. Jill explained the precautions needed because of the absence of sensation. The staff brainstormed on ideas to decrease David's complaints of being cold.

1. Which of the following would be feasible?

    a. wrapping lower extremities in bath blankets
    b. using K-pads on arms and legs
    c. placing the bed away from the air duct
    d. getting a long sleeved gown
    e. making sure IV solution is out of refrigerator half an hour before being hung
    f. warming sheets for upper or lower frame before turning

1. a, c, e, f
(b—would cause greater loss of heat by ↑vasodilation
d—not feasible with IV's)

2. What is the main cause for David's being cold?

2. ↓sympathetic discharge causes vasodilation which allows for escape of body heat

Frame 14

Four days after his injury David was transferred out of the intensive care unit. His neurologic status was unchanged except that his hand grasp was stronger.

1. Why has his grasp improved?

    a. nerve tracts are healing after the trauma
    b. spinal shock persists
    c. edema is subsiding
    d. circulation in the extremities is improved

1. c
(See Chapter 13, Frame 4.)

PART II
INTERMEDIATE CARE

Case Presentation

After the initial phase with its life-threatening problems was managed, the team turned its attention to preventing complications and preparing David for rehabilitation.

Managing David's bladder problems was an important decision. Two types of catheterization were being debated:

Continuous drainage with a Foley catheter

Intermittent catheterization every 4–6 hours with a sterile, straight catheter. This method has been shown to reduce the incidence of urinary tract infections, urethral irritation and damage, stone formation and hydronephrosis. Muscle tone in the bladder is maintained, as urine accumulates in the bladder between catheterizations. This method also promotes feelings of normalcy in the patient.

It was decided to use the intermittent catheterization procedure for David and to teach him how to catheterize himself as soon as he was able to learn.

A cystometrogram was done to check David's bladder function. Measured amounts of sterile solution were introduced into his bladder until spontaneous emptying took place or total filling of 500–700 ml was reached. This tests the muscle tone and capacity of the bladder. Figure 16.1 shows a cystometric graph with representative curves for a normal, spastic and flaccid bladder.

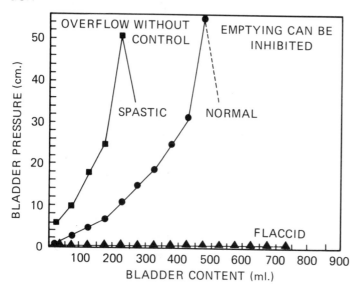

Figure 16.1. *Cystomatric graph*

David's cystometrograms showed some reflex contractions with 150 ml of filling.

A bowel program was also begun. A bisacodyl (Dulcolax) rectal suppository was inserted at 6:30 P.M. The time was chosen to take advantage of the gastro-colic reflex that is stimulated after meals, as well as the turning schedule. David was lying on his abdomen from 6–7 P.M. and would be turned at 7:00 and placed on the bedpan.

David was gradually advanced from clear liquids to a regular diet. The dietician planned a meal pattern with him to include: foods he enjoyed, small frequent meals, adequate protein, and sufficient fiber. Foods which were eliminated were gas-formers and foods rich in calcium that are thought to precipitate renal stone formation.

Discussion

Use the Response Indicator below to evaluate signs and symptoms of complications David might have.

Problem 1

Choose the signs and symptoms of autonomic hyperreflexia. Squares numbered _____.

Problem 2

Choose the signs and symptoms of situations which could *cause* autonomic hyperreflexia. Squares numbered _____.

Response Indicator			
Hypertension—sudden onset 1	Moist breath sounds 2	Urine cloudy with sediment 3	Redness and warmth of skin on right calf 4
Abdominal distention 5	Frequent small voidings between catheterizations 6	Nausea 7	Small liquid stools 5 x per day 8
Throbbing headache 9	Thick, yellow-green sputum 10	Elevated temperature 11	Sweating above the level of lesion 12
Increased respiratory rate 13	Blurred vision 14	Small decubitus ulcer area on coccyx 15	Increased ventilatory effort 16
Slow pulse rate 17			

Problem 3

Which signs and symptoms would indicate a pulmonary infection? Squares numbered _____ .

Problem 4

Which are the signs of fecal impaction? Squares numbered _____ .

Comments

Problem 1—Signs of autonomic hyperreflexia (AH)

Suggested responses: 1, 7, 9, 12, 14, 17

O [1 ⟩

Impulses from the sensory receptors are interrupted in travel up the cord. The autonomic reflex is intact and uninhibited, causing spasm of arterioles and hypertension which may be life-threatening.

O [7, 9, 14, 17 ⟩

Nausea, headache and blurred vision are associated with hypertension. The heart slows and beats more forcefully to overcome higher resistance in cerebral vessels.

O [12 ⟩

Because impulses to the sympathetic neurons are blocked, compensatory vasodilation and sweating cannot occur to relieve the hypertension. Arterioles remain constricted below the lesion, resulting in pallor and cold, clammy skin.

I [3, 5, 6, 8 ⟩

These may be *causes* of AH but are not symptoms of excessive autonomic response.

Problem 2 – Causes of AH
Suggested responses: 3, 4, 5, 6, 7, 8, 15

O [3, 6 ⟩

These are signs of urinary infection and bladder distention with overflow. Both are common causes of AH.

O [5, 7, 8 ⟩

These signs point to fecal impaction as a cause of AH. Small, frequent liquid stools are often a sign of impaction higher in the colon and if abdominal distention and nausea are also present, seriously consider the lower intestine the trigger site.

O [4, 15 ⟩

Pain stimuli and skin irritation and breakdown also trigger AH.

I [11 ⟩

If you included fever because it sometimes accompanies urinary infection and venous thrombosis, you were correct in your thinking.

I   2, 10, 13, 16 >

These respiratory problems are not considered causes of AH. Look for visceral distention, stimulation of pain receptors, and cutaneous stimuli as causes.

Problem 3 – Pulmonary Infection

Suggested responses: 2, 10, 11, 13, 16

O   2, 10, 11 >

Retained secretions are detected by moist breath sounds. These secretions become infected, thick and purulent. Fever usually follows.

O   13, 16 >

As more alveoli are filled with secretions, less area is available for O_2 and CO_2 exchange. Respiratory rate will increase to take in more O_2 and blow off more CO_2. The patient will work harder at breathing to overcome resistance in clogged airways. This increased effort uses up more O_2 and adds to the problem.

I   1 >

Hypertension can sometimes be caused by pulmonary problems of long standing. This would not be expected in David's case.

I   17 >

In pulmonary infection, pulse rate increases as the heart tries to compensate for low O_2 levels.

Problem 4 – Fecal impaction

Suggested Responses: 5, 7, 8

O   5, 7 >

Fecal impaction causes back-up of intestinal contents and gas, resulting in distention of the intestinal wall. This obstruction of the lumen can also cause reverse peristalsis and nausea.

O   8 >

If the impaction does not completely block the lower intestine, liquid stool can leak around the fecal mass. Distention prevents the normal absorption of water through the intestinal wall, leaving a large volume of liquid stool behind the fecal mass.

I   13, 16 >

If you included these signs of ventilatory problems because abdominal distention decreases ventilatory adequacy, you were correct in your thinking.

I   9 >

Fecal impaction may cause headache and malaise, but it is usually not the throbbing, severe headache associated with AH.

Case Presentation

The amount of weight on the tongs was increased, but the physicians were still not able to maintain David's spine in alignment. They decided that surgery was needed to establish stability of the vertebrae. It was not anticipated that surgery would improve David's neurologic status, but rehabilitation would be aided if the spine were stable.

A laminectomy and a spinal fusion were performed. Bone from the iliac crest was used to fuse the vertebral areas. The procedure was done with David lying on the Stryker frame with the tongs in place.

David's neurologic status did not change following surgery. He was able to hold items in his hands and raise his arms off of the bed. While he remained very quiet, David did ask some questions about his condition. David's family came to visit regularly. Every evening his girlfriend came to visit. David looked forward to her visits, but he always seemed depressed and withdrawn after she left.

One month after admission David was fitted with a cervical brace to be worn until x-ray demonstrated bone healing. This usually takes 6–12 weeks. David was transferred to a regular bed and began going to the physical therapy department.

Discussion

Recovery From Spinal Shock

Frame 15

About four weeks after the accident, David's mother came running to the nurses' station crying out, "He's moving his toes. He can move. He's better. It's a miracle." Other family members were at his bedside trying to have David move his toes again. Only when his foot was stroked vigorously did his toes move.

True or False:

1. _____ The cervical fusion has reduced pressure on the cord and voluntary movement is returning.

2. _____ The movement of the toes indicates that the reflex arc is intact.

3. _____ The movement indicates that spinal shock is ending.

4. _____ One can expect an increase in reflex movement when noxious stimuli are present.

5. _____ David will soon have return of sensation in his legs.

1. False

2. True

3. True

4. True

5. False

Frame 16

One morning while the nurse was bathing David's abdomen, he had an erection. They had been having a conversation about David's work and he was not aware that he was having an erection. David previously stated, "I'm not a man any more. I can't walk, I can't work, I can't have sex."

1. What would be a therapeutic action for the nurse to take in this situation?

    a. continue on with the bath ignoring the erection
    b. cover David and tell him you'll return later to finish his bath
    c. Tell him he's having an erection and that this means he has the capability for reflex erections
    d. Tell David he's having an erection but it doesn't mean he can control them

1. c
(a—neglects a teaching opportunity
b—shows own embarrassment
d—negative approach)

Frame 17

David comments, "It's good my girlfriend has a child. We won't be able to have any. Or will we be able to have children?"

1. Which is the best response?

    a. You'll be able to have intercourse, but frequently ejaculation is absent.
    b. It would be best not to have children because of your disability.
    c. You have as much of a chance to have children as anyone does.

1. a

Patient and Family Teaching

Frame 18

Learning about self care was important for David. The nurse tried to assess David's readiness to learn.

1. What signs show that David may be psychologically ready to begin learning?

    a. At bedside rounds, he has no suggestions, but says "you know what is best."
    b. He often seems sad and depressed.
    c. When goals for the future are discussed he says, "I'll never be able to do that."

1. d, e
(shows an active interest)

d. He is starting to ask questions about his care and his condition.

e. He is carefully observing other patients and comparing disabilities.

2. Note, however, that depression was a dominant feature of his behavior. How can the nurse begin teaching David?

    2. a

a. Answer his questions clearly, giving the information he requests.

b. Embark on the routine teaching program with the hope that information will dispel depression.

c. Request a psychiatric consultation.

3. What factors should the nurse assess before teaching David self-catheterization?

    3. all

a. his ability to tolerate sitting up

b. his interest in learning the procedure

c. the strength of his grip in both hands

d. concentration span and fatigue level

e. how much he understands about the anatomy of the urinary tract

4. David's family spends much time at the hospital. Eventually they will have to learn some of the aspects of David's care. Which factors should be considered in including the family in a teaching plan?

    4. all

a. how much responsibility David is willing to assume

b. what David thinks about having various family members help with his care

c. the time and effort required from the family

d. motivation and readiness of various family members

5. Why might David be depressed after visits from his girlfriend?

    5. c, d
    (maybe a)

a. He feels jealous that she is normal and well and he can't move.

b. Her visits tire him as they talk a lot.

c. He's worried about his ability to provide a living for her in his present state.

d. He's afraid she will lose interest in him.

Frame 19

The nurse writes "acceptance of condition" as a goal on the care plan.

1. Do you agree with including this goal? Why or why not?

1. Your choice, but we disagree because it is too soon to expect this of David. He has many new demands to cope with and will have much frustration to overcome

Frame 20

Plans were made to transfer David to a rehabilitation center. David didn't want to transfer, "I like it here. Anyway, what can they teach me to do? If I can't walk, there's nothing I can do."

1. These statements probably indicate David is:

    a. denying his condition
    b. regressing
    c. depressed
    d. in shock

1. b, c

2. Which of the following responses would be most therapeutic?

    a. I'll check and see if you can stay with us a week longer.
    b. Walking is very important. I'm not sure what I'd do if I couldn't walk.
    c. You're young. You'll get along fine.
    d. Rehab will be good for you. They don't let you feel sorry for yourself and they help you to find ways to do the things that are important to you.

2. d
(a—encourages regression
b—sympathy which is depressing
c—lacks understanding)

David transferred to the Rehab Unit where he stayed for three months. His neck brace was removed and he learned to transfer independently to a wheelchair and back to bed. He assumed responsibility for much of his care but would not consider any type of vocational counseling at this time. David's family made some adaptations in their home so David could move about in his wheelchair. His girl friend continued to visit, and he found her friendship and support a great source of strength.

APPENDIX A
Sample Nursing Care Plan

Problem	Goal	Nursing Orders
Increased intracranial pressure	1. Decrease pressure	1. Elevate head of bed 30° Administer stool softener If diet allows, increase bulk Monitor fluid intake carefully to prevent overhydration

	2. Promote compensatory mechanisms	2. Reduce demands for O_2 by
		  a. decreasing activity
		  b. decreasing anxiety, explain procedures and care
		    to patient and family
		  c. temperature control (See Chapter 9.)
		  d. quiet atmosphere, allowing for rest

	3. Early detection of changes	3. Assess for indicators of increasing pressure: LOC pupils motor sensory

Impairment of respiratory function	Maintain normal levels of
	O_2
	CO_2
	pH
		1. Monitor blood gases
		2. Assess
		    rate, rhythm
		    muscles used
		    depth
		3. Suction to maintain patent airway
		4. Position on side with head of bed elevated
		5. Turn patient at least q2h and deep breathe

Impairment of sensory acuity—skin	Maintain skin integrity	1. Turn at least q2h 2. Teach patient and family to observe skin for redness 3. Modify surface of bed with sheepskin, alternating pressure mattress, foam, etc. 4. Keep skin dry especially where skin surfaces meet

Impairment of sensory acuity—vision	Ability to communicate, mental acuity	1. Place articles in visual field 2. Teach to move head to see 3. Utilize radio, tapes, etc., to supply stimuli
Impaired motor function	1. Prevent complications	1. a. Range of motion exercises at least tid. b. Reduce calcium in diet c. Weight bearing if possible d. Use appropriate splints and supports
	2. Promote return of function	2. a. Range of motion exercises b. Incorporate activities patient can perform c. Allow time for patient to complete activities without pressure
Confusion	1. Ability to communicate effectively	1. Assign same personnel to provide care 2. Talk distinctly 3. Orient patient 4. Place familiar objects in visual field 5. Assess for possible causes of confusion 　—electrolytes 　—sensory overload or deprivation 　—ICP 6. Assist family to understand patient—give time to express feelings and concerns 7. Remove unsafe objects from environment 8. Have family member stay if possible 9. Restrain only if absolutely necessary
	2. Safety of patient	

APPENDIX B

NEUROLOGIC   CLINICAL FLOW SHEET

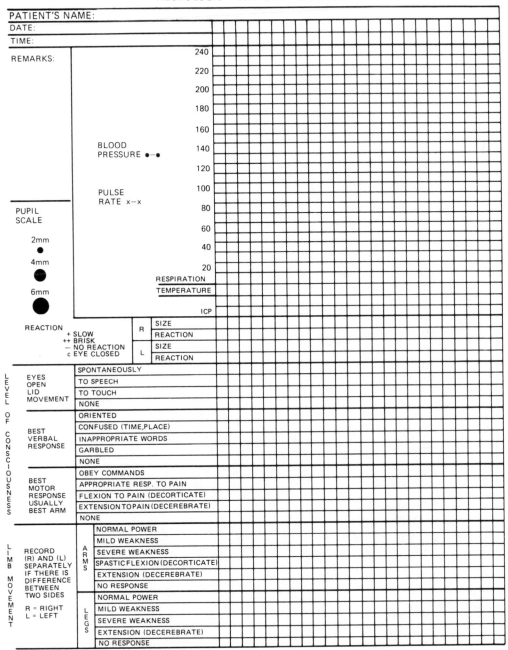

PATIENT'S NAME:

DATE:

TIME:

REMARKS:

BLOOD PRESSURE ●—●

PULSE RATE x—x

PUPIL SCALE

2mm
●

4mm
●

6mm
●

REACTION
+ SLOW
++ BRISK
− NO REACTION
c EYE CLOSED

	R	SIZE	
		REACTION	
	L	SIZE	
		REACTION	

240
220
200
180
160
140
120
100
80
60
40
20
RESPIRATION
TEMPERATURE
ICP

LEVEL OF CONSCIOUSNESS

EYES OPEN LID MOVEMENT
- SPONTANEOUSLY
- TO SPEECH
- TO TOUCH
- NONE

BEST VERBAL RESPONSE
- ORIENTED
- CONFUSED (TIME, PLACE)
- INAPPROPRIATE WORDS
- GARBLED
- NONE

BEST MOTOR RESPONSE USUALLY BEST ARM
- OBEY COMMANDS
- APPROPRIATE RESP. TO PAIN
- FLEXION TO PAIN (DECORTICATE)
- EXTENSION TO PAIN (DECEREBRATE)
- NONE

LIMB MOVEMENT

RECORD (R) AND (L) SEPARATELY IF THERE IS DIFFERENCE BETWEEN TWO SIDES

R = RIGHT
L = LEFT

ARMS
- NORMAL POWER
- MILD WEAKNESS
- SEVERE WEAKNESS
- SPASTIC FLEXION (DECORTICATE)
- EXTENSION (DECEREBRATE)
- NO RESPONSE

LEGS
- NORMAL POWER
- MILD WEAKNESS
- SEVERE WEAKNESS
- EXTENSION (DECEREBRATE)
- NO RESPONSE

INDEX

Abdomen, distension of, 372, 373, 374
Abdominal muscle(s), paralysis of, 366, 369
Abscess, brain, 102, 105
Absence seizure(s), features of, 248
Absolute refractory period, defined, 34
Acceleration/deceleration
  brain tissue damage from, 70, 71, 75
  effect on brain stem, 71, 72, 75
Acetaminophen, 274, 280, 286
Acetylcholine, 35, 73
Acid(s), in blood, effect on respiration, 133
Acid-base balance, see pH
Acidosis, signs of, 167
Acromegaly, 81
Adenohypophysis, 80
Adrenal cortex, 269
Adrenal hormone, disruption of production of,
  212
Adrenalin, 177
  action of, 329
Afferent nerve fiber(s), 14
  function of, 14
Agnosia, 85, 88
Airway obstruction, 136, 282
  prevention of, 369
Airway patency, 139
Alcoholic(s), subdural hematoma in, 69
Alertness, 152, 159
  decreased, 16
    nursing management of, 234-235
  defined, 155, 159
Alkalosis, signs of, 167
Amnesia, 157, 160
  types of, 157
Anaerobic metabolism, 47
Anastomoses, 99
Aneurysm(s), 101, 351
  causes of, 91
  diagnosis of, 90
  repair of, 93
  rupture of, 93
  sites of, 91, 92
  stages of development of, 91
  symptoms of, 89, 90
Angiogram, 280
  cerebral, see Cerebral angiogram
  femoral, 121
  use of, 266
Annulus, 307
  damage to, 307
Anoxia, 49, 57, 58, 59
Antacid(s), use with corticosteroid therapy, 268
Anterior cerebral artery, brain areas supplied by,
  95
Anterior corticospinal tract, 324
Anterior root, 325
Antibiotic therapy, 291, 408
  for meningitis, 104, 105

Anticoagulant therapy, 127
  subdural hematoma and, 69
Anticonvulsant(s), 253
Antidiuretic hormone (ADH), deficiency in, 82
Anxiety, 225, 264
  reduction of, 253
Aphasia, 228
  classification of, 237-239, 241-242
  expressive, 10
  fluent, see Fluent aphasia
  nursing management of, 239-240, 242
  receptive, 10, 237
Apnea, 133
Apneustic breathing, features of, 135-136
Apraxia, 85, 88
Aprosoline, see Hydralazine
Arachnoid, 67, 309
  membrane, 19, 20
  villi, 22
Arousal, 152
Arterial blood gas(es), 280, 285
  normal values of, 368, 369
  respiratory status and, 265
Arterial blood supply, 142
Arterial pressure, decrease in, 44
Arteriography, 175
Arteriosclerotic vascular disease (ASVD), cranial
    pathology from, 93, 101
  hematoma, 94-95
  infarction, 93, 96-99
Arteriovenous (AV), malformation, cerebral
    dysfunction from, 99, 100, 101
Artery(ies), 312
  brachial, 121
  carotid, 24, 118, 312
  cerebral, 99
  occlusion of, 101
Artificial life support, 174
Ascending reticular activating system (ARAS),
  234
  function of, 153, 159
  pressure in, 154
Association area(s), of cerebrum, function of, 8
Association tract, damage to, 229, 233
Astereognosis, 85 88
Ataxia, 87, 88
Ataxic breathing
  features of, 135
  slow, 138
Atlas, 301, 302
  function of, 301
Atrophy, cerebral, 68
Atropine, 143, 272
Attention span, lessened, 228, 232, 233
Auditory stimuli, for treatment of decreased
    alertness, 234, 235
Autonomic hyperreflexia, following spinal cord
    injury, 374, 379

mechanism of 375-376
nursing assessment of, 376-378, 379
signs and symptoms of, 374-375, 379, 412, 413
situations causing, signs and symptoms of, 412, 413
Autonomic nervous system, 297, 299, 329
disruption of, 376
function of, 3, 332
regulation of, 332
systems of
parasympathetic, 331
function of, 332
sympathetic, 329-330
Autonomic reflex, 413
Autonomic reflex arc, 375
Axis, 301, 302
function of, 301

Babinski reflex
determination of, 162, 165
indications of, 162
Baroreceptor(s), 375
Basal ganglia, 324
Basal metabolic rate (BMR), 224
Baseline, assessment of, 130
Baseline information, obtaining of, 221
Basilar artery(ies), 24
Behavior, of closed head injury patient, 294
Biot's breathing, see Ataxic breathing
Bladder, 206
contraction of, 375
distention of, 375, 379, 413
causes of, 376-377
function of, following spinal cord injury, 360-363, 365, 366
infections, 132, 138
immobility and, 206, 208
prevention of, 209
problems, following spinal cord injury, management of, 411-412
Bleeding
gastrointestinal, 276
intracranial, 231, 277
venous, 67
see also Hemorrhage
Blood
acid accumulation in, 133
aspiration of, 249
carbon dioxide levels in, 133
circulating
effects of immobility on, 202, 203, 204
interference with, 337
extravascular, 65
flow
cerebral, see Cerebral blood flow
vascular changes preventing, 94
intravascular, 38, 39, 41
oxygenation, adequacy of, 136
pools, in lungs, 204, 206
redirection of, 41

supply
to brain, 24
pathways for, 24
patterns of, 26
to spinal cord, 312-313
venous stasis of, 371
volume, increase in, 39
Blood-brain barrier
antibiotic passage through, 104, 105
cerebral edema and, 50, 58
function of, 50, 104
Blood gas(es), 280
arterial, 280, 285
disturbances in, 282
Blood pressure, 130, 170
decrease in, 202, 203, 204, 375, 377, 378
effect of immobility on, 195, 201
rise in, 93, 131, 138, 222, 225, 255, 375
Blood vessel(s), 47
clamping of, 351
damage to, 65
effect of immobility on, 203
vasodilation of, see Vasodilation
Body heat, conservation of, 216-217
Body image, effects of immobility on, 211, 212, 214
Body fluid(s), balance of, assessment of, 165, 167
of disturbances in, 166
Body system(s), reactions in, 27
Body temperature, see Temperature
Bone(s), loss of calcium from, 193, 194
prevention of, 193
Bone graft, 401
Bony prominence(s), pressure on
decrease in, 198
decubitus ulcers from, 195, 196-197, 201
Bowel(s), spinal cord injury and, 412
distention of, 414
function of, 360-363, 365
motility, nursing management of, 373, 374
Bowel sound(s), 404
observation of, 373, 374
Brace(s), 386, 392
Brain, 3
capillary membrane of, 50
cerebrospinal fluid in, 22-24
circulatory supply to, 24-27
compression of, 65
damage, 174
dysfunction, diagnostic tests for, see Diagnostic tests
metabolic demand of, 42
interference with, 43-45
oxygen supply to, 249, 250
protection of, 19
structure of, 5, 12
brain stem, 15-17
cerebellum, 13, 14-17
cerebrum, 5-14
cranial nerves, 17-19
meningeal, 19-22
ventricles of, see Ventricles

Brain abscess, 102, 105
Brain cell(s), damage to, 88
Brain death, 175
  criteria for, 174-175, 176
  occurrence of, 43, 45
Brain stem, 5, 12, 19, 72, 153, 158
  ARAS in, 234
  body function centers in, 16-17
  compression in, 56
  contusion of, 280
  cranial nerves originating from, 17
  dysfunction of, effect on respiration, 133, 138
  effect on acceleration/deceleration on, 71, 72, 75
  hemorrhage in, 56
  injury to, 65
    nursing care for, 279
    see also Closed head injury
  ischemia in, 56
  nourishment of, 42
  pressure on, 16, 255
  reflexes, absence of, 174, 175, 176
  respiratory control center in, 133
  structure of, 15-16
Brain tissue, 38, 41
  destruction of, 78
  displacement of, 40, 41
  expansion of, 39
Brain tumor(s), 108
  benign, features of, 76, 88
  brain tissue expansion from, 39
  craniotomy for, see Craniotomy
  growth rate of, 79
  histological classification of, 78
  metastatic, 76, 78
  nursing assessment of, 259
  nursing care plan in, 260-271
  pre-operative period in, 258
  symptoms of, 257
    generalized, 78, 88
    location-related, 79
      of cerebellar tumors, 86-88
      of parietal lobe tumors, 84-86, 88
      of pituitary gland tumors, 79-84, 88
    pathologic mechanisms of, 78, 88
  types of, 76, 88
Breath sound(s), 134, 138, 139, 414
  in cervical spine injury, 368, 389
Breathing exercise(s), 265
Broca's area, 96, 238
  damage to, 10

Calcium
  balance of, 166
  bone loss of, 193
  serum levels of, 194
Capillary membrane, effect of corticosteroids on, 267
Carbohydrate(s), 286, 406
Carbon dioxide (CO_2), 139, 174, 282
  blood levels of, 136, 139

effect on respiration, 133, 138
  exchange, 204, 414
  retention of, 368
Cardiac arrest, 222
Cardiac dysrhythmia(s), 203, 204, 222
Cardiac function, spontaneous, 174
Cardiovascular regulation, for spinal cord injury patient, 370-371, 374
Cardiovascular system, effect of immobility on, 201-203
Carotid artery, 24, 118, 312
Catheter, 265, 376
Catheterization, for spinal cord injury patient, 411
Cauda equina, 310
Cell(s)
  anoxia of, 58
  function, hindrance of, 74
  membrane, 32
Central nervous system (CNS), 16
  excitation, 167
  organs of, 3
  respiratory control centers in, 367
Central neurogenic hyperventilation (CNH), features of, 134
Central venous pressure, monitoring of, 177
Cerebellar tonsil(s), herniation of, 57, 59
Cerebellar tumor(s), symptoms of, 86, 87-88
Cerebellum, 5, 153
  function of, 14
  location of, 21
  nerve fibers of, 13, 14
  structure of, 14
Cerebral angiogram
  allergic reactions in, 117
  complications from, 120, 121
  information obtained from, 119
  post procedure care in, 120-121, 122
  procedure for, 117, 118-119, 120
Cerebral artery(ies), 99
Cerebral atrophy, 68
Cerebral blood flow, 44
  collapse in, 44
  factors affecting, 46
    cerebral vasodilation, 47, 48
    increased intracranial pressure, 46, 48
Cerebral blood pressure, increase in, 93
Cerebral bulk, increased, treatment of, 269-270
Cerebral cortex, 98, 152
Cerebral death, see Brain death
Cerebral edema, 49, 61, 78, 95, 101, 266, 269
  associated with infarcts, 99
  causes of, 49, 51, 58
  from closed head injury, 70-71, 75
  decreased, 272
  defined, 49, 58
  effect of, 58
    on blood-brain barrier, 50, 58
  rebound, 269, 270
  use of corticosteroids for, 266-269, 270
Cerebral infarction, from ateriosclerotic vascular disease, 93

loss of function from, 98, 99
  recovery of function in, 99
  symptoms of, 97
Cerebral metabolism, 44
Cerebral trauma, 134, 157, 175
Cerebral vascular resistance, 46
  defined, 47
Cerebral vasodilation, occurrence of, 47
Cerebral water balance, upset of, 61
Cerebrospinal fluid (CSF), 20, 38, 90
  absorption of, 39, 41
  analysis of, by lumbar puncture, 122-128
  blockage of, 88
  channels for, compression of, 88
  continued formation of, 78
  drainage of, 103, 105, 178
  escape of, 391
  flow of, interference with, 56, 59, 86, 88
  function of, 22
  location of, 22
  normal components of, 22
  volume of, 41
    increase in, 38, 39
Cerebrospinal rhinorrhea, 103, 105
Cerebrum, 5, 54, 153
  associaton areas of, 8
  corpus callosum of, 13
  division of, 21
  dysfunction of, confusion from, 230
  lobes of, 6, 7
  location of, 21
  motor-sensory areas of, 10, 12
  pathways for communication in, 236
  speech centers in, 10
Cervical brace, 415
Cervical spine injury, respiratory status
    following, see Repiratory status
Cervical vertebrae
  function of, 301, 302
  injury to, 336
Chemical pump, 50
Chest, expansion of, 264
Cheyne Stokes respiration (CSR), 176
  features of, 133, 135
Choroid plexes, 22
Circle of Willis, 24, 99
  aneurysms in, 92
  function of, 24
Ciliospinal reflex, 174
Cimetidine, action of, 269
CircOlectric bed, 370, 386, 393, 398
  plugging of, 396, 401
  turning of, 394
Circulation, 264
  changes in, 57
  promoting of, 265
Clinical flow sheet, 130
  use of, 170
    for closed head injury, 285
Closed head injury, 279
  cerebral edema from, 70-71

critical phase of, 280
medical regimen in, 280
nursing assessment in, 281-283
nursing goals and interventions in, 283-284
  maintaining skin integrity, 288-291
  preventing infections, 291-292
  promote responsiveness, 291
  providing adequate nutrition, 293-295
recovery phase of
  clinical flow sheet for, 285
  medical orders for, 286
  medical plan of care in, 286-288
  nursing goals and intervention in, 282
types of, 71
  concussion, 72-74, 75
  contusion, 74-75
Coccyx, 303, 304, 305, 310
Codeine, 128, 274, 275
  use of, 260
Cold caloric reflex, see Oculovestibular reflex
Coma, 56, 57, 167, 234
  cause of, 174, 279
  occurrence of, 43, 44, 45
Comatose, defined, 155
Comfort, promoting of, for spinal cord patient,
    408-410
Communication
  brain areas for, 236
  structural, 254
Communication problem(s)
  in closed head injury patient, 295
  nursing management of
    for dysarthria, 241
    types of aphasia, 236-240, 241-242
Compensation, state of, 170, 176
Compression
  of spinal column, 340-341
  of spinal cord, 354
    causes of, 336
    relief of, 336, 341
Computerized axial tomography (CAT) scan, 115,
    280
  advantages of, 108, 109
  mechanism of, 108
  patient preparation for, 109-110
  use of, 266
Concentration, inability in, 232, 233
Concussion, symptoms of, 72, 75
  see also Post concussion syndrome
Confusion, 66, 157, 229, 239, 368, 409
  causes of, 229-230, 233
  occurrence of, 43, 45, 156
Connective tissue, 187
  effect of immobilization on, 187-188, 194
Consciousness
  components of, 152
  impairment of, 212, 246-247, 250
  levels of, see. Levels of consciousness
  loss of, see Coma, Unconsciousness
  maintenance of, 16
Constipation, 373
  alleviation of, 265

prevention of, 277
Contracture, of joints, *see* Joints
Contralateral dysfunction, 13
Contusion, 72, 337
  features of, 74, 75
  signs and symptoms of, 75
  sites of, 74
  of spinal cord
    causes of, 336
    characteristics of, 336, 341
Conus medullaris, 310
Convulsion(s), *see* Seizure
Coordination, 14
Corneal reflex
  in brain tumor patient, 262
  presence of, determination of, 162-163, 165
Corpus callosum, 13
  function of, 13
Cortex, motor nerves of, 328
Cortical function, 174
Cortical lesion(s), detection of, 115
Corticosteroid(s), 337
  effect of
    on capillary membrane, 267
    on metabolism, 267
  side effects of, 268, 269, 282
  use in cerebral and spinal edema, 266-269, 270
  see also Dexamethasone
Cough, coughing, 264, 408
  difficulty, 366, 369
Crackles, 136
Cranial content(s), increase in, 56, 65
Cranial nerve(s), 3
  V, 162
  IV, 148, 258
  involved in eye movement, 148
  IX, 241
  origin of, 17
  reflexes affected by, 18
  VI, 148, 258
  VII, 162
  X, 241, 331
  III, 54, 59, 141, 142, 144, 148, 255, 258
  XII, 241
Cranial tumor(s), *see* Brain tumor
Craniotomy, 257, 272
  family concerns in, 272
  frontal, 251
  post-discharge plans in, 278
  post-operative period
    clinical course in, 275-278
    medical regimen for, 274
    nursing regimen for, 274
  pre-operative care for, 272
  procedure for, 272, 273
Crutchfield tong(s), insertion of, 387
Cuffed tube, 280
Cyanosis, 136, 138, 282, 368
Cycloplegic drug(s), effect on pupils, 143
Cystometrogram, for spinal cord injury patient, 411-412
Cytoplasm, 32

Death, 57
  legal definition of, 174
  see also Brain death
Decadron, *see* Dexamethasone
Deceleration, *see* Acceleration/deceleration
Decerebrate posturing, 285, 294
Decerebrate response, indicators of, 158, 160
Decerebrate rigidity, 292
Decompensation, of neuro status, 171, 176
Decorticate response, indications of, 157-158, 160
Decubitus ulcer(s), 265
  causes of, 195, 196-197, 198, 199, 201
  patient characteristics for, 200, 201
  prevention of, 198, 231
Dehydration, symptoms of, 166
Delirium, in immobilized patient, 212
Dendrite(s), 31
Denial, following spinal cord injury, 381
  nursing care for, 381-382, 384
Dentate ligament, 309
Depolarization, 35
  defined, 33
  wave of, 33, 34
Depression, 417
  following spinal cord injury, therapeutic interventions for, 383, 384
Dermatome(s), 320
Dexamethasone, 266, 272, 274, 280, 283, 286
  dosage for, 269
  rash from, 288
Dextrose, 274, 280
Diagnostic test(s), for brain dysfunction, 107
  invasive procedures
    cerebral angiogram, 117-122, 128
    lumbar puncture, 122-128
  non-invasive procedures
    computerized axial tomography, 108-110, 115
    electroencephalogram, 110-115, 116
Diaphoresis, 203, 282, 375, 379
  initiation of, by hypothalamus, 216, 217
  lack of, 282
Diaphragm
  movement of, 264
  paralysis of, 366
Dioctyl, 277
Diet
  liquid, 275
  for spinal cord injury patient, 406
  see also Nutrition
Dilantin, *see* Phenytoin
Disorientation, 228
  defined, 156
Displacement, sensitivity to, 20
Disuse phenomena, 185
  immobility and, *see* Immobility
  prevention of, 265, 385
Dizziness, 202, 203
Doll's eyes, *see* Oculocephalic reflex
Drowsiness, 66
Drug(s), 209, 230, 233

effect on pupil size, 143
  see also Medication
Drug reaction(s), fever and, 218
Dura, 67, 309
Dura mater, 19
Dysarthria, 228, 241, 242
  nursing management of, 241, 242
Dyspnea, 203

Edema, 55, 58, 59, 65, 89, 151, 153, 276, 283, 336
  cerebral, *see* Cerebral edema
  post operative, 277
  pulmonary, 134, 407
  rebound, 281
  spinal cord, 266, 337
  tissue, 278
Efferent nerve fiber(s), 14
  function of, 14
Elastic hose, 272, 370
Electrochemical gradient(s), 44
Electroencephalogram (EEG), 110, 116, 175
  features of, 110-112, 116
  patient preparation for, 114, 116
  post procedure care in, 115
  procedure for, 113-114
  uses of, 115
Electrolyte(s), 32, 50
  balance of
    assessment of, 166, 167
    problems in, 281, 282
  imbalances in, 82, 230, 233
Emboli, embolism
  cerebral dysfunction by, 101
  pulmonary, 371
Emotional behavior, 246, 247
Energy
  production of, 47
  regeneration of, 331
Environment, 233
  for aphasia patient, 239, 242
  for judgment deficit patient, 231-232
Epidural hematoma, 63
  causes of, 63
  pathology of, 64-65
  sites of, 64
Epileptic focus, cells in, 244
Equilibrium, maintenance of, 14
Excitatory cardiovascular center, 17
Exercise, 265
Expressive aphasia, *see* Nonfluent aphasia
Extension injury(ies), 338
  of spinal cord, 339, 340, 342
Extracellular fluid, 32
Extradural tumor, of spinal column, 349
Extra-pyramidal tract(s), features of, 324
Extravascular blood, 65
Eye(s)
  corneal reflex in, 162-163, 165
  see also Pupils, Visual field
Eye movement(s)

abnormal, 148
cranial nerves controlling, 148
reflex
  oculocephalic, 149
  oculovestibular, 150-151

Falx cerebri, 21
  function of, 21
Family
  of comatose patient, nurse relationship with, 284
  of spinal cord injury patient, education of, 416-418
Fat-soluble substance(s), dissolving of, 50
Fatigability, 232, 233, 295
Fecal impaction, 373
  autonomic hyperreflexia and, 377, 379
  signs of, 412, 413, 414
Femoral angiogram, patient care in, 121
Fever, 105, 282, 288, 408, 413
  causes of, 132, 138, 255
    extracranial, 218-219
      treatment of, 218-219
    intracranial, 216-218, 219
  in closed head injury patient, 292
  effects of, 215
    on metabolic demand of brain, 44, 45
  treatment of, *see* Hypothermia, Hypothermia blanket
Fifth cranial nerve, dysfunction of, 162
Filum terminale, 310
  injury to, 128
Fissure(s), 6
Flaccid paralysis, 358, 366
  following spinal cord injury, 359, 365
Flexion
  deformity, 189
  fractures
    of spinal column, 338, 341
    processes involved in, 338-339
  injury, 338
Fluent aphasia
  features of, 237-238, 241-242
  nursing management of, 239
Fluid
  balance, 19
    problems in, 281, 282
  imbalances in, 82
  intake, monitoring of, 265, 407
  loss of, calculation of, 282
  presence of, hypothermia and, 224
  restriction of, 264
  retention of, symptoms of, 166
  see also Body fluid
Focal seizure(s), *see* Partial seizure
Foley catheter, 272, 275, 280, 404
Foramen magnum, 40, 57, 59, 72
Foramen spinosum, 63
Foramina, 304
Foreign substance(s), sensitivity to, 20

Foster frame, 386
Fourth cranial nerve, 148, 258
Fracture(s)
    of cervical spinal column, categories of,
        338-340, 341-342
    skull, see Skull fractures
Frontal craniotomy, seizure following, 251
Frontal lobe, 152
    damage to, 233, 238
    motor area of, 10
    motor strip of, 10, 323, 328
Frostbite, prevention of during hypothermia, 224
Frustration, in aphasia patient, 239, 240
Fungal infection(s), of mouth, treatment of, 291

Gag reflex, 258
Ganglionic blocking agent(s), 378, 379
Gardner-Wells tongs, 404
    insertion of, 388
Gastrointestinal (GI) tract
    effect of immobility on, 209
    motility, for spinal cord injury patient, 372-373,
        374
        assessment of, 373, 374
Generalized seizures(s)
    absence, 248, 250
    features of, 244
    status epilepticus, 249, 250
    tonic-clonic, 248-249, 250
Glioma(s), 79, 349
Global aphasia, defined, 237, 242
Glucose, 50, 153
    brain consumption of, 42, 44, 45, 46
        interference in, 42, 45
    energy from, 44
    lack of, 43-44
Grand mal seizure, see Tonic-clonic seizure
Guiac test(s), 268
Gyrus, gyri, 6
    post central, 8
    precentral, 8

Hallucination(s), in immobilized patient, 213, 214
Halo brace, 292
Head elevation of, 264
    hyperflexion of, 338
    injury, see Closed head injury
Head trauma, 63
    cerebral edema from 70-71
    types of, 63
        closed head injury, 71-75
        epidural hematoma, 63-66
        subdural hematoma, 66-70
Headache, 78, 89, 275, 368, 379, 413, 414
    following lumbar puncture, 128
Heart
    effect of immobility on, 203, 204

pulsation, 181
rate, slowing of, 375
Hematoma, 121, 258, 266
    from arteriosclerotic vascular disease, 94
        symptoms of, 95
    epidural, see Epidural hematoma
    post operative, 276, 277
    subdural, see Subdural hematoma
Hemiplegia
    defined, 160, 164
    indication of, 163
Hemiplegic posturing, 188
Hemorrhage, 84, 101
    brain stem, 56
    petechial, 336
    prevention of, 120
    subarachnoid, 99, 178, 218
    venous, 74
Herniated intervertebral disc, 307, 350, 351
    symptoms of, 350
Herniation
    infratentorial, 57, 58
    tentorial, 55-56
Hip, flexion of, 264
Homeostatic balance, assessment of, 165
    of blood electrolyte, 166, 167
    of body fluid, 165-166, 167
    of pH, 166-167
Homonymous hemianopsia, 85, 97
Hydration, 265
Hydrogen peroxide (H_2O_2), 391, 392
Hydralazine, 378
Hygiene, 409
Hyperextension, of spine, 400, 401, 404
    patient position for, 400
Hypernatremia, 282
    fever in, 217
Hyperosmolar solution(s), 178, 270, 282, 283
    side effects of, 217, 218
Hypertension, 58, 93, 258, 379, 413, 414
    arterial, 49
Hyperthermia, see Fever
Hyperventilation
    central neurogenic, 134, 286
    regular rhythm of, 134
Hypophysis, see Pituitary gland
Hypotension, in spinal cord injury patient, 370,
    374
    see also Orthostatic hypotension
Hypothalamus, 282
    body temperature control by, 225, 282
        areas of, 216-217, 219
        dysfunction of, 217, 218-219
    damage to, 132
    dysfunction of, 82
    function of, 19
Hypothermia, induction of, 221
    automatic setting, 221-222, 226
    manual setting, 222, 226
    nursing observation and assessment in,
        224-226
Hypothermia blanket, 219, 220, 280, 206

controls of, 222
methods for use, 220-221
nursing observations in, 225, 226
Hypothermia unit
components of, 220-221
induction phase in, 220-222
Hypoxia, 265
signs of, 368

Ice bag(s), 219
Ileus, paralytic, 372
Immobility, immobilization, 354, 271, 380, 398,
409
effects of, 265
on cardiovascular system, 201-204
on gastrointestinal tract, 209
on kidneys, 206-208
on lungs, 204-206
on musculoskeletal system, 186-195
psychological, 210-213, 214
prevention of, 214
on skin, 195-201
for spinal cord injury patient, 386
Impaction, see Fecal impaction
Impulse(s), transmission of, 24, 315, 318
see also Nerve impulse
Increased intracranial pressure (↑ICP), 37, 57, 61,
65, 71, 89, 94, 102, 143, 151, 165, 225,
231, 257, 261, 280
causes of, 78, 264, 283
cerebellar tumors and, 86
cerebral edema and, 49-50
compensation for, 255
in brain tumors, 88
in concussion, 72
cranial components for, 38-39, 41
adjustment to, 39-41
effects of, 58-59, 131, 138
on cerebral blood flow, 46, 48
cerebral vasodilation and, 47, 48
on eye movement, 148
following craniotomy, 277
interference with nutrient supply to brain, 42
lumbar puncture and, 127
monitoring of, waves encountered by, 181,
182, 184
papilledema from 151, 152
parameters of, 254-255
prevention of, 283
progression of, 52
signs and symptoms of, 78, 79, 176, 281, 282
tissue damage by, 51
treatment of, 269-270
Infarction, see Cerebral infarction
Infection, 127, 136, 413
in brain stem injury, prevention of, 291-292
fungal, 291
intracranial, 255
prevention of, 266, 409
pulmonary, 412

Infectious process, cranial dysfunction by, 102,
104
by meningitis, 102
Information, processing of, 294
Infratentorial herniation, 57, 58
lesions of, 57
Infratentorial pressure, increased, results of, 57,
58, 59
Inhibitory cardiovascular center, 17
Inspiratory respiratory center, 17
Integration, interference with, 153
Intercostal muscle, paralysis of, 366, 369
Internal capsule, 98
Interstitial fluid, increased, 71
Intervertebral disc
features of, 307
herniated, see Herniated intervertebral disc
Intracranial bleeding, 231, 277
Intracranial contents, volume of, 41
Intracranial lesion(s), 260
expansion of, 163, 165
Intracranial pressure (ICP), 285
determination of, 41
increased, see Increased intracranial pressure
monitoring of, 177-178, 254, 255, 261
accuracy of readings in, 182, 184
equipment for, 177, 178-182, 184
nursing care for, 183, 184
normal range of, 184
reduction of, 122
nursing care plan for, 263-264
Intradural tumor(s), 349
Intramedullary tumor(s), characteristics of,
349-350
Intravascular blood, 38
volume of, 41
increase in, 39
Ionic change(s), nerve impulse and, 33, 34
Ipsilateral function, 13
Irritability, 232, 233
Ischemia, 49, 56

Jacksonian seizure, characteristics of, 246, 250
Joint(s)
contracture of, 188, 194
prevention of, 189, 190, 191-192
results of, 189
motion in, 188
Judgment, 230
deficits
causes of, 233
nursing management of, 231-232, 233

Kernig's sign, 90, 105
testing for, 90
Kidney(s), 348
effect of immobility on, 206-208, 209
Kidney stone(s), 194

from immobility, 209
 prevention of, 209
 symptoms of, 208
 prevention of, 194
Kinesthetic stimulation, 265

Laboratory work, for brain tumor, 262
Laceration, of spinal cord, 337, 341
Lactic acid, 47
 accumulation of, 72
Lamina, fracture of, 338
Laminectomy, 415
Language ability, assessment of, 238
Lateral spinothalamic tract (LST), 318
Lateral sulci, 12
Lesion(s), 55
 EEG detection of, 115
Lethargy, 368
 defined, 155
Level of consciousness, 260
 assessment of, 154-155, 159
  appropriateness of motor response in,
    157-158, 160
  memory and, 157, 160
  of response to pain, 158, 160
 change in, 172
 components of, 152, 159
 decreased, 56, 153, 154, 228, 264, 265-266
  infection occurrence and, 218, 219
 factors affecting, 155
 recording of
  orientation and, 156, 159
  terms for, 155-156, 159
Ligament(s), 340
 of spinal column, 306, 309
Light, pupil response to, see Pupil
Limbic area(s), pathology of, 250
Limbic system, 246
Longitudinal fissure, 12
Lower motor neuron (LMN), 326, 327
Lumbar puncture (LP)
 procedure for, 123-125, 128
  contraindications to, 127.
  patient care in, 127-128
  Queckenstedt test in, 126
 purpose of, 122
Lumbar vertebrae, structure of, 303, 304
Lung(s), 282, 348
 effect of immobility on, 204, 206
 expansion of, decreased, 372
 infection in, fever from, 218, 219
 oxygenation of, 264
Lymphoma(s), 348

Malignant tumor(s), 257, 276
 brain, features of, 76, 88
 growth rate of, 79
 of spinal column, 348-349

Mannitol, 272, 280, 281, 283
 action of, 269-270
 administration of, 270
Mechanical respiration, 174
Mechanical ventilator, 280
Medication, administration of, during
   hypothermia, 225, 226
Medulla, 15, 319, 323
 body function centers in, 17
 compression of, 57
 damage to, 135, 136
 herniation of, 57, 59
Memory, 160, 232
 brain areas for, 157
 loss of, 228, 230, 233
  see also Amnesia
Meninges, 19, 20, 309
 covering, 38
 damage to, 65
 irritation of, 90, 158
 structure of, 309, 310
  layers of, 19-20
   nerve endings of, 20
   tentorium cerebelli, 21-22
Meningioma(s), 79
 of spinal column, 349
Meningitis, 102
 course of, 102-103
 symptoms of, 104, 105
Mental cloudiness, 78
Mental status, in hypoxia, 368, 369
Metabolic waste(s), removal of, 71
Metabolism
 anaerobic, 47
 cerebral, 44
 effect of corticosteroids on, 267
Metastatic brain tumor(s), origin of, 76, 88
Microcirculation, interference with, 71
Midbrain, 15, 55, 134, 158, 372
 compression of, 59
Middle cerebral artery
 brain areas supplied by, 96, 98
 infarct of, 98
Middle meningeal artery, damage to, 63, 236, 237
Mineral(s), 286, 406
Minerva jacket, 391-392
Miosis
 drug induced, 143, 152
 light and, 144
 parasympathetic pathways for, 141, 151
Monoplegia, defined, 160
Mood, shifts in, 232, 233
Morphine sulfate, contraindications for, 260
Motor activity(ies), 13
Motor fiber(s), 326
 disruption of, 158
Motor impulse(s), transmission of, 328
Motor neuron(s), 326
 origin of, 328
Motor response(s)
 as indication of level of consciousness,
    157-158, 160

loss of, 176
travel of, 326
Motor-sensory area(s), anatomy of, 10
Motor and sensory function
    assessment of, 160, 161, 164
        of Babinski reflex, 162, 165
        of corneal reflex, 162-163, 165
    dysfunction of
        indications of, 163
        progression of, 163, 165
        terms for, 160, 164
Motor strip, see Precentral gyrus
Motor weakness, 120
Mucous membrane(s), cyanosis of, 136
Multiple myeloma, 349
Muscle(s), 323, 326
    atrophy of, 186
    contraction of, 250
    effect of immobility on, 186, 188, 194
    fibrillation of, 349
    incoordination of, see Ataxia
    irritability, 167
    paralysis, 371
    spasticity of, 349
    tone, maintenance of, 14
Muscular effort, 139
Musculoskeletal system
    effect of immobility on, 186, 194
        on bone, 193
        on connective tissue, 187-188, 194
        contracture formation, 188, 189, 194
        nursing intervention in, 189, 190, 191, 193,
            194, 196
        range of motion exercises for, 191, 192
    mobility of, 187
Mydriasis, 65, 176, 255
    drug induced, 143, 152
    single, 176
    sympathetic pathway for, 140
Myelin sheath, 29
    function of, 30
    structure of, 30

Nailbed(s), cyanosis of, 222
Narcotic(s), 225
    use for neurogenic patient, 260
Nasogastric feeding, for comatose patient, 293
    procedure for, 293
Nasogastric (NG) tube, 268, 275, 286
Nausea, 78, 202, 379, 413
Necrosis, 58, 59
Nerve(s)
    cells
        depolarization of, 244, 250
        function of, 27
        polarized, 32
    fibers
        afferent, 14
        efferent, 14
    innervation of, loss of, 188

root
    compression of, 350
    in spinal column, 308, 309
    stimulation of, 188
    loss of, 186
    see also Spinal nerve
Nerve impulse(s)
    propagation of, 32-34
    refractory period in, 34
    transmission of, 44
        interference in, 64, 73
        synaptic, 35-36
Nervous system
    divisions of, 13
        see also Autonomic nervous system, Central
            nervous system, Peripheral nervous
            system
    neurons of, 27-31
Neural impulse, see Nerve impulse
Neurilemma, function of, 30
Neuro check, 274, 280, 294, 389
Neuro deterioration, prevention of, 405-406
Neuro flow sheet, 130, 137, 155
Neuro sign(s), progression of, 172
Neurohypophysis, 80
Neurologic assessment, 129, 221
    of baseline, 130
    determining significance of change in, 169-176
    of homeostatic balance, 165-167
    of levels of consciousness, 152-159
    of motor and sensory function, 160-165
    of visual field deficits, 151
    of vital signs, 130, 136
        of apneustic breathing, 130
        of Biot's or ataxic breathing, 130
        of central neurogenic hyperventilation, 134
        of Cheyne Stokes respiration, 133-134
Neurologic function, nursing assessment of, see
            Neurologic assessment
Neurologic status, deterioration of, 172
Neuron(s), 326
    excitation of, 44
    function of, 27
    resting, 32
    supporting tissue of, 28-30
    synapses of, 30-31
Neurotransmitter(s), 35
    types of, 35
Ninth cranial nerve, 241
Nodes of Ranvier, function of, 30
Nonfluent aphasia
    defined, 10
    features of, 238, 242
    nursing management of, 238, 242
Nose, cerebrospinal fluid drainage from, 103, 105
Nuchal rigidity, 89
Nursing care, for seizures, see Seizure
Nutrient(s)
    demand for, 42, 224
    malabsorption of, 209
    transport of, 71
Nutrition, for comatose patient, 293

see also Diet
Nystagmus, defined, 148

Obtunded, defined, 155
Occipital lobe, function of, 8
Oculocephalic reflex (doll's eyes), 174
  features of, 149-150
Oculomotor nerve, see Third cranial nerve
Oculovestibular reflex, 174
  features of, 150-151
Olfactory nerve, 17
Olfactory stimuli, for treatment of decreased
        alertness, 234, 235
Opisthotonus position, 158
Optic chiasm, 82
  features of, 19
Optic nerve, 17
Optic tract(s), 84
Oral hygiene, for closed head injury patient, 291,
        292
Orientation, 152, 156, 159
  defined, 156
  determination of, 156
  interference with, 156
  see also Disorientation
Orthostatic hypotension, 204
  causes of, 202
  prevention of, 202, 204
  in spinal cord injury patient, 370, 374
  symptoms of, 202, 204
Oscilloscope, 179
Overhydration, 264
Oxygen (O₂), 136, 153, 274, 282, 285
  brain consumption of, 42, 44, 45, 46, 74, 249,
        250
    effect of fever on, 44
    interference in, 42, 45
  delivery of, increase in, 47
  demand for, 224
  energy from, 44
  exchange, 204, 414
  lack of, 43, 47
  levels of, 282
    in blood, 136, 139
      effect on respiratory control center,
          133, 134
    maintenance of, 264
  transport of, 71

Pain, 105
  decreased, 163
  response to, assessment of, 158, 160
  stimuli, 413
Pain receptor(s), stimulation of, 375, 376
Pallor, 202, 203
Papilledema, features of, 151, 152
Paralysis, 163, 350, 351, 366, 371
  defined, 160, 164
  from interruption of blood supply, 361

see also Flaccid paralysis
Paraplegia
  defined, 160, 164
  indications of, 163
Parasympathetic fiber(s), in pupils, action of,
        141, 142, 151
Parasympathetic system
  function of, 330
  structure of, 331
Paresis, defined, 160
Parietal lobe, 96, 99, 246
  function of, 8, 85, 319
  lesions in, 237
  sensory area of, 10
Parietal lobe tumor(s), symptoms of, 84, 85, 88
Partial seizure
features of, 244
Jacksonian, 246, 250
psychomotor, 246-247, 250
Peduncle(s), cerebellar, 14
Perception, brain areas for, 8
Perceptual problem(s)
  immobility and, 211
  nursing management for
    for confusion, 229-230, 233
    for judgment deficits, 231-232, 233
    for loss of memory, 230, 233
    of post concussion syndrome, 232-233
Peripheral nerve, ganglia of, 372
Peripheral nervous system, 297, 299
  organs of, 3
Peristalsis, decrease in, 209
  prevention of, 209
Personality change(s), in aphasia
Perspiration, see Diaphoresis
Peterson brace, 392
Petit mal seizure(s), see Absence seizure pH, 74
  monitoring of, 166-167
Phenytoin, 246, 247, 249
Phrenic nerve, 366
  pacing, 369
Photophobia, 90, 105
Pia mater, 19, 20, 309, 310
Pituitary gland
  lobes of, 80
  location of, 81
Pituitary gland tumor(s), 79
  location-related symptoms of, 81, 82-83, 88
Plaque, dislodgment of, 120
Pneumonia, 132, 138, 218, 282
  hypostatic, immobility and, 205
    death from, 205, 206
    prevention of, 205, 206
Pneumotaxic center(s), 17
Polarization-depolarization cycle, 34
Pons, 15, 134
  body function centers in, 17
Position sensation(s), travel of, 319
Post central gyrus, function of, 8
Post concussion syndrome
  nursing care for, 232-233
  symptoms of, 232, 233

Posterior cerebral artery, 55
  compression of, 59
Posterior root, 325
Potassium (K+)
  balance of, 166
  repolarization and, 33
Precentral gyrus, 96, 158, 328
  disruption of, emergency care for, 354
  features of, 323
  function of, 8
  pathology of, 246, 250
  pressure on, 163
Pre-frontal area
  function of, 8
  lesions in, 230
Pressure, 89, 190
Pre-synaptic vesicle(s), 35
Primary brain tumor(s)
  histological classification of, 78
  origin of, 76, 88
Proprioception, 319, 357
Protein, 23, 286, 293
Psychomotor seizure, features of, 246-247, 250
Pulmonary edema, 134, 407
Pulmonary embolism, 371
Pulmonary infection, signs and symptoms of, 412
Pulmonary problems, 366
  respiratory sounds indicating, 136
Pulpulus, 307
Pulse, 130
  pressure
    narrowing of, 176
    widening of, 176
  rise in, 255
  rate
    increased, 202, 203, 222
    slowing of, 131, 176
Pupil(s), 294
  changes in, 172
  constriction of, see Miosis
  dilation of, see Mydriasis
  fixation, 176
  neurologic assessment of, 140, 143, 144, 146,
    147
    of parasympathetic fibers, 141, 142, 151
    of response to light, 144, 152
    of sympathetic fibers, 140-142, 151
  response to light, 176, 258, 283, 294
  size of, 258

Quadriplegia, defined, 160
Queckenstedt test, for cerebrospinal fluid
    blockage, 126

Radiation therapy, for brain tumor, 277-278
Radicular artery(ies), 312
Radioisotope(s), 175
Range of motion exercise(s), 264, 399

movements for, 191, 192, 194
Rapid eye movement(s) (REM), interruption of,
    212
Rebound edema, 269, 281
  causes of, 270
Receptive aphasia, 237
  defined, 10
Rectal thermometer probe, 221
Rectum
  contraction of, 375
  distention of, 375, 379
Reflex(es), 326
  cranial nerves affecting, 18
  following spinal cord injury
    absence, 366
    bowel and bladder function, 360, 365
    spasticity and flaccid paralysis, 359, 365
    spinal shock, 358-359, 365
  occurrence of, 325
  pathways for, 326
Refractory period, defined, 34
Regression, following spinal cord injury, 382
  nursing care for, 383, 384
Rehabilitation center, transfer to, 418
Relative refractory period, defined, 34
Renal calculi, see Kidney stones
Renal output, decrease in, 222
Repolarization, 35
  defined, 33
  wave of, 34
Respiration(s), 130, 221
  adequacy of, 264
    nursing care for, 286-287
  disturbances in, 265, 337
    parameters indicating, 281-282
  following cervical spine injury
    factors affecting, 366-367
    nursing assessment of, 368, 369
    nursing plan for, 369
    respiratory muscle paralysis, 367
  following spinal cord injury, 372, 407
  mechanical, 174
  nursing assessment of, 132-133, 136, 138-139
    for apneustic breathing, 135-136
    of Biot's or ataxic breathing, 135
    of central neurogenic hyperventilation, 134
    of Cheyne Stokes respiration, 133, 135
  patterns of, changes in, 176
  rate of, 255
    increase in, 414
  spontaneous, absence of, 174, 175, 176
  support of, 284
Respirator, 174
Respiratory arrest, 57
Respiratory control center, 367
  action of, 133, 138
  damage to, 136
Respiratory cycle, 181
Respiratory disease(s), 134
Responsiveness
  absence of, 175
  promoting of, 291

Resting neuron(s), 32
Restlessness, 368, 409
Reticular activating system (RAS), 16, 115, 152
  function of, 16
Rhinorrhea, cerebrospinal, 103, 105
Richmond screw, 255, 261, 272, 280
Rolando fissure, 95
Roto rest bed, 393, 399
  benefits of, 399
  nursing care for, 399
Rubrospinal tract, 324

Sacral vertebrae, 303, 304, 305
Saliva, aspiration of, 249
Secretion(s), 136
  aspiration of, 264, 265
  infected, 282
  pooling of, 369
  retained, 414
Sedative(s), 225
  use for neurogenic patient, 260
Seizure(s), 99, 117, 167, 243, 276
  causes of, 244, 250
  classification of, 244
    generalized, 248-249, 250
    partial, 246-247, 250
  diagnosis of, 115
  nursing care for, 243, 251-253
    case studies for, 254-255
  threshold, decrease in, 222
Self-care, for spinal cord injury patient, 416-418
Self-image, effect of immobility on, 211, 212
Sensation
  following spinal cord injury, testing of, 357, 365
  loss of, 88, 380
  perception of, 19
  segmental distribution of, 321
  transmission of, 316
Sense(s), integrity of, orientation and, 156
Sensory activity(ies), 13, 98
Sensory deficit(s), 228, 233, 238, 246
  immobility and, 211, 214
Sensory disturbance(s), patterns of, 322
Sensory fiber(s), crossing of, 316
Sensory function, see Motor and sensory
    function
Sensory input, 238
  alertness increase by, 234
  increase in, 398
Sensory modalities, 8, 326
Sensory stimulation, for closed head injury
    patient, 295
Sensory tract(s), 96, 315, 317
  body areas specific to, 320, 321
  disruption of, emergency care for, 354
  fibers of, 316
  impulse travel through 318, 319
  names of, 320
  pressure on, 163
Sensory overload, 230, 233

immobility and, 211, 214
Seventh cranial nerve, dysfunction of, 162
Sexual function, 19
  following spinal cord injury, 364, 365
Shearing force, decubitus ulcers from, 198, 199,
    201
Shivering, from hypothermia, nursing care for,
    224-225, 226
Shock following spinal cord injury
  nursing assessment of, 380, 384
  psychological, 403, 405
  see also Spinal shock
Sight, perception of, 8
Sixth cranial nerve, 148, 258
Skeletal traction, for spinal cord injury patient,
    386
  position for, 390
  use of tongs for, see Tongs
Skin, 221, 258, 282
  assessment of, in spinal cord injury patient,
    380
  breakdown of, 265, 413
    prevention of, 380
  care, 265
  color, in hypoxia, 368
    see also Cyanosis, Pallor
  effect of immobility on, 195
    decubitus ulcers, 195-198
  flushing of, 117
  integrity of, maintenance of, 288-291, 406
  irritation of, 413
  sensations from, 326
  stimulation of, 375, 376
Skull, 19, 38, 39
  capacity, 41
  contents, increased volume of, 88
  fracture, 280
    infection from, 102, 104
    x-ray, 108, 280
Sleep deprivation, in immobilized patient, 212
Smoking, 407
Sodium (Na+)
  balance of, 166
  depolarization and, 33
  retention of, 282
Soft tissue, stimulation of, 188
Sound, perception of, 8
Spasm, 121, 136
  arterial, 120
  pilomotor, 379
Spasticity, 349
  defined, 160, 164
  following spinal cord injury, 359, 365
Speech, 278
  problems, 120
Speech center, location of, 10
Spinal column, 301
  fractures of, categories of, 338-340, 341-342
  function of, 306
  nerve roots in, 308, 309
  intervertebral disc in, 307
  structure of, 300

trauma to, 336
  results of, 340, 342
  tumors of, see Spinal column tumors vertebrae
    of, 301-305, 308
Spinal column tumor(s), 351
  characteristics of, 347
  classification of, 345, 348-350, 351
  location and frequency of, 346
Spinal cord, 3, 22, 299
  blood supply to, 312-314
    interruption of, 351, 352
  compression of, 354
  dysfunction of, 297
  fibers of, 328
  function of, 315
  nerve tracts of
    extra-pyramidal, 324
    motor, 323-324
    sensory, 315-323
  parts of, 315
  pathways to, 16
  pressure on, 349
  protective structure of
    meninges, 309-311
    vertebral column, 300-309
  transection, 359
    effects of, 367
  trauma to, 354
    results of, 336-337, 341
Spinal cord edema, use of corticosteroids for,
  266-269, 270
Spinal cord injury, 335, 353
  autonomic hyperreflexia following, 374-379
  bowel and bladder function following,
    360-363, 365
  cardiovascular regulation in, 370-371, 374
  clinical manifestation of, 343
  emergency care for, 354, 365
  gastrointestinal motility in, 372-373, 374
  initial care for, 404-405
    prevention of neuro deterioration, 405-406
    prevention of respiratory complications,
      407-408
    promoting comfort, 408-410
    spinal shock following, diagnosis of, 405
  intermediate care in
    evaluation of signs and symptoms of
      complications, 412-415
    goals of therapeutic plan in, 411-412
    patient and family teaching, 416-418
    for spinal shock recovery, 415-416
  level of, determination of, 356
  maintenance of skin integrity, 406
  nursing care plan for, 419-420
  prevention of, 340
  psychological reactions to, 380, 384, 403, 408
    denial, 381-382, 384
    depression, 383-384
    regression, 382-383, 384
    shock, 380-381, 384
  sexual function following, 364, 365
  skin assessment in, 380

spastic and flaccid paralysis following, 359,
  365
spinal shock following, 358-359, 365
temperature control in, 372, 374
testing of sensation in, 357, 365
testing of voluntary movement in, 355, 365
treatment of, see Spine, stabilization of
Spinal nerve(s), 3, 304, 312, 355
  roots of, 325
  structure of, 308, 309
Spinal shock, 366, 372
  following spinal cord injury, 358-359, 365
    diagnosis of, 405
    recovery from, 415-416
Spinal tap, fever from 218
Spine, stabilization of, 385
  by hyperextension of spine, 400, 402
  by skeletal traction, 386-392
  by surgical fusion, 401, 402
  by turning frames, 393-399, 401
Status epilepticus, characteristics of, 249, 250
Steroid(s), 283
  see also Corticosteroids
Stimulus, stimuli
  processing of, post concussion syndrome and,
    232
  response to, 28
  withdrawal from 326
Stress, response to, 408
Structural communication, 254
Stryker frame, 386, 393, 404
  turning of, 394-395
Stuperous, defined, 155
Subarachnoid hemorrhage, 99, 178
  fever from, 218
Subarachnoid screw, 177, 182
  flushing of, 179
  insertion of, 178, 179
  nursing care for, 180
  purpose of, 178
Subarachnoid space, 20, 22, 68, 93, 122, 151, 177,
    261, 391
  infection in, 183, 184
Subdural hematoma
  causes of, 67-69
  classification of, 69
  features of, 66
  sites of, 69
  symptoms of, 69
Subsynaptic membrane, 35
Suctioning, 280, 285
Sulci, 6
Supratentorial compartment, 55
Supratentorial lesion(s), detection of, 115
Supratentorial pressure, increased, 59
Surgery, 178, 247
Surgical fusion, 392, 415
  indications for, 401, 402
  procedure for, 401, 402
Sweating, see Diaphoresis
Sympathetic fiber(s), of pupils, action of, 140,
  142, 151

Sympathetic system, 330, 331
  function of, 329
  structures innervated by, 330
Synapse(s), 31
  defined, 30
  impulse transmission across, 35
  quantity of, 31
  types of, 31
Synaptic cleft, 30, 35
Synaptic knob, 35
Systolic pressure, increase in, 283

Tactile stimulant(s), for treatment of decreased
      alertness, 234, 235
Temperature, recording of, 130, 132
  see also Fever
Temperature control, 19
  for spinal cord injury patient, 372, 374, 404,
      409-410
Temperature control center, 132
Temperature impulse(s), travel of, 318
Temporal bone, fracture through, 63
Temporal fossa, bleeding into, 63
Temporal lobe, 96, 246
  damage to, memory loss from, 230, 233
  function of, 8
  lesions in, 237
  pathology of, 250
  uncus of, 54, 55
    herniation of, see Tentorial herniation
  Wernicke's center in, 10
Temporal lobe seizure, see Psychomotor seizure
Tenth cranial nerve, 241, 331
Tentorial herniation, 55, 59, 142, 165, 266
  effects of, 56, 59
    on consciousness, 154
Tentorial notch, 40, 54, 55, 57, 163
Tentorium, 54
  location of, 142
Tentorium cerebelli, function of, 21
Testape, 103, 105
Thalamus, function of, 19, 319
Thinking problem(s), 247, 250
Third cranial nerve, 55, 142, 255, 258
  compression of, 59
  effect on eye movement, 148, 152
  function of, 141
  position of, 54
Thoracic vertebrae, structure of, 303
Thrush, 291
Tilt table, 370
Tissue
  compression of, 65
  damage to, from increased intracranial
      pressure, 51
  edema, 278
Tongs, use for skeletal traction, 398, 401, 414
  insertion of, 386-389, 392
  nursing assessment of, 389-391, 392
  nursing care for, 391-392

weight of, 414
Tonic-clonic seizure(s), 250, 251
  nursing care for, 251
  phases of, 248-249
  treatment of, 249
Touch, 156
  perception of, 8
Tracheostomy, 280, 285, 294
  nursing care following, 287
Traction, 354, 386
  see also Skeletal traction
Traction weight(s), 389, 396, 401
Transducer, 179, 182
Trauma, 49, 58, 68, 84, 178, 351
  cerebral, 157, 175
  to spinal column, results of, 340, 342
  to spinal cord, 336-337, 341, 354
  see also Head trauma
Tumor(s), 49, 58
  see also Brain tumors, Malignant tumors,
      Spinal column tumors
Turning frame, for spinal cord injury patient
  nursing considerations in, 398, 399, 401
  types of, 393
  use of, 393, 401
    of circOlectric bed, 394
    methods for, 396
    of Roto rest bed, 399
    safety considerations in, 396, 401
    of Stryker frame, 393
    turning schedule for, 397, 401
Twelfth cranial nerve, 241
Twitching, following craniotomy, 275
Tylenol, see Acetaminophen

Unconsciousness, 16, 20, 176, 246, 250
Uncus, 54
  herniation of, see Tentorial herniation
Upper motor neuron (UMN), 327, 328
Urinary tract infection(s), 413
  fever from, 218, 219
Urine, 282
  excessive excretion of, 82
  flow of, effect of mobility on, 206, 297, 209
  retention of, 358
  voiding of, problems in, 128
Urologic complication(s), from immobility
  prevention of, 209
  symptoms of, 208

Vagus, see Tenth cranial nerve
Vagus system, 18
Valsalva maneuver, 93, 103, 277
Vascular lesion(s), brain dysfunction from, 89,
      101
  aneurysms, 89-93, 101
  by arteriosclerotic vascular disease, 93-99, 101
  by arteriovenous malformation, 99, 100, 101

methods of, 101
Vascular resistance, 46, 47
Vascular surgery, 351
Vascular system, disruption of, 89
Vasoconstriction, 224
   effects of, 225
   from hypothermia, 221, 222
Vasodilation, 225, 370, 407
   cerebral, 47
   initiation of, by hypothalamus, 216, 217
Vasomotor reflex, loss of, 370, 371
Venous network, 68
Venous stasis, 204, 380
Venous thrombosis, 204, 413
   in spinal cord injury patient, 371, 374
Ventilation, 264
   accessory muscles for, 368, 369
   adequacy of, 136, 139
   artificial, 369
   decreased, 366
   effect of immobility on, 204, 206
   problems in, 414
Ventilator, 280, 285
Ventricle(s), 22, 86, 177
Ventricular system, 122
   cerebrospinal fluid flow from, 22
Vermis, 14
Vertebrae, 339
   alignment of, 386
      use of hyperextension for, 400
   fractures of, 339
   stabilization of, 340, 415
   structure of, 303-304

surgical removal of, 401
Vertebral column, *see* Spinal column
Vestibulospinal tract, 324
Vibration sensation(s), travel of, 319
Vision, blurred, 379, 413
Visual field defect(s), 88, 138, 398
   nursing evaluation of, 151, 152
   parietal lobe function and, 85, 88
   related to pituitary tumors, 82-83
Visual stimuli, for treatment of decreased
      alertness, 234, 235
Vital capacity (VC), measurement of, in cervical
      spine injury, 368, 369
Vital sign(s), 258, 404
   changes in, 172
   nursing assessment of, 130-133, 221
Vitamin(s), 280, 286, 406
Voluntary motor system, dysfunction of, 162
Voluntary movement(s)
   control of, 8
   following spinal cord injury, testing of, 355, 365
   impulses for, 323

Weakness, 66, 163, 164, 202, 258, 294, 404
Wernicke's center, damage to, 10
White matter, effect of contusion on, 336

X-ray(s), 391
   skull, 108, 280